# Geriatric Cardiology

# Books Available in Cardiovascular Clinics Series

# Geriatric Cardiology

**David T. Lowenthal, M.D., Ph.D.** / Editor

Professor of Medicine, Pharmacology, and Exercise Science
University of Florida College of Medicine
Director of Geriatric Research, Education, and Clinical Center
VA Medical Center
Gainesville, Florida

## CARDIOVASCULAR CLINICS

**Albert N. Brest, M.D.** / Editor-in-Chief

James C. Wilson Professor of Medicine
Jefferson Medical College
Philadelphia, Pennsylvania

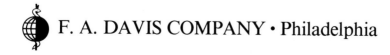 F. A. DAVIS COMPANY · Philadelphia

Last digit indicates print number: 10 9 8 7 6 5 4 3 2 1
Acquisitions Editor: Robert H. Craven
Production Editor: Gail Shapiro

As new scientific information becomes available through basic and clinical research, recommended treatments and drug therapies undergo changes. The author(s) and publisher have done everything possible to make this book accurate, up to date, and in accord with accepted standards at the time of publication. The authors, editors, and publisher are not responsible for errors or omissions or for consequences from application of the book, and make no warranty, expressed or implied, in regard to the contents of the book. Any practice described in this book should be applied by the reader in accordance with professional standards of care used in regard to the unique circumstances that may apply in each situation. The reader is advised always to check product information (package inserts) for changes and new information regarding dose and contraindications before administering any drug. Caution is especially urged when using new or infrequently ordered drugs.

**Library of Congress Cataloging in Publication Data**

Cardiovascular clinics.
  Philadelphia, F. A. Davis, 1969–
    v. ill. 27 cm.
    Editor: v. 1– A. N. Brest.
    Key title: Cardiovascular clinics, ISSN 0069-0384
  1. Cardiovascular system—Diseases—Collected works   I.   Brest, Albert N., ed.
    [DNLM: WI CA77N]
RC681.A1C27    6.6.1                          70-6558
ISBN 0-8036-5653-X                        MARC-S

# Preface

This text, a compilation of material relevant to the understanding of aging and cardiac function in health and disease, is not the first instance recognizing the combinations of age and disease.

Both in Leviticus 3:14–17 and in Perek Moshe (Jerusalem 1959, M. Sussman, ed.) the great physician and Hebraic Scholar, Maimonides, sagaciously speaks of the evils of and warnings against consuming animal fats. As promulgated in Exodus (31:6 and 36:1), the heart was thought to be the chamber of all emotions: love, rage, courage, understanding, and wisdom. Thus the scenario was laid in place millennia ago for what we accept today as atherosclerosis and the type A or hot reactor. The aspiration for longevity was first articulated in the pragmatism of the 5th Commandment (Exodus 20:12). Although unrelated to dietary prohibitions, the concept of long life was appreciated by our forebears.

Secularly, Shakespeare's recognition of aging was best recited by Edgar in *King Lear* V, "The oldest hath borne most; we that are young shall never see so much nor live so long." Later, Robert Browning penned in "Rabbi Ben Ezra", "Grow old along with me! The best is yet to be. . . ."

Today we can readily refer to the amalgam of religion, philosophy, and poetry to help us cope with the wishes for successful aging. Realistically the art and science of medicine superimposed on one's genetic predisposition is what really dictates the facts relating to the heart in health, disease, and age.

To regard this text as seminal to an understanding of "Geriatric Cardiology" is naive. As stated, our sages, secular and biblical, were avant-garde. To regard this text as a current reference source to help buttress the burgeoning knowledge of geriatric medicine is more appropriate. The tables of contributors and contents attest to the near completeness of this text, leaving open the possibility for a future edition as the population continues to age and expand. To paraphrase the play, *I'm Not Rapaport,* "We [the authors and readers] are the coming generation."

Thus, this text, Volume 22, Number 2, aptly fits into the niche of topical material published in Cardiovascular Clinics since 1969. I am most grateful to my friend and colleague, Albert N. Brest, M.D. and to F.A. Davis for acknowledging the subject of Geriatric Cardiology to be an integral part of this series of textbooks.

David T. Lowenthal

# Editor's Commentary

Elderly patients with heart disease present special diagnostic challenges. Aging per se causes physiologic changes in the cardiovascular system and other vital organs and these alterations can substantially influence the course and management of heart disease in the elderly. Additionally, older patients may exhibit certain clinical disorders that are not ordinarily encountered in younger persons. Lifestyle, socioeconomic, and quality-of-life considerations also may affect clinical decisions. These factors can effect material differences in the diagnosis and treatment of the elderly as compared with younger individuals. This book explores all of these issues in detail. I am extremely grateful to my friend, David Lowenthal, for his guidance in the development of this book. Both of us are indebted to each of the contributing authors for their exemplary efforts.

Albert N. Brest, M.D.
Editor-in-Chief

# Contributors List

Frederick R. Armenti, M.D.
*Assistant Professor of Surgery*
*Cardiothoracic Surgery*
*Department of Surgery*
*Thomas Jefferson University Hospital*
*Philadelphia, Pennsylvania*

Richard J. Backes, M.D.
*Cardiology Fellow*
*Mayo Medical Center*
*Rochester, Minnesota*

Albert N. Brest, M.D.
*James C. Wilson Professor of Medicine*
*Jefferson Medical College*
*Philadelphia, Pennsylvania*

Stephen E. Borst, Ph.D.
*Assistant Research Scientist*
*Department of Pharmacology*
*University of Florida*
*College of Medicine*
*Staff Pharmacologist, Geriatric Research, Education and Clinical Center*
*VA Medical Center*
*Gainesville, Florida*

Joan F. Carroll, M.A.
*Doctoral Student*
*Department of Exercise and Sport Science*
*Center for Exercise Science*
*University of Florida*
*Gainesville, Florida*

Simon C. Chakko, M.D.
*Associate Professor of Medicine*
*University of Miami School of Medicine*
*Chief, Non-Invasive Cardiac Laboratory*
*Department of Veterans Affairs Medical Center*
*Miami, Florida*

Raymond T. Coward, Ph.D., M.S.W.
*Professor of Medicine*
*University of Florida College of Medicine*
*Director, Center for Rural Health and Aging*
*Associate Director, Center for Health Policy Research*
*J. Hillis Miller Health Science Center*
*Gainesville, Florida*

Richard N. Edie, M.D.
*Professor of Surgery*
*Chief, Division of Cardiothoracic Surgery*
*Thomas Jefferson University*
*Philadelphia, Pennsylvania*

Bernard J. Gersh, D. Phil., M.B., Ch.B.
*Professor of Medicine*
*Mayo Medical School*
*Consultant in Cardiovascular Diseases*
*Mayo Clinic*
*Rochester, Minnesota*

Nanette Barbara Hoffman, M.D.
*Clinical Assistant Professor*
*Department of Medicine*
*University of Florida College of Medicine*
*Medical Director, Nursing Home Care Unit*
*Gainesville VA Medical Center*
*Gainesville, Florida*

Claydell Horne, M.S.N.
*Doctoral Candidate*
*University of Florida*
*Graduate Research Assistant*
*Center for Health Policy Research*
*J. Hillis Miller Health Science Center*
*Gainesville, Florida*

Larry E. Jacobs, M.D.
*Director, Echo-Doppler Laboratory*
*Albert Einstein Medical Center*
*Assistant Professor of Medicine*
*Temple University School of Medicine*
*Philadelphia, Pennsylvania*

William B. Kannell, M.D., M.P.H.
*Professor of Medicine and Public Health*
*Boston University*
*Senior Researcher*
*Framingham Heart Study*
*Framingham, Massachusetts*

Kenneth M. Kessler, M.D.
*Professor of Medicine*
*University of Miami School of Medicine*
*Chief, Cardiology Section*
*Department of Veterans Affairs Medical Center*
*Miami, Florida*

Morris N. Kotler, M.D.
*Professor of Medicine*
*Temple University*
*Chief of Cardiology*
*Albert Einstein Medical Center*
*Philadelphia, Pennsylvania*

Peter R. Kowey, M.D.
*Professor of Medicine*
*Thomas Jefferson University*
*Chief, Division of Cardiovascular Diseases*
*Lankenau Hospital and Medical Research Center*
*Wynnewood, Pennsylvania*

Marian C. Limacher, M.D.
*Associate Professor of Medicine*
*Division of Cardiology*
*University of Florida College of Medicine*
*Director, Preventive Cardiology Program*
*Shands Hospital at the University of Florida*
*Gainesville, Florida*

Jannet F. Lewis, M.D.
*Associate Professor of Medicine*
*Howard University College of Medicine*
*Director of Echocardiography*
*Department of Medicine (Cardiology)*
*Howard University Hospital*
*Washington, DC*

David T. Lowenthal, M.D., Ph.D.
*Professor of Medicine, Pharmacology, and Exercise Science*
*University of Florida College of Medicine*
*Director, Geriatric Research, Education, and Clinical Center*
*VA Medical Center*
*Gainesville, Florida*

John D. Mannion, M.D.
  *Assistant Professor of Surgery*
  *Department of Surgery*
  *Division of Cardiothoracic Surgery*
  *Thomas Jefferson University*
  *Philadelphia, Pennsylvania*

Roger A. Marinchak, M.D.
  *Associate Professor of Medicine*
  *Thomas Jefferson University*
  *Director, Cardiac Electrophysiology Laboratory*
  *The Lankenau Hospital and Medical Research Center*
  *Wynnewood, Pennsylvania*

Barry J. Maron, M.D.
  *Senior Investigator*
  *National Heart, Lung, and Blood Institute*
  *National Institutes of Health*
  *Bethesda, Maryland*

Anne Pepine, B.S.
  *University of Florida*
  *College of Medicine*
  *Gainesville, Florida*

Carl J. Pepine, M.D.
  *Professor of Medicine*
  *Department of Medicine*
  *Division of Cardiology*
  *University of Florida College of Medicine*
  *Gainesville, Florida*

Michael L. Pollock, Ph.D.
  *Professor of Medicine and Exercise and Sport Sciences*
  *Director, Center for Exercise Science*
  *Department of Medicine*
  *University of Florida College of Medicine*
  *Gainesville, Florida*

Seth J. Rials, M.D., Ph.D.
  *Clinical Assistant Professor of Medicine*
  *Thomas Jefferson University*
  *Director, Basic Cardiovascular Research*
  *The Lankenau Hospital and Medical Research Center*
  *Wynnewood, Pennsylvania*

Dennis Tighe, Jr., M.D.
*Division of Cardiology*
*Thomas Jefferson University Hospital*
*Philadelphia, Pennsylvania*

Nanette K. Wenger, M.D.
*Professor of Medicine (Cardiology)*
*Emory University School of Medicine*
*Director, Cardiac Clinics*
*Grady Memorial Hospital*
*Atlanta, Georgia*

Leonard Williams, M.D.
*Clinical Instructor in Medicine*
*University of Florida College of Medicine*
*Geriatric Research, Education, and Clinical Center*
*VA Medical Center*
*Gainesville, Florida*

T. Franklin Williams, M.D.
*Director*
*National Institute on Aging*
*National Institutes of Health*
*Bethesda, Maryland*

# Contents

# PART 1

# Epidemiologic Considerations

# CHAPTER 1

# Demographics of Aging

*T. Franklin Williams, M.D.*

Virtually everyone now, and especially those of us in the health professions, is aware of the rapid increases in numbers and proportions of older persons—already a major fact of life in most developed countries but also rapidly occurring world-wide. By the year 2000, there will be at least 580 million persons older than the age of 60, of whom almost two thirds will be in underdeveloped countries. Even more important, in particular from the point of view of needs for healthcare, the "oldest old" is the most rapidly growing group of older persons: there are already 1 million or more people aged 80 or older in each of eight developed nations, and at least 6 more nations will reach such population numbers within the next 30 years.

Our changes in the United States are similar to those worldwide: there are already more than 31 million persons older than the age of 65, that is, 12% of our population; by the year 2020 or 2025, this figure will rise to 20%—well within the lifetime of most of the readers of this chapter. By the year 2000, eight years from now, the numbers of those aged 85 and older, already 2.5 million, will almost double, and there will be more than 100,000 persons aged 100 and older. These predictions are based on information from the 1980 census and further census-developed data. Given the progress that we are seeing in preventive and health maintenance practices as well as progress in treatment and rehabilitation in older persons, in particular with cardiovascular diseases, my own expectation is that the results of the 1990 census, soon to be available, will show even higher numbers and projections.

Among those in the United States aged 65 and more, 60% are women; among those older than the age of 70, 72% are women. Most older men—75%—are living with a spouse compared with only 36% of older women. As of 1987 in the United States, 52% of women older than the age of 85 were living alone, compared with only 29% of men of that age;[1] these numbers are considerably higher than in other comparably developed countries such as Canada and New Zealand and reflect the numbers of very old persons in our country who are at high risk of chronic diseases and disabilities and who do not have immediate access to help in the home. About 10% of older persons in the United States are non-white, a lower percentage than non-whites in the total population, but the numbers in this age group are increasing similar to increases among white persons.

3

## LIFE EXPECTANCY

Life expectancy has progressively increased; the most recent (1986) figures are 71.3 years at birth for men, 78.3 years for women, and 74.8 years overall.[2] At age 65, life expectancies are 14.7 additional years for men, 18.6 years for women, or 16.8 years overall. Non-whites have lower life expectancies than whites.

## VARIABILITY

Within the past few years, with more attention devoted to the demographic and epidemiologic characteristics of our older population, we have been able to learn in more detail the challenges presented. In the first place, the great variation among older persons must be emphasized: Those in their 80s and 90s are different in many ways from those in their 60s; and each older person, with a life history unique to her or him, is truly a unique individual with a special (and usually quite complex) constellation of functional capabilities and disabilities, diseases, life experiences, and preferences for what is next. Approaching each person as an individual, regardless of age, is of course the basic intent and responsibility of every physician and other healthcare professional. This is even more important in the case of older patients; there has been an unfortunate tendency among the medical profession to think and talk about "the elderly" as if older people were all alike.

## GOOD HEALTH AND FUNCTIONING

Secondly, we have learned that many older persons can and do maintain high degrees of health and functioning, even into very late years. Among subjects in the Baltimore Longitudinal Study on Aging (BLSA) who do not have even occult evidence of coronary artery disease—and about 50% of those aged 60 to more than 80 do not—there is no evidence of decline in maximal cardiac output on standard stress tests, compared with younger subjects.[3] In repeated longitudinal measurements in BLSA subjects, there is virtually no change in personality characteristics,[4] and one third or more show no decline in renal function as measured by repeated creatinine clearances.[5] In other studies of healthy older persons, there is no decline in brain glucose metabolism as measured by positron emission tomography (PET) scans;[6] and in virtually all tests of cognitive function, 15% to 30% or more of subjects in later years perform as well as average, much younger subjects. Furthermore, there is now ample evidence of the restorability of such functions as maximal aerobic capacity and muscle mass and strength, even in persons in their 80s and 90s,[7] who have lost such functions by disuse. The rehabilitative potential of older persons, even in the face of disease conditions, must be kept constantly in mind.

## DISABLING CONDITIONS

Third, despite the important optimistic perspective just stated, we also know that most older persons do acquire one or more chronic and potentially disabling conditions that can complicate their response to, or management of, other problems like an acute cardiovascular illness. Almost 50% of persons older than the age of 65 report some symptoms of arthritis—usually typical of osteoarthritis;[8] other very commonly reported conditions (in order of descending frequency) are hypertension, hearing loss, some form of heart disease, an orthopedic impairment, chronic sinusitis, visual impairments, and diabetes. Most of these conditions, except for hearing impairment, are more common in women than men. Not reported by the persons affected but as ascertained by careful surveys is the marked increase in numbers and percentages of persons with dementing conditions in very old age; the latest careful study in one population-based study concludes that 45% or more of persons older than the age of 85 probably have dementia of the Alzheimer's type.[9]

## NEED FOR PERSONAL ASSISTANCE

In association with such chronic conditions, there is an increasing likelihood of need for personal assistance. A major contribution to our ability to understand and develop approaches to meet the health needs of frail older persons has been the development and use of measures of activities of daily living (ADL)—the daily activities of personal care that every person needs to carry out for herself or himself or to have someone carry out for her or him (e.g., eating, toileting, bathing, dressing)—and the instrumental activities of daily living (IADL)—the necessary activities that go beyond personal care, including shopping for food and other necessities as well as managing money, housecleaning, and medications.

Careful national health surveys of persons living in the community, which look at such characteristics, indicate progressive increases with age in the percentages of older persons with problems with ADL and IADL and consequent needs for personal assistance. Overall, among persons aged 85 and older, these studies show that 45% are disabled to the point of needing some help from another person every day (Fig. 1–1).[10] The most common causes of this degree of disability, in descending order, are dementia, arthritis, peripheral vascular disease, cerebrovascular disease or stroke, and fractures particularly of the hip.[8] It is noteworthy that the two major causes of death in older persons, namely coronary artery disease and cancer, appear to contribute little to the chronic morbidity requiring daily assistance.

## NEED FOR NURSING HOME AND SIMILAR CARE

Increasing disability is associated with the increasing likelihood of moving into a nursing home or other type of assisted living setting. In the United States, about 5.7% of persons older than the age of 65 currently reside in such settings. But this figure does not give an adequate picture of the lifetime likelihood of spending some time in a nursing home. A recent analysis[11] of national data indicates that 17% of persons dying between the age of 65 and 74 will have lived some time in a nursing home, with sharply rising percentages with survival into later years: 36% of those dying between ages 65 and 74 and 60% of those dying between ages 85 and 94. The study authors projected that 43% of persons who become 65 years old in 1990 will spend some portion of their remaining years in a nursing home.

## ACTIVE LIFE EXPECTANCY

The concepts of "active life expectancy" and "disabled life expectancy" have been developed to describe the portion of a lifetime that can be expected to be lived

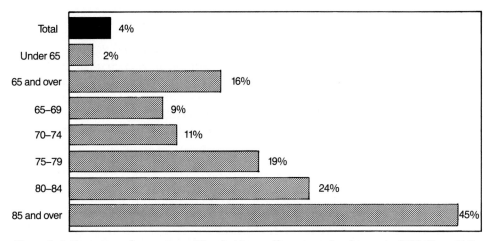

**Figure 1–1.** Percentage of persons age 15 and older needing personal assistance in 1986 (From U.S. Department of Commerce Bureau of the Census. SB-12-90, December 1990).

essentially independently versus the portion during which the person will be dependent on others for some help—at home or in an institution. Current estimates are that men, at age 65, have an active life expectancy of about 7 years followed by a dependent life expectancy of 7.7 years; comparable figures for women at age 65 are 9 years and 9.5 years respectively.[12] These figures do not take into account the fact that some persons who become sufficiently dependent to be counted as such in these studies and/or to enter nursing homes do regain independence; we need more information on such reversals and of course need to accomplish it whenever possible.

## HEALTH AND RETIREMENT

In this country, despite progressive improvement in the health of older persons in recent years, the percentage of persons retiring from active employment at age 65 has increased; currently less than 20% of persons older than age 65 are in paid employment. This fact is probably much more related to economic factors including social security and retirement benefits than to health changes; and studies of "productive" activities by older persons, including in that term activities to which a price could be attached such as painting one's own house or babysitting with grandchildren while the middle generation works, indicate that on average older persons are contributing more to society than they are receiving from it at least up to age 75. The important interrelations between health and retirement are the subject of a newly initiated longitudinal study.

## GEOGRAPHIC REDISTRIBUTIONS

A final aspect of the demography of aging is that of the geographic distribution and redistributions of older persons. A number of substantial changes and trends have been documented in recent years:[13] The obvious movements of retiring persons to the "sunbelt" states (and the reverse migration of a number of such persons, as they have become even older and more frail, back to be near their families[14]);

the development of various types of retirement living, including continuing-care retirement communities; and concentrations of poorer older persons in certain urban and rural areas. These movements create special challenges for physicians and all aspects of healthcare. A related interest is in the development of suitable designs for housing and communities to support "aging in place" as more and more persons go through their own transitions from fully independent existence to needs for environmental modifications as well as some personal assistance.

## REFERENCES

1. Kasper, JD: Aging alone. Profiles and Projections. A Report of the Commonwealth Fund Commission on Elderly People Living Alone. Johns Hopkins School of Public Health, Baltimore, 1987.
2. National Center for Health Statistics: Health, United States, 1988. DHHS Pub. No. (PHS) 89-1232. Public Health Service, U.S. Government Printing Office, Washington, D.C., March 1989, p 53.
3. Rodeheffer, RJ, Gerstenblith, G, Becker, LC, et al: Exercise cardiac output is maintained with advancing age in healthy human subjects: Cardiac dilatation and increased stroke volume compensate for a diminished heart rate. Circulation 69:203–213, 1984.
4. McRae, RR and Costa, PT: Emerging Lives, Enduring Dispositions: Personality in Adulthood. Little Brown, Boston, 1984.
5. Lindeman, RD, Tobin, J, Shock, N: Longitudinal studies on rate of decline in renal function with age. J Am Geriatr Soc 33:278–285, 1985.
6. Creasy, H and Rapoport, SI: The aging human brain. Ann Neurol 17:2–10, 1985.
7. Fiatarone, MA, Marks, EC, Ryan, ND, et al: High-intensity strength training in nonagenerians: Effects on skeletal muscle. JAMA 263:3029–3034, 1990.
8. Brody, JA, Brock, DB, Williams, TF: Trends in the health of the elderly population. Annual Review of Public Health 8:211–234, 1987.
9. Evans, DA, Funkenstein, HH, Albert, MS, et al: Prevalence of Alzheimer's disease in a community population of older persons. JAMA 262:2551–2556, 1989.
10. U.S. Department of Commerce, Bureau of the Census. Statistical Brief: Persons needing assistance with everyday activities. SB-12-90, December 1990.
11. Kemper, P and Murtaugh, CM: Lifetime use of nursing home care. N Engl J Med 324:595–600, 1991.
12. Suzman, R: Demography of older populations in developed countries. In Evans, JG and Williams, TF (eds): Oxford Textbook of Geriatric Medicine. Oxford University Press, Oxford, in press.
13. Golant, SM, Rowles, GD, Meyer, JW: Aging and the aged. In Gaile, GL and Willmott, CJ (eds): Geography in America. Merrill Publ. Co., Columbus, Ohio, 1989, pp 451–466.
14. Longino, CF Jr.: Going home: Aged return migration in the United States, 1965–1970. J Gerontology 34:736–745, 1979.

# CHAPTER 2

# Epidemiology of Cardiovascular Disease in the Elderly: An Assessment of Risk Factors*

*W. B. Kannel, M.D., MPH*

Cardiovascular disease is the leading cause of death and a prominent cause of disability that takes the joy out of reaching a venerable stage of life. Coronary heart disease is the major lethal cardiovascular outcome and a prominent contributor to disability in the elderly.[1] With an aging population of increased size, it is becoming increasingly necessary to keep the elderly healthy and productive in the work force. Coronary heart disease and stroke mortality have been declining dramatically in the United States, Australia, Canada, and New Zealand, and the elderly have shared in the decline.[2] Hence, it is evident that cardiovascular morbidity and mortality are not inevitable and that risk factor modification has potential even for the elderly.

## INDIVIDUAL RISK FACTORS

Four decades of epidemiologic research have identified innate and acquired cardiovascular risk factors that contribute to the major atherosclerotic disease outcomes.[3] Nontrivial differences in their impact on specific cardiovascular events exist.[4] Whereas all the major cardiovascular risk factors contribute powerfully to coronary heart disease, for stroke, hypertension predominates and lipids play little role. For peripheral arterial disease, cigarettes and glucose intolerance are most influential. For cardiac failure, hypertension, left ventricular hypertrophy, coronary disease, and diabetes are paramount.[4]

These common risk factors operate in both sexes at all ages but with different strengths. Diabetes and a low HDL cholesterol eliminate the favorable advantage of women over men.[5] Cigarette smoking has a greater influence in men and is non-

*Supported by: Charles A. Dana Foundation, Merck, Sharpe & Dohme. NIH Grants Nos. N01-HV-92922 and N01-HV-52971.

cumulative and reversible on quitting.[6] Fibrinogen is a major independent risk factor for coronary heart disease, stroke, and peripheral arterial disease in both sexes.[7]

Some risk factors, such as blood lipids, impaired glucose tolerance, and fibrinogen diminish in impact with advancing age.[4,7,8] Decreased risk ratios are offset by a high absolute risk resulting in a large excess risk. All risk factors are relevant in the elderly. Obesity and weight gain promote all the major atherogenic traits,[9] and physical indolence promotes risk factors and coronary heart disease at all ages.[10] Systolic blood pressure and isolated systolic hypertension are major risk factors.[11-13] The total/HDL cholesterol ratio provides the best and most convenient lipid risk profile.[14]

Risk factors seldom occur in isolation and, when they cluster, they greatly augment the risk associated with any particular risk factor, making it necessary to deal with any risk factors as an ingredient of a cardiovascular risk profile.[14]

## PREVALENCE OF RISK FACTORS

Cardiovascular risk factors that predispose to lethal and disabling events in the elderly are very common. Beyond age 65 years, 20% to 50% of men and women respectively have cholesterol values exceeding 240 mg/dl (Table 2–1). Some 7.5% of women and 20% of men have reduced ($< 35$ mg/dl) high density lipoprotein (HDL) cholesterol values. About 2.5% have electrocardiogram–left ventricular hypertrophy (ECG-LVH) and 20% to 30% are obese. Smoking occurs at a 15% prevalence in women and 20% in men. All these risk factors are more common in persons with hypertension. Less than 10% of hypertensive elderly persons were free of other major cardiovascular risk factors (Table 2–2).

## LIPIDS

National cholesterol treatment guidelines recommend detection, investigation, and treatment of all persons older than age 20 years with serum total cholesterol

**Table 2–1.** Prevalence of
Risk Factors at Age 65*

|  | Percent Prevalence | | |
|---|---|---|---|
|  | Total | Men | Women |
| Hypertension |  |  |  |
| 140–159 | 31 | 30 | 31 |
| > 160 | 23 | 19 | 26 |
| ECG-LVH | 2.2 | 2.4 | 2.1 |
| Cholesterol |  |  |  |
| 200–239 | 32 | 36 | 30 |
| > 240 | 39 | 25 | 49 |
| Glucose |  |  |  |
| 125–174 | 5.6 | 6.6 | 4.9 |
| ≥ 175 | 2.0 | 2.4 | 1.7 |
| NRW ≥ 130 | 28 | 24 | 31 |
| Cigarettes ≥ 20 | 17 | 23 | 13 |

*Data from the Framingham Study.

**Table 2–2.** Prevalence of Cardiovascular Risk Factors in the
Elderly Aged 65–89 Years*

| | Hypertensive Status (%) | | | | | |
| | Men | | | Women | | |
| | Normal | BHBP† | Definite | Normal | BHBP† | Definite |
|---|---|---|---|---|---|---|
| Cholesterol | 21 | 25 | 26 | 44 | 50 | 52 |
| HDL < 35 | 27 | 21 | 14 | 9 | 8 | 8 |
| Diabetes | 14 | 15 | 20 | 10 | 12 | 15 |
| ECG-LVH | 2 | 3 | 10 | 3 | 2 | 6 |
| Cigarettes | 21 | 20 | 21 | 16 | 15 | 12 |
| Obesity | 20 | 22 | 22 | 23 | 30 | 34 |

*Data from the Framingham Study.
†BHBP = Borderline or mild hypertension

levels exceeding 240 mg/dl and low density lipoprotein (LDL) cholesterol more
than 160 mg/dl, with no stated upper age limit.[15] In the Framingham Study, the
impacts of serum total cholesterol and LDL cholesterol were found to weaken with
advancing age, but continued to predict coronary heart disease up to age 75 years
(Table 2–3). LDL cholesterol was noted to offer little advantage over serum total
cholesterol as a predictor of coronary heart disease (see Table 2–3). Serum triglyceride was found to be a significant age-adjusted predictor in elderly women, but not
in men (see Table 2–3). The impact of the total/HDL cholesterol ratio, which
reflects the joint effect of the two-way traffic of cholesterol entering and leaving the
tissues, appears to exhibit a consistent excess risk across all age groups of the elderly
of both sexes. In women, the impact of this risk profile diminishes progressively

**Table 2–3.** Comparison of Lipid-Lipoprotein Associations
with Incidence of Coronary Heart Disease (Framingham
Study, Subjects Aged 50–80 Years)

| | Total Cholesterol | LDL Cholesterol | HDL Cholesterol | Triglyceride | Total/HDL Cholesterol | LDL/HDL Cholesterol |
|---|---|---|---|---|---|---|
| Age-Adjusted Standardized Regression Coefficient | | | | | | |
| Men | .174† | .200† | −.256‡ | .119§ | .280‡ | .294‡ |
| Women | .190† | .257‡ | −.343‡ | .240‡ | .303‡ | .340‡ |
| Age-Adjusted $Q_1/Q_5$ Hazard Ratios | | | | | | |
| Men | 2.0† | 1.7* | 0.5‡ | 1.4§ | 2.2‡ | 2.2‡ |
| Women | 1.5 | 2.2‡ | 0.5† | 2.4‡ | 2.6‡ | 2.6‡ |

*$P < 0.08$
†$P < 0.01$
‡$P < 0.001$
§NS = not significant

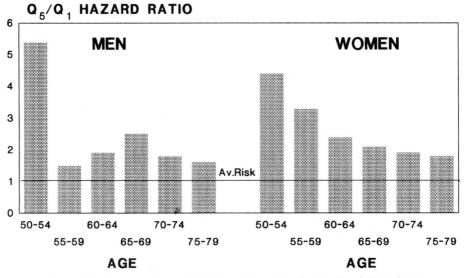

Figure 2–1. Age trends in total/HDL cholesterol risk ratio. The Framingham Study.

with advancing age, whereas in men there is an abrupt decline beyond age 55 years (Fig. 2–1). Serum total cholesterol levels measured in middle age prior to attaining age 65 years were found to predict cardiovascular events better after achieving age 65 years than cholesterol values measured on attaining age 65 years (Table 2–4). Although coronary heart disease risk ratios for LDL cholesterol and total choles-

**Table 2–4.** Risk of Coronary Heart Disease in the Elderly* by Average Serum Cholesterol Over 12 Years Prior to Age 65 (Framingham Study 32-Year Follow-up)

| KAPLAN-MEIER AGE-ADJUSTED RATES/1000 | | |
|---|---|---|
| | 10-Year | |
| Cholesterol (mg/dl) | Men | Women |
| < 200 | 158 | 49 |
| 200–239 | 214 | 86 |
| 240–279 | 225 | 122 |
| 280+ | 321 | 160 |

| COX PROPORTIONAL HAZARDS REGRESSIONS | | | |
|---|---|---|---|
| | Beta | Standard Error | P value |
| Men | 0.00466691 | 0.00167446 | 0.0053 |
| Women | 0.00799060 | 0.00147539 | 0.0001 |

*After attaining age 65 years.

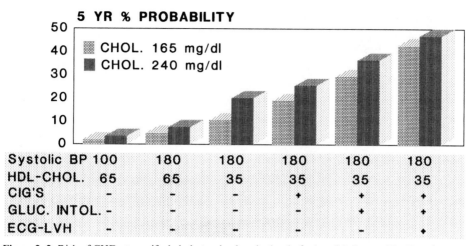

**5 YR % PROBABILITY**

CHOL. 165 mg/dl
CHOL. 240 mg/dl

| Systolic BP | 100 | 180 | 180 | 180 | 180 | 180 |
|---|---|---|---|---|---|---|
| HDL-CHOL. | 65 | 65 | 35 | 35 | 35 | 35 |
| CIG'S | - | - | - | + | + | + |
| GLUC. INTOL. | - | - | - | - | + | + |
| ECG-LVH | - | - | - | - | - | + |

**Figure 2–2.** Risk of CHD at specified cholesterol values by level of other risk factors. The Framingham Study, 70-yr-old women.

terol diminish with advancing age, this relationship is offset by an increased excess risk because of a higher absolute risk in advanced age.

The impact of any lipid varies widely, depending not only on the balance of LDL and HDL but also on the profound influence of associated cardiovascular risk factors (Fig. 2–2). Multivariate cardiovascular risk profiles composed of the other risk factors and HDL cholesterol predict coronary heart disease better in men than those including either serum total cholesterol or LDL cholesterol. In women, all of the lipids perform equally well in the context of the comprehensive risk profile.

Thus, the blood lipids appear to have relevance in the elderly. However, those with lower total/HDL cholesterol ratios or who are free of other risk factors can be spared needless therapy. Because there is no controlled trial evidence demonstrating the efficacy of controling lipids in the elderly, therapy can be justified only by extrapolating from data in the middle aged in whom both dietary and drug treatment of disordered lipids have been shown to be efficacious.[16] A clear answer will have to await evidence of slowing of lesion growth by treatment in advanced age.

## HYPERTENSION

Blood pressure and the prevalence of hypertension tends to rise progressively with advancing age.[11,12] Owing to a disproportionate rise in systolic blood pressure as age advances, the prevalence of isolated systolic hypertension increases sharply with age.[11,12] In the elderly, this variety of hypertension comprises 60% to 65% of all elevated blood pressure.[11] This isolated systolic hypertension is not an innocuous accompaniment of the loss of arterial compliance in old age. It is associated with more than a twofold increased risk of atherosclerotic cardiovascular disease (Fig. 2–3).[11,12] The high systolic pressure appears to be a direct cause of this cardiovascular morbidity and mortality rather than only a sign of the diseased rigid artery.[12] Systolic hypertension is a persistent risk factor even when arterial rigidity is taken into account.

The chief determinant of systolic hypertension in the elderly is prior elevated pressure within the normal range in middle age.[11] All components of the blood

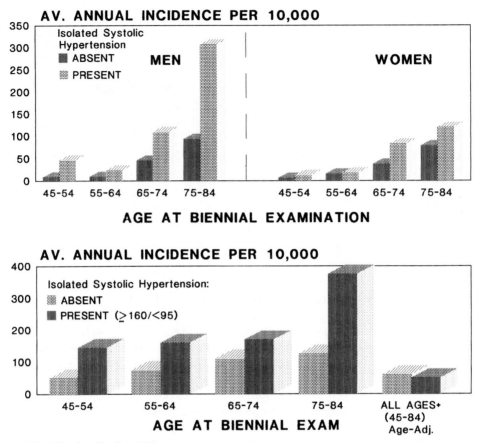

**Figure 2–3.** *Top,* ABI risk in isolated systolic hypertension by age and sex. The Framingham study, 24-yr follow-up. *Bottom,* Risk of myocardial infarction with isolated systolic hypertension (160/<95 mmHg). The Framingham Study, 24-yr follow-up, new age 45–84.

pressure appear to affect risk, particularly prior systolic pressure, although about a third of isolated systolic hypertension appears to evolve from prior diastolic or combined hypertension.[11]

Hypertension tends to occur in association with various atherogenic risk factors that either promote its occurrence or influence its impact on cardiovascular health (Table 2–5). The propensity of the hypertensive patient to develop cardiovascular sequelae is markedly influenced by these coexistent cardiovascular risk factors.[13] Judgement as to the need for treatment and regarding the choice of antihypertensive agent must be dependent on these coexistent factors. Drugs that lower blood pressure at the expense of raised LDL cholesterol, blood sugar, uric acid, and triglyceride levels and reduced HDL cholesterol may not lower risk of coronary heart disease because of failure to improve the comprehensive risk profile.

## HYPERGLYCEMIA AND ATHEROSCLEROSIS

Three decades of epidemiologic research from the Framingham Study indicate that diabetes is a powerful predisposing factor for atherosclerotic disease in general

**Table 2–5.** Risk of a Cardiovascular Event in 70-year-old Men with Hypertension* by Associated Risk Factors†

| Risk Factors | 8-Year Rate of Cardiovascular Disease per 1000 | | | | |
|---|---|---|---|---|---|
| | 281 | 309 | 403 | 547 | 804 |
| Cholesterol | 185 | 260 | 260 | 260 | 260 |
| Glucose Intolerance | — | — | + | + | + |
| Cigarettes | — | — | — | + | + |
| ECG-LVH | — | — | — | — | + |

*Systolic blood pressure 165 mm Hg.
†Framingham Study—26-year follow-up

and coronary heart disease in particular. For all age groups, in both sexes the incidence of cardiovascular disease is higher in diabetics: an average twofold for men and threefold for women (Table 2–6). This impact diminishes somewhat with advancing age, suggesting that late-onset diabetes may be less atherogenic. At all ages, the impact of diabetes is substantially greater for women in whom it eliminates their advantage over men (see Table 2–6). The relative impact (risk ratio) in women is greatest for stroke and cardiac failure, but coronary heart disease is the most common and most lethal sequela of diabetes in both sexes (Fig. 2–4).[4]

Impaired glucose tolerance predicts cardiovascular events whether manifested by a diagnosis of diabetes, hyperglycemia (130 mg/dl), glycosuria, or abnormal glucose tolerance. Blood glucose levels are an independent risk factor for cardiovascular disease in women, even within relatively normal blood sugar ranges.[17] Diabetics have higher levels of atherogenic risk factors than nondiabetics, including blood pressure, blood sugar, total/HDL cholesterol ratio, triglyceride, very low density lipoprotein (VLDL) cholesterol, uric acid, LVH, hematocrit, and fibrinogen.[17] The impact of diabetes on atherosclerotic cardiovascular disease is not entirely attributable to associated higher levels of cardiovascular risk factors, indicating

**Table 2–6.** Risk of Cardiovascular Disease* from Diabetes by Age (30-Year Follow-up—Framingham Study)

| | AGE-ADJUSTED RISKS | | | | | |
|---|---|---|---|---|---|---|
| | Absolute Risk Rate per 1000 | | Risk Ratio Diabetes/Non-diabetes | | Excess Risk Diabetes/ Nondiabetes | |
| Age | Men | Women | Men | Women | Men | Women |
| 35–64 | 38 | 30 | 2.4† | 3.8† | 22† | 22† |
| 65–94 | 65 | 48 | 1.9† | 2.0† | 30† | 24† |

*Cardiovascular disease = coronary heart disease, stroke, peripheral vascular disease, coronary heart failure
†$P < 0.001$

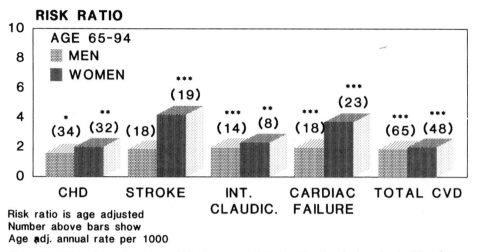

Risk ratio is age adjusted
Number above bars show
Age adj. annual rate per 1000

**Figure 2–4.** Risk of vascular disease, diabetics vs. nondiabetics. The Framingham Study, 30-yr follow-up.

some additional unique effect. Cardiovascular risk factors do not appear to operate with greater potency in diabetics than nondiabetics.[17] However, cardiovascular risk in diabetics is not uniform and varies widely depending on the level of associated risk factors (Fig. 2–5).

This unique influence of diabetes, independent of the often accompanying atherogenic risk factors, may involve an effect on thrombogenesis. Diabetics have higher mean fibrinogen values, which have been shown to enhance risk of cardiovascular disease in general and coronary heart disease in particular.[7] The excess risk of cardiovascular disease in the diabetic patient persists on adjustment for fibrinogen level, but the coronary heart disease risk seems to be predominantly in those with high fibrinogen values.

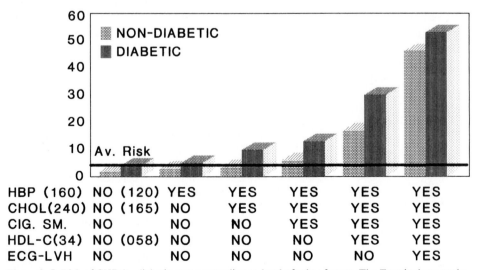

**Figure 2–5.** Risk of CHD by diabetic status according to level of other factors. The Framingham study, 50-yr-old women.

**Table 2–7.** Prognostic Outlook for Glucose Intolerance Following Myocardial Infarction (30-Year Follow-up—Framingham Study)

| SUBJECTS 65–94 YEARS OF AGE | | | |
| --- | --- | --- | --- |
| | | Coronary | |
| | Cardiovascular | Heart Disease | Myocardial | Cardiac |
| | Mortality | Mortality | Infarction | Failure |
| Men | 1.3* | 1.3* | 1.6* | 0.7* |
| Women | 3.1‡ | 2.9† | 3.2† | 4.7† |

*NS = not significant
†*P* < 0.01
‡*P* < 0.001

In those who have already sustained a myocardial infarction, diabetes imposes an added risk of recurrence, cardiac failure, and cardiovascular mortality, especially in women (Table 2–7).

Late-onset noninsulin-dependent diabetes mellitus (NIDDM) is common. In the Framingham Study, 7.8% of men and 6.2% of women developed diabetes.[17] The incidence increased sharply with age. A positive family history and obesity (especially abdominal obesity) were the strongest predisposing factors. Diabetes tended to arise from those in the high end of the normal distribution of blood sugars. Blood sugar tended to increase with age in both sexes. Examination of secular trends in the prevalence of diabetes during the past 3 decades indicates an increasing occurrence. Thus, we need more efforts at primary prevention such as weight control and exercise. Also, inasmuch as elevation of triglycerides and VLDL precedes diabetes, control of lipids may be of value.

In persons who have already developed diabetes, optimization of risk would appear to require a multifactorial approach. Inasmuch as the high risk of coronary heart disease in the diabetic patient is concentrated in those with one or more associated risk factors, prevention requires more than normalization of the blood sugar. Rational preventive measures include weight reduction, exercise, a fat-modified diet, cessation of smoking, lowering blood pressure, raising HDL cholesterol, and lowering LDL cholesterol. These measures also will lower fibrinogen.

## LEFT VENTRICULAR HYPERTROPHY

Left ventricular hypertrophy (LVH) is an important feature of the evolution of cardiovascular disease at all ages.[18] The prevalence increases with age. Its incidence increases with blood pressure and body weight.[18]

X-ray, ECG, and echocardiographic indications of LVH are frequent manifestations of organ involvement in hypertension.[18] This is not an incidental finding in the course of hypertension as the heart attempts to cope with the increased workload. Once it appears, the risk induced by hypertension escalates threefold.[18] In persons who exhibit ECG-LVH, clinical manifestations of atherosclerosis occur at about two to three times the rate of the general population (Table 2–8). The risk of coronary events and mortality in persons with ECG-LVH rivals that of persons

**Table 2–8.** Risk of Cardiovascular Events from ECG-LVH (30-Year Follow-up)

| | SUBJECTS 65–94 YEARS OF AGE | | | | | |
|---|---|---|---|---|---|---|
| | Absolute Risk Rate Per 1000* | | Risk Ratios Def. LVH/None | | Excess Risk ECG-LVH/None | |
| Cardiovascular Sequelae | Men | Women | Men | Women | Men | Women |
| Coronary heart disease | 69 | 55 | 3.0† | 3.7† | 46† | 40† |
| Stroke | 32 | 42 | 3.2† | 5.3† | 22† | 34† |
| Peripheral vascular disease | 13 | 8 | 1.9‡ | 2.7‡ | 6‡ | 5‡ |
| Cardiac failure | 51 | 40 | 6.4† | 6.7† | 43† | 34† |

*Annual rate
†P < 0.001
‡NS = not significant

with ECG evidence of myocardial infarction (MI).[18] The risk of stroke or cardiac failure associated with ECG-LVH is actually greater in women than that following appearance of ECG-MI. Left ventricular hypertrophy induces potentially lethal arrhythmias, which predispose to sudden death.[18]

Other ECG abnormalities that are more common in the elderly, such as non-specific repolarization abnormality, are also associated with an increased rate of cardiovascular events, except possibly for blocked intraventricular conduction (Table 2–9).

## LIVING HABITS

It is well recognized that diets rich in calories, saturated fat and cholesterol and deficient in fiber and fish oils are atherogenic, promoting dyslipidemia and hypertension. This appears to apply in the young as well as the old.[19,20] Weight gain also tends to promote all the major cardiovascular risk factors, and weight loss tends to correct them. Obesity promotes hypertension, a poor total/HDL cholesterol ratio,

**Table 2–9.** Risk of Coronary Heart Disease by ECG Abnormality (30-Year Follow-up—Framingham Study)

| | SUBJECTS 65–94 YEARS | | | | | |
|---|---|---|---|---|---|---|
| | Absolute Risk Rate Per 1000 | | Risk Ratio Abnormal/Normal | | Excess Risk Abnormal/Normal | |
| ECG Abnormality | Men | Women | Men | Women | Men | Women |
| ECG-LVH | 69 | 55 | 3.0* | 3.7* | 46 | 40 |
| IV-Block | 31 | 23 | 1.3† | 1.4† | 7 | 9 |
| NSA-ECG | 35 | 28 | 1.5‡ | 2.0* | 12 | 14 |

*P < 0.001
†NS = not significant
‡P < 0.05

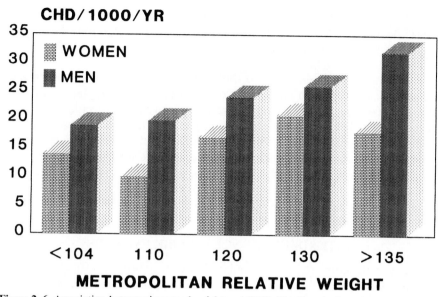

**Figure 2–6.** Association between increased weight and CHD. The Framingham Study, ages 65–94.

glucose intolerance, hyperuricemia, hypertriglyceridemia, insulin resistance, hypertension, and elevated fibrinogen.[9]

Abdominal obesity seems to be an especially disadvantageous variety of adiposity.[9,21] Largely, but not entirely, as a result of its adverse atherogenic influence on risk factors, obesity is associated with an increased risk of cardiovascular events in young and old individuals (Fig. 2–6).

Exercise exerts a protective effect against coronary heart disease in young and old, at any level of other risk factors.[10] It raises HDL cholesterol, lowers blood pressure, improves glucose tolerance, and helps control weight gain.[10] It is clearly a useful adjunct for a comprehensive risk reduction program at any age. Inasmuch as moderate exercise confers benefit, a vigorous walking program is a feasible option for the elderly.

Cigarette smoking is unhealthy at all ages. It makes platelets aggregate, lowers HDL, decreases the oxygen-carrying capacity of the blood, raises fibrinogen, and causes release of catecholamines making the myocardium more irritable.[6] As a result of these influences, cigarette smoking has a powerful influence on coronary heart disease precipitating coronary attacks and sudden deaths in those who have other risk factors and a compromised coronary circulation. There is evidence suggesting that risk of cardiovascular events such as coronary heart disease and peripheral arterial disease can be lowered by reducing by half the amount of cigarettes of those who continue to smoke.[6] This is possible regardless of how long persons have previously smoked.[6] The efficacy of quitting smoking after age 65 is not as well established as for stopping in middle age.

## MULTIVARIATE RISK

For a long time, it was considered axiomatic that virtually all disease had a single etiology that was necessary, and in most instances, sufficient to produce a particular disease. Three decades of epidemiologic research in the field of atherosclerosis have emphasized the multifactorial causality of coronary heart disease. The disease has proven to be the result of a complex interaction of atherogenic traits promoted by faulty living habits.

The formulation of causation is that certain life styles promote atherogenesis in susceptible persons culminating in overt disease during a long latent period. For example, overeating leads to obesity, which promotes atherogenic dyslipidemia, hypertension, diabetes, and elevated fibrinogen, leading to a compromised coronary circulation and, finally, a clinical event. Risk factors tend to cluster and are very common in the elderly. In every instance, the risk associated with any particular atherogenic risk factor varies widely depending on the associated risk factors present. This has implications for selection of candidates for preventive management and for comprehensive preventive measures to optimize risk.

## INTERDEPENDENCE OF RISK FACTORS

Major contributors to cardiovascular disease have been identified as a result of epidemiologic research. These risk factors fall into a number of interdependent categories: atherogenic personal attributes, living habits that promote them, signs of a compromised coronary circulation, and host susceptibility to those risk factors.

Atherogenic risk attributes include blood lipids, blood pressure, glucose intolerance, and fibrinogen. Risk associated with each is markedly affected when the others coexist. In addition, living habits such as cigarette smoking or lack of exercise can affect the risk as can innate susceptibility signified by a family history of premature vascular disease. Also at a given level of total cholesterol, risk varies depending on total/HDL ratio, providing a practical means for assessing the joint effect of the two-way traffic of total cholesterol. Diabetes on average doubles cardiovascular mortality, imparting substantially greater risk in women than men and exerting an independent effect. The risk varies widely for diabetes, hypertension, and dyslipidemia, depending on the coexisting risk factors.

Preclinical indicators of ischemic myocardial involvement greatly augment the risk in persons with a poor cardiovascular risk profile. These include ECG evidence of LVH, blocked intraventricular conduction, abnormal repolarization, and abnormal response to exercise.

Optimal risk predictions require a quantitative synthesis of risk factors into a composite estimate. For office use handbooks (Table 2–10), hand calculators, and PC software have been devised based on multiple logistic risk formulations. These have been shown to accurately predict disease in a variety of American population samples, and in old as well as young coronary candidates.

Preventive management as well as risk estimation should be multifactorial if optimal results are to be achieved. Preventive strategies should include public health measures to alter the ecology so as to shift the distribution of risk factors to a more favorable level, health education to enable people to protect their own health, and preventive medicine for high-risk candidates. Greater skill must be developed to carry out such interventions.

## SUMMARY

The major risk factors apply in the elderly as well as the young, including hypertension, dyslipidemia, impaired glucose tolerance, physical indolence, and

**TABLE 2–10.** Multivariate Risk Estimation (Framingham Study—30 Years)

| PTS: | 0 | 1 | 2 | 3 | 4 | 5 | 6 | 7 | 8 | 9 | 10 |
|---|---|---|---|---|---|---|---|---|---|---|---|
| SBP | 100 | 110 | 120 | 130 | 140 | 150 | 160 | 170 | 180 | 190 | 200 |
| HDL | 65 | 62 | 58 | 55 | 51 | 48 | 44 | 41 | 38 | 34 | 31 |
| SEX | FEM | | | | | | | MALE | | | |
| GLUC | NONE | | MALE | | | FEM | | | | | |
| CIGS | NO | | YES | | | | | | | | |
| LVH | NO | | | | | | | YES | | | |

| Age*Chol Points | 36 | 38 | 40 | 42 | 44 | 46 | 48 | 50 | 55 | 60 | 65 | 70 |
|---|---|---|---|---|---|---|---|---|---|---|---|---|
| 165 | 3 | 4 | 5 | 6 | 7 | 8 | 9 | 10 | 12 | 14 | 17 | 19 |
| 180 | 4 | 5 | 6 | 7 | 8 | 9 | 9 | 10 | 13 | 15 | 17 | 20 |
| 195 | 5 | 6 | 7 | 8 | 9 | 9 | 10 | 11 | 13 | 16 | 18 | 20 |
| 210 | 6 | 7 | 8 | 9 | 9 | 10 | 11 | 12 | 14 | 16 | 18 | 21 |
| 225 | 7 | 8 | 9 | 9 | 10 | 11 | 12 | 13 | 15 | 17 | 19 | 21 |
| 240 | 8 | 9 | 10 | 10 | 11 | 12 | 13 | 14 | 16 | 18 | 20 | 22 |
| 255 | 9 | 10 | 11 | 11 | 12 | 13 | 14 | 14 | 16 | 18 | 20 | 22 |
| 270 | 10 | 11 | 11 | 12 | 13 | 14 | 15 | 15 | 17 | 19 | 21 | 23 |
| 285 | 11 | 12 | 12 | 13 | 14 | 15 | 15 | 16 | 18 | 20 | 22 | 23 |
| 300 | 12 | 13 | 13 | 14 | 15 | 15 | 16 | 17 | 19 | 20 | 22 | 24 |
| 315 | 13 | 14 | 14 | 15 | 16 | 16 | 17 | 18 | 19 | 21 | 23 | 24 |

| PTS | 10-Year Probability | PTS | 10-Year Probability | PTS | 10-Year Probability |
|---|---|---|---|---|---|
| 3 | 0.004 | 16 | 0.023 | 30 | 0.146 |
| 4 | 0.005 | 17 | 0.027 | 31 | 0.165 |
| 5 | 0.005 | 18 | 0.030 | 32 | 0.187 |
| 6 | 0.006 | 19 | 0.035 | 33 | 0.211 |
| 7 | 0.007 | 20 | 0.040 | 34 | 0.237 |
| 8 | 0.008 | 21 | 0.045 | 35 | 0.266 |
| 9 | 0.009 | 22 | 0.052 | 36 | 0.297 |
| 10 | 0.010 | 23 | 0.059 | 37 | 0.332 |
| 11 | 0.012 | 24 | 0.068 | 38 | 0.368 |
| 12 | 0.013 | 25 | 0.077 | 39 | 0.408 |
| 13 | 0.015 | 26 | 0.088 | 40 | 0.449 |
| 14 | 0.018 | 27 | 0.100 | 41 | 0.492 |
| 15 | 0.020 | 28 | 0.114 | 42 | 0.537 |
| | | 29 | 0.129 | | |

| PTS | 10-Year Probability |
|---|---|
| 43 | 0.583 |
| 44 | 0.628 |
| 45 | 0.674 |
| 46 | 0.718 |
| 47 | 0.760 |
| 48 | 0.799 |
| 49 | 0.835 |
| 50 | 0.867 |
| 51 | 0.895 |
| 52 | 0.919 |
| 53 | 0.939 |
| 54 | 0.955 |
| 55 | 0.968 |
| 56 | 0.977 |

**10 Year Average Probability by Age and Sex (%)**

| Age | Men | Women |
|---|---|---|
| 35–44 | 5 | 1 |
| 45–54 | 11 | 4 |
| 55–64 | 19 | 10 |
| 65–74 | 23 | 14 |

cigarette smoking. These risk factors are highly prevalent in the elderly and are not inevitable consequences of aging and genetic makeup. With aging, there is a longer exposure to risk factors and diminished capacity to cope with them, resulting in a doubled incidence of cardiovascular sequelae at any level of risk factors compared with younger candidates for cardiovascular disease.

The predisposing modifiable risk factors for coronary disease, stroke, cardiac failure, and peripheral arterial disease are virtually the same in younger and older candidates for cardiovascular disease. Multivariate cardiovascular risk profiles predict cardiovascular disease as efficiently in the elderly as in the young. There is also evidence that recurrent cardiovascular events are influenced by the same risk factors that predispose to initial events.

Although proof of the efficacy of modifying risk factors in older persons is limited to hypertension control, recent declines in coronary and stroke mortality in the United States have included the elderly. This justifies extrapolations of data from the middle aged until sorely needed data become available on the efficacy of modifying risk factors in the elderly.

## REFERENCES

1. Lerner, DJ and Kannel, WB: Patterns of coronary heart disease morbidity and mortality in the sexes: A 26-year follow-up of the Framingham population. Am Heart J 3:383–390, 1986.
2. Thomas, TJ and Kannel, WB: Downward trend in cardiovascular mortality. Annu Rev Med 32:427–434, 1981.
3. Kannel, WB: Contributions of the Framingham Study to the conquest of coronary artery disease. Am J Cardiol 62:1109–1112, 1988.
4. Cupples, LA, D'Agostino, RB, Kiely, T: Some risk factors related to the annual incidence of C.V. disease and death. Framingham Study 30-year follow-up. NIH Public. No. 87-2703. US Dept. Commerce, National Technical Information Service, Springfield, Va, 1987.
5. Kannel, WB: New perspectives in cardiovascular risk factors. Am Heart J 114:213–219, 1987.
6. Kannel, WB, McGee, DL, Castelli, WP: Latest perspective on cigarette smoking and cardiovascular disease: The Framingham Study. Journal of Cardiac Rehabilitation 4:267–277, 1984.
7. Kannel, WB, Wolf, PA, Castelli, WP, et al.: Fibrinogen and risk of cardiovascular disease. The Framingham Study. JAMA 258:1183–1186, 1987.
8. Harris, T, Cook, EF, Kannel, WB, et al: Proportional hazards analysis of risk factors for coronary heart disease in individuals aged 65 or older. The Framingham Heart Study. J Am Geriatr Soc 36:1023–1028, 1988.
9. Higgins, M, Kannel, WB, Garrison, R, et al: Hazards/obesity. The Framingham Experience. Acta Med Scand (Suppl) 723:23–36, 1987.
10. Kannel, WB, Wilson, PWF, Blair, SN: Epidemiologic assessment of the role of physical activity and fitness in development of cardiovascular disease. Am Heart J 109:876–885, 1985.
11. Wilking, S, Van, B, Belanger, A, et al: Determinants of isolated systolic hypertension. JAMA 260:3451–3455, 1988.
12. Kannel, WB, Dawber, JR, McGee, DL: Perspectives in systolic hypertension: The Framingham Study. Circulation 61:1179–1182, 1980.
13. Kannel, WB: Hypertension: Relationship with other risk factors. Drugs (Suppl 1):1–11, 1986.
14. Kannel, WB: High-density lipoproteins: Epidemiologic profile and risks of coronary artery disease. Am J Cardiol 52:93–123, 1983.
15. The Expert Panel: Report of the national cholesterol education program expert panel on detection, evaluation, and treatment of high blood cholesterol in adults. Arch Intern Med 148:36–39, 1988.
16. Tikkanen, MJ: Hypercholesterolemia in the elderly. Is drug treatment justified? Am Heart J 9(Suppl 1):79–82, 1988.
17. Kannel, WB and McGee, DL: Diabetes and glucose intolerance as risk factors for cardiovascular disease. The Framingham Study. Diabetes Care 2:110–126, 1979.
18. Kannel, WB, Dannenberg, AL, Levy, D: Population implications of electrocardiographic left ventricular hypertrophy. Am J Cardiol 60:851–931, 1987.
19. Report of intersociety commission for heart disease resources. Optional resources for primary prevention of atherosclerotic disease. Circulation 70:155A–205A, 1984.
20. Grundy, SM, Bilheimer D, Blackburn, H, et al: Rationale of the diet-heart statement of the American Heart Association. Report of the nutrition committee. Circulation 65:839A, 1982.
21. Bjorntorp, P: Regional patterns of fat distribution. Ann Intern Med 103:994–995, 1985.
22. Leaverton, PE, Sorlie, PD, Kleinamen, JC, et al: Representativeness of the Framingham risk model for coronary heart disease mortality: A comparison with a national cohort study. J Chronic Dis 40:775–785, 1987.
23. Anderson, KM, Wilson, PWF, Odell, PM, Kannel, WB: An updated coronary risk profile. A statment for health professionals. Circulation 83:356–362, 1991.

# PART 2

# Clinical Considerations

# CHAPTER 3

# Cardiovascular Consequences of the Aging Process

*Jannet F. Lewis, M.D.*
*Barry J. Maron, M.D.*

The average life span for Americans has increased substantially during the past several decades. This improved longevity has resulted in marked growth in the elderly segment of the population. As a consequence, there has been considerable interest and investigation into the "normal" physiologic processes that are associated with aging, apart from the pathologic changes that occur with the development of disease.[1-6] Indeed, to understand the physiologic consequences of cardiovascular disease in the elderly, it is first necessary to have an understanding of those physiologic changes that occur as part of the normal aging process in order to establish the "baseline" upon which pathologic conditions are superimposed.

## CHANGES IN CARDIOVASCULAR STRUCTURE

### LEFT VENTRICULAR MYOCARDIUM

A number of echocardiographic and necropsy studies, evaluating large numbers of patients stratified for age in a cross-sectional fashion (and excluding individuals with obesity, systemic hypertension, or clinically apparent valvular or coronary artery disease), have shown relatively mild increases in left ventricular wall thickness and cardiac mass concomitant with the aging process.[7-13] However, the wall thickness values reported as part of these studies in apparently normal elderly individuals are usually within generally accepted normal limits in absolute terms, that is, $\leq 11$ mm.

Kitzman and associates[10] performed postmortem examinations on more than 700 normal hearts in subjects ranging in age from 20 to 99 years and found ventricular septal thickness to increase with advancing age; however, these differences were statistically significant only when youthful individuals in the third decade of life and elderly subjects in the tenth decade were compared. Similarly, investigations employing M-mode echocardiography have assessed the relationship between aging and myocardial hypertrophy (Fig. 3–1).[8,9,11,12] Most such studies also have

25

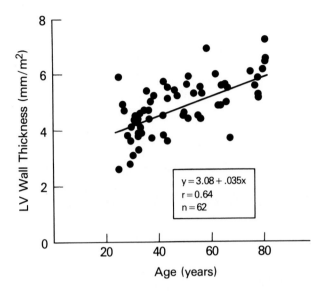

**Figure 3–1.** Linear regression plot demonstrating the relationship between age and diastolic left ventricular wall thickness (indexed to body surface area). Advancing age is associated with increasing wall thickness. (Adapted from Gerstenblith, G et al, Circulation 1977; 56:273 and reproduced with permission of the American Heart Association.)

shown a modest but statistically significant increase in left ventricular wall thickness and mass with aging. Of note, in each of these studies, absolute increases in ventricular septal and posterior wall thicknesses were usually modest, and statistically significant differences also were found only when comparing the oldest with the youngest age groups. For example, in the study by Gerstenblith and coworkers[8] in 105 subjects ranging in age from 25 to 84 years, mean wall thickness in individuals ≥ 65 years was 11 mm, compared with a mean of 9 mm in those < 45 years. More than 90% of elderly subjects ≥ 65 years of age had wall thickness between 10 and 12 mm. Similarly, Gardin and colleagues[9] studied 136 subjects ranging in age from 20 to 96 years. Individuals in the oldest age group (older than 70 years) had mean ventricular septal and free wall thicknesses of 12 mm, which were significantly greater than subjects in the youngest age group (30 years or younger). However, between these extremes in age, wall thickness showed very minimal changes, so that the mean values for septal and free wall thicknesses increased by only 0.3 mm for each decade between ages 30 and 70. In each of the echocardiographic studies cited, left ventricular cavity dimension showed little or no change with increasing age.[8–10]. Thus, increases in left ventricular mass associated with aging were due largely to increases in wall thickness rather than to cavity enlargement. It would appear from most of these studies cited that it is unusual for elderly individuals without underlying cardiovascular disease to have wall thickness > 13 mm. This observation is relevant to the distinction between the normal aging heart and certain pathologic states. For example, when obstructive hypertrophic cardiomyopathy is identified in elderly patients, only a relatively modest increase in ventricular septal thickness (15 to 16 mm) is usually present.[14,15] Thus, in elderly patients suspected of having hypertrophic cardiomyopathy, it is unlikely that septal thickness ≥ 15 mm, in the absence of another cardiovascular disease capable of producing left ventricular hypertrophy (e.g., systemic hypertension or aortic valvular stenosis), is a normal concomitant of the aging process. Rather, it is more likely (particularly in the presence of symptoms) that wall thicknesses of this magnitude represent primary cardiac disease.

The mechanism by which wall thickness and mass increase with aging is not known. However, several potential explanations have been offered. For example, increased stiffness of the aorta occurring as a consequence of the aging process may result in the modest myocardial hypertrophy observed in the elderly.[16,17] It has been proposed that reduced distensibility of the aortic wall results in increased systolic blood pressure,[18-20] and consequently increased impedance to left ventricular ejection, which in turn causes secondary left ventricular hypertrophy.

Owing to the lack of histologic data in healthy elderly individuals, it is not known to what extent the observed increase in wall thickness and mass are due to cellular hypertrophy. On the other hand, there are data showing increased connective tissue elements of the aging myocardium.[21-23] Schaub[21] reported that the collagen concentration in normal rat hearts (as assessed by measurement of hydroxyproline) increased threefold with aging. Therefore, it is possible that increased collagen content may account, in part, for the increased left ventricular wall thickness and mass that has been observed with aging.

## CARDIAC VALVES

The size of the cardiac valves appears to increase with aging. Although careful morphometric studies measuring the leaflet area and length have not been performed, age-related changes in valve circumference have been reported. In an examination of 765 autopsy specimens, Kitzman and coworkers[10] found that mean valve circumferences for each of the four cardiac valves increased progressively throughout life. In younger subjects, the atrioventricular valves were substantially larger than the semilunar valves, with the aortic valve the smallest of the four valves. However, with advancing age, the aortic valve showed the greatest increases in valvular circumference; by the fourth decade of life, the aortic valve exceeded the pulmonic valve in size, and by the tenth decade, aortic valve size approached that of the mitral valve. These changes in cardiac valve size did not appear to be associated with important valvular dysfunction.

Aging is also associated with thickening and calcification of the aortic and mitral leaflets.[24-26] Sahasakul and colleagues[26] measured both aortic and mitral leaflet thicknesses at autopsy in 200 hearts without evidence of cardiovascular disease. Leaflet thicknesses increased substantially with age, so that ultimately (in subjects older than 60 years of age) the valves were more than twice the thickness of those in subjects younger than age 20 years.

In another necropsy study of 200 normal hearts (without clinically significant aortic or mitral stenosis),[24] calcification of the aortic valve (usually limited to the aortic surfaces of the cusps, but not involving the commissures) was more common and occurred earlier in life than did mitral valve calcification. These age-related structural changes in the aortic and mitral valves appear to be due to similar processes, that is, degeneration of the collagen fibers and decreased size and number of nuclei, followed by lipid accumulation and calcification.[24]

Calcification in the aging heart is commonly situated in the potential space between the posterior mitral leaflet and the mural endocardium of the left ventricular wall.[25,27-29] Of note, this submitral calcification, commonly known as "mitral annular calcification," occurs more commonly in women[27-29] and appears to be associated with an increased prevalence of cardiac conduction defects and atrial fibrillation even in the absence of structural cardiovascular disease.[28,29] Calcification

in the submitral region is usually not associated with clinically significant mitral regurgitation or stenosis, unless particularly severe.

It is possible, however, that submitral calcification may influence the clinical expression of other cardiovascular diseases. For example, development of submitral calcification is common in elderly patients with hypertrophic cardiomyopathy,[14,30] and may be, in part, responsible for obstruction to left ventricular outflow and severe cardiac symptoms in older patients with this disease.[14] It has been proposed that deposition and accumulation of calcium beneath the posterior mitral leaflet may gradually displace the valve apparatus anteriorly within the left ventricular cavity, closer to the ventricular septum. Such narrowing of the left ventricular out-flow tract may create the circumstance whereby systolic contact between the mitral valve and septum (and subaortic obstruction)[31–33] develops for the first time rela-tively late in life.

## Aorta

With advancing age, the aorta undergoes enlargement associated with a reduc-tion in compliance.[8,9,17,19,34] Nichols and associates[17] studied 45 subjects with con-trast angiography and found the internal systolic radius of the ascending aorta to increase significantly with advancing age. Specifically, in individuals ranging in age from 19 to 65 years, the aorta showed almost a 10% increase in radius (20% increase in cross-sectional area) for each decade studied. Similarly, M-mode echocardio-graphic studies have shown a progressive increase in aortic root diameter with advancing age. Gerstenblith and associates[8] demonstrated a modest, but statisti-cally significant increase in aortic root diameter in subjects 65 years of age or older (mean 33 mm) compared with subjects younger than 45 years (mean 31 mm). Gar-din and coworkers[9] also showed larger aortic root diameter in individuals older than age 70 years (mean 34 mm) compared with that in younger individuals under 30 years (mean 27 mm). Of note, absolute values for aortic root dimension are only modestly increased in normal elderly subjects, rarely exceeding 40 mm.

Aging changes in aortic size are associated with progressive thickening of the aortic media and intima.[6,18] On histologic examination, this increase in aortic thick-ness appears to be associated with elastin fragmentation, calcification, and increased amounts of collagen.[20] These structural changes are associated with mea-surable decreases in aortic distensibility as evidenced clinically by increases in pulse wave velocity.[16,17,19,34,35]

The changes in the aortic wall that have been described with aging are believed to occur independent of coexistent atherosclerosis. In this regard, Avolio and col-leagues[16] showed that pulse wave velocity (a measure of aortic stiffness) increased with aging in native Chinese, despite the low prevalence of atherosclerosis in that population.

## CHANGES IN LEFT VENTRICULAR FUNCTION

### Systolic Function

The preponderance of data show that left ventricular systolic function under basal conditions is not altered by the aging process. In recent investigations using volunteer subjects who were carefully screened for the presence of coexistent car-

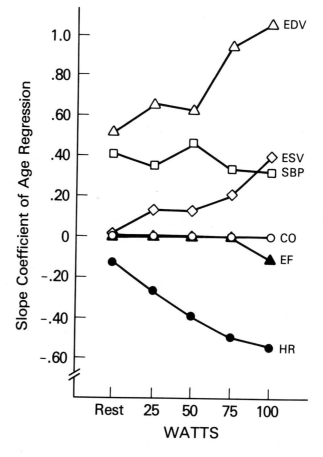

**Figure 3–2.** Relation of effects of aging on hemodynamic parameters elicited with exercise. Vertical axis is slope coefficient of age, and horizontal axis is level of exercise workload. For each of the hemodynamic parameters studied, an increase or decrease in the slope coefficient with increasing workloads indicates a respective increase or decrease in that parameter with advancing age. CO = cardiac output; EDV = end-diastolic volume; EF = ejection fraction; ESV = end-systolic volume; HR = heart rate; SBP = systolic blood pressure. (Adapted from Rodeheffer, RJ et al, Circulation 1984; 69:203 and reproduced with permission of the American Heart Association.)

diovascular disease, neither cardiac output nor ejection fraction showed a relationship to age (Fig. 3–2).[8,9,36–38] In addition, certain experimental data appear to support these observations. In a study using isolated rat cardiac muscle, measures of myocardial contractility did not differ between adult and senescent animals.[39,40]

Similarly, systolic function with exercise also does not appear to be impaired by the aging process. Rodeheffer and coworkers[36] used radionuclide angiography to study the effect of aging on left ventricular volume and function with exercise in 61 subjects who were carefully screened for the presence of underlying cardiac disease. Elderly subjects showed less increase in ejection fraction with exercise than did younger individuals; however, absolute values for ejection fraction at maximal exercise in elderly individuals rarely decreased from the basal levels. In addition, cardiac output appeared to be maintained at maximal exercise, largely by virtue of an increase in left ventricular diastolic volume.

Of note, early invasive studies described lower cardiac output at rest in elderly subjects (compared with younger individuals) as well as decreased cardiac output and increased filling pressures with exercise.[41–43] Julius and associates[42] showed that cardiac output was 25% less in study subjects older than 50 years of age compared with those younger than 35 years. However, because the subjects in these invasive studies did not undergo coronary arteriography or treadmill exercise testing, these reports may have inadvertently included individuals with occult coronary artery

disease, and therefore these data may not be entirely applicable to healthy individuals.

## DIASTOLIC FUNCTION

In contrast to the absence of important changes in systolic function associated with aging, several investigators have demonstrated age-related alterations in measures of left ventricular diastolic performance.[9,37,38,44–51] Using invasive techniques to measure intracardiac pressures, Harrison and coworkers[44] demonstrated prolongation of left ventricular relaxation in elderly men without clinical or angiographic evidence of cardiovascular disease. More recently, a variety of noninvasive techniques have been used to show abnormalities of left ventricular filling associated with aging in subjects without cardiovascular disease.[9,37,46–51] For example, radionuclide angiographic studies have demonstrated an age-related reduced rate of early diastolic rapid filling, prolonged time to peak filling, and an increased compensatory contribution of late diastolic (or atrial) filling.[37,48,51]

Similar findings have been reported using pulsed Doppler echocardiography to assess the pattern of transmitral flow-velocity. Several such reports show that advancing age is associated with decreased early diastolic flow-velocity as well as reduced rate of decline of early diastolic flow-velocity, associated with augmentation of late diastolic flow-velocity; therefore, the relative contribution of late flow-velocity to total transmitral flow-velocity is increased (Figs. 3–3 and 3–4).[46,49,50] Indeed, the strong relationship between age and the relative contribution of atrial systole to total left ventricular filling often creates difficulty in the clinical interpretation of Doppler-derived indexes of diastolic filling in the elderly. This pattern of reduced early diastolic flow-velocity, slowed rate of decline of flow-velocity in early diastole, and increased late diastolic flow-velocity closely resembles abnormal diastolic filling patterns observed in patients with a variety of cardiovascular diseases[52–57] (see Fig. 3–4).

The exact mechanisms responsible for these age-related diastolic changes are not completely understood. It is possible that alterations in diastolic filling are due, in part, to the modest increase in left ventricular wall thickness and mass that often

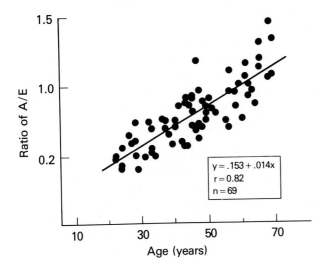

$$y = .153 + .014x$$
$$r = 0.82$$
$$n = 69$$

**Figure 3–3.** Relation between the ratio of late diastolic and early diastolic flow-velocities (A/E) and age. Advancing age is associated with an increase in the peak late diastolic flow-velocity (A) relative to peak early diastolic flow-velocity (E). (Adapted from Miyatake, K et al, Am J Cardiol 1984; 53:586 and reproduced with permission of the American Journal of Cardiology.)

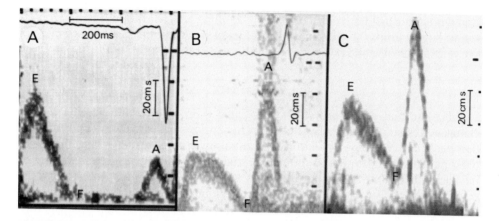

**Figure 3–4.** Transmitral diastolic flow-velocity waveforms in three subjects. *A*) From a 30-year-old man without evidence of cardiovascular disease. Peak early diastolic flow-velocity (*E*) is substantially greater than peak late flow-velocity (*A*), and rate of decline of flow-velocity in early diastole (*EF* slope) is normal. *B*) From a 72-year-old healthy woman without evidence of cardiovascular disease. Peak early diastolic flow-velocity (*E*) is reduced compared to *Panel A*, and peak late flow-velocity (*A*) is increased. Rate of decline flow-velocity in early diastole is prolonged. *C*) From a 40-year-old man with systemic hypertension and moderate left ventricular hypertrophy. Waveform from this hypertensive patient is virtually identical to normal healthy elderly patient in *Panel B*. Each vertical division represents a 20 cm/s increment in flow-velocity; horizontal time-lines are 40 ms apart.

accompanies aging.[8,9,58] However, several investigations have shown little correlation between indexes of left ventricular filling in elderly patients and wall thickness.[37,38] Alternately, such diastolic filling alterations could be due to aging-induced changes in left ventricular compliance that are not entirely a consequence of increased myocardial mass. The progressive increase in left atrial size that occurs with advancing age[8–10] probably also reflects such changes in left ventricular compliance.

Certain cellular mechanisms may play an important role in production of diastolic alterations that occur in the aging myocardium. For example, the aging process is associated with slowing of the rate at which calcium is sequestered by the sarcoplasmic reticulum following myocardial excitation.[39] It has been suggested that accumulation of calcium at the onset of diastole may impair left ventricular relaxation and filling.[39,59]

Finally, increased myocardial collagen content[21,22] may contribute to alterations in diastolic filling by virtue of increasing left ventricular stiffness. In addition to increased amounts of collagen, it also has been suggested that qualitative changes in the cross-linking of collagen (which increase the rigidity of the intercellular collagenous fibers) also may impact on the overall myocardial stiffness.[21,22]

Regardless of the precise mechanisms by which left ventricular diastolic filling alterations occur with aging, recognition that these changes are part of the normal aging process is essential to the reliable interpretation of noninvasively obtained parameters of diastolic filling in elderly patients. For example, in normal elderly individuals, the transmitral flow-velocity waveforms obtained by Doppler echocardiography are often indistinguishable from those in symptomatic (and asymptomatic) patients with a variety of cardiovascular diseases—e.g., systemic hypertension, coronary artery disease, and hypertrophic cardiomyopathy—known to be associated with abnormal left ventricular diastolic filling and relaxation.[52-57] This observation largely limits the clinical utility of Doppler echocardiographic assessment of left ventricular diastolic performance in this age group.

## SUMMARY

The normal aging process is associated with a variety of cardiovascular changes. Recognition of these alterations in cardiovascular structure and function that occur in the aging population is essential for assessment of cardiac disease in older patients. For example, a number of studies show that aging is associated with increasing left ventricular wall thickness and mass. However, these changes are gradual and relatively mild, and absolute wall thickness measurements in individual elderly subjects rarely exceed generally accepted normal values.

Parameters of left ventricular systolic function (either under basal conditions or with exercise) change little with aging. In contrast, apparent alterations in left ventricular diastolic filling patterns often accompany advancing age. Investigations in normal elderly subjects have shown that the early filling phase is prolonged, and the rate and volume (as well as flow-velocity) of rapid filling are decreased. These alterations are associated with a compensatory increase in late diastolic filling with atrial systole. The aging changes in left ventricular filling identified by noninvasive tests (such as Doppler echocardiography or radionuclide angiography) may mimic in appearance those observed in a number of cardiovascular diseases, making interpretation of their clinical significance difficult in an elderly population.

## REFERENCES

1. Lakatta, EG: Alterations in the cardiovascular system that occur in advanced age. Fed Proc 38:163–167, 1979.
2. Fleg, JL: Alterations in cardiovascular structure and function with advancing age. Am J Cardiol 57:33C–44C, 1986.
3. Lakatta, EG and Yin, FCP: Myocardial aging: Functional alterations and related cellular mechanisms. Am J Physiol 242:H927–H931, 1982.
4. Walsh, RA: Cardiovascular effects of the aging process. Am J Med 82(Suppl 1B):34–40, 1987.
5. Lakatta, EG, Mitchell, JH, Pomerance A, et al: Human aging: Changes in structure and function. J Am Coll Cardiol 10:42A–47A, 1987.
6. Safar, M: Aging and its effects on the cardiovascular system. Drugs 39(Suppl 1):1–8, 1990.
7. Sjögren, AL: Left ventricular wall thickness determined by ultrasound in 100 subjects without heart disease. Chest 60:341–346, 1971.
8. Gerstenblith, G, Frederiksen, J, Yin, FCP, et al: Echocardiographic assessment of a normal adult aging population. Circulation 56:273–278, 1977.
9. Gardin, JM, Henry, WL, Savage, DD, et al: Echocardiographic measurements in normal subjects: Evaluation of an adult population without clinically apparent heart disease. Journal of Clinical Ultrasound 7:439–447, 1979.
10. Kitzman, DW, Scholz, DG, Hagen PT, et al: Age-related changes in normal human hearts during the first 10 decades of life. Part II (maturity): A quantitative anatomic study of 765 specimens from subjects 20 to 99 years old. Mayo Clin Proc 63:137–146, 1988.
11. Henry, WL, Gardin, JM, Ware, JH: Echocardiographic measurement in normal subjects from infancy to old age. Circulation 62:1054–1061, 1980.
12. Marcomichelakis, J, Withers, R, Newman, GB, et al: The relationship of age to the thickness of the interventricular septum, the posterior left ventricular wall and their ratio. International Journal of Cardiology 4:405–415, 1983.
13. Maron, BJ: Living with the septal to free wall thickness ratio. International Journal of Cardiology 4:417–419, 1983.

14. Lewis, JF and Maron, BJ: Elderly patients with hypertrophic cardiomyopathy: A subset with distinctive left ventricular morphology and progressive clinical course late in life. J Am Coll Cardiol 13:36–45, 1989.

15. Spirito, P and Maron, BJ: Relation between extent of left ventricular hypertrophy and age in hypertrophic cardiomyopathy. J Am Coll Cardiol 13:820–823, 1989.

16. Avolio, AP, Chen, S-G, Wang, R-P, et al: Effects of aging on changing arterial compliance and left ventricular load in a northern Chinese urban community. Circulation 68:50–58, 1983.

17. Nichols, WW, O'Rourke, MF, Avolio, AP, et al: Effects of age on ventricular-vascular coupling. Am J Cardiol 55:1179–1184, 1985.

18. O'Rourke, MF: Arterial function in health and disease. Edinburgh, Churchill Livingstone, 1982, pp 53–66, 153–169, 196–252.

19. Merillon, JP, Motte, G, Masquet, C, et al: Relationship between physical properties of the arterial system and left ventricular performance in the course of aging and arterial hypertension. Eur Heart J 3(Suppl A):95–102, 1982.

20. Yin, FC: The aging vasculature and its effects on the heart. In Weisfeldt, ML (ed): The aging heart. Raven Press, New York, 1980, pp. 137–213.

21. Schaub, MC: The aging of collagen in the heart muscle. Gerontologia 10:38–41, 1964–1965.

22. Verzar, F: The stages and consequences of aging collagen. Gerontologia 15:233–239, 1969.

23. Weisfeldt, ML, Loeven, WA, Schok, HW: Resting and active mechanical properties of trabeculae carnae from aged male rats. Am J Physiol 22:H1921–7, 1971.

24. Sell, S and Scully, RE: Aging changes in the aortic and mitral valves. Am J Physiol 46:345–355, 1965.

25. Roberts, WC: The senile cardiac calcification syndrome. Am J Cardiol 58:572–574, 1986.

26. Sahasakul, Y, Edwards, ED, Naessens, JM, et al: Age-related changes in aortic and mitral valve thickness: Implications for two-dimensional echocardiography based on an autopsy study of 200 normal human hearts. Am J Cardiol 62:424–430, 1988.

27. Fulkerson, PK, Beaver, BM, Auseon, JC, et al: Calcification of the mitral annulus. Etiology, clinical associations, complications and therapy. Am J Med 66:967–977, 1979.

28. Nair, CK, Aronow, WS, Sketch, MH, et al: Clinical and echocardiographic characteristics of patients with mitral annular calcification. Comparison with age- and sex-matched control subjects. Am J Cardiol 51:992–995, 1983.

29. Savage, DD, Garrison, RJ, Castelli, WP, et al: Prevalence of submitral (annular) calcium and its correlates in a general population-based sample (The Framingham Study). Am J Cardiol 51:1375–1378, 1983.

30. Motammed, HE and Roberts, WC. Frequency and significance of mitral annular calcium in hypertrophic cardiomyopathy: An analysis of 200 mecropsy patients. Am J Cardiol 60:877–884, 1987.

31. Henry, WL, Clark, CE, Griffith, JM, et al: Mechanism of left ventricular outflow obstruction in patients with obstructive asymmetric septal hypertrophy (idiopathic hypertrophic subaortic stenosis). Am J Cardiol 35:337–345, 1975.

32. Pollick, C, Rakowski, H, Wigle, ED: Muscular subaortic stenosis: The quantitative relationship between systolic anterior motion and the pressure gradient. Circulation 69:43–49, 1984.

33. Maron, BJ, Gottdiener, JS, Arce, J, et al: Dynamic subaortic obstruction in hypertrophic cardiomyopathy: Analysis by pulsed Doppler echocardiography. J Am Coll Cardiol 6:1–8, 1985.

34. Learoyd, BM and Taylor, MG: Alterations with age in the viscoelastic properties of human arterial walls. Circ Res 18:278–292, 1966.

35. Gonza, ER, Marble, AE, Shaw, A, et al: Age related changes in the mechanics of the aorta and pulmonary artery of man. J Appl Physiol 36:407–411, 1974.

36. Rodeheffer, RJ, Gerstenblith, G, Becker, LC, et al: Exercise cardiac output is maintained with advancing age in healthy human subjects: Cardiac dilatation and increased stroke volume compensate for a diminished heart rate. Circulation 69:203–213, 1984.

37. Bonow, RO, Vitale, DF, Bacharach, SL, et al: Effects of aging on asynchronous left ventricular regional function and global ventricular filling in normal human subjects. J Am Coll Cardiol 11:50–58, 1988.

38. Arora, RR, Machac, J, Goldman, HE, et al: Atrial kinetics and left ventricular diastolic filling in the healthy elderly. J Am Coll Cardiol 9:1255–1260, 1987.

39. Lakatta, EG, Gerstenblith, G, Angell, CS, et al: Prolonged contraction duration in the aged myocardium. J Clin Invest 55:61–68, 1975.

40. Spurgeon, HA, Thorne, PR, Yin, FCP, et al: Increased dynamic stiffness of trabeculae carnae from senescent rats. Am J Physiol 232:H373–80, 1977.

41. Granath, A, Jonsson, B, Strandell, T: Circulation in healthy old men studied by right heart catheterization at rest and during exercise in supine and sitting positions. Acta Med Scand 176:425–446, 1964.

42. Julius, S, Avery, A, Whitlock, LS, et al: Influence of age on the hemodynamic response to exercise. Circulation 36:222–230, 1967.

43. Conway, J, Wheeler, R, Hammerstedt, R: Sympathetic nervous activity during exercise in relation to age. Cardiovasc Res 5:577–581, 1971.

44. Harrison, TR, Dixon, D, Russell, RO, et al: The relation of age to the duration of contraction, ejection, and relaxation of the normal human heart. Am Heart J 67:189–199, 1964.

45. Weisfeldt, ML: Left ventricular function. In Weisfeldt ML (ed): The Aging Heart. Raven Press, New York, 1980, pp. 297–316.

46. Miyatake, K, Okamoto, M, Kinoshita, N, et al: Augmentation of atrial contribution to left ventricular inflow with aging as assessed by intracardiac Doppler flowmetry. Am J Cardiol 53:586–589, 1984.

47. Nixon, JV, Hallmark, H, Page, K, et al: Ventricular performance in human hearts aged 61 to 73 years. Am J Cardiol 56:932–937, 1985.

48. Miller, TR, Grossman, SJ, Schectman, KB, et al: Left ventricular diastolic filling and its association with age. Am J Cardiol 58:531–535, 1986.

49. Kuo, LC, Quinones, MA, Rokey, R, et al: Quantitation of atrial contribution to left ventricular filling by pulsed Doppler echocardiography and the effect of age in normal and diseased hearts. Am J Cardiol 59:1174–1178, 1987.

50. Spirito, P and Maron, BJ: Influence of aging on Doppler echocardiographic indices of left ventricular diastolic function. Br Heart J 59:672–679, 1988.

51. Sinak, LJ and Clements, IP: Influence of age and sex on left ventricular filling at rest in subjects without clinical cardiac disease. Am J Cardiol 64:646–650, 1989.

52. Gardin, JM, Dabestani, A, Glasgow, GA, et al: Echocardiographic and Doppler flow observations in obstructed and nonobstructed hypertrophic cardiomyopathy. Am J Cardiol 56:614–621, 1985.

53. Maron, BJ, Spirito, P, Green, KJ, et al: Noninvasive assessment of left ventricular diastolic function by pulsed Doppler echocardiography in patients with hypertrophic cardiomyopathy. J Am Coll Cardiol 10:743–747, 1987.

54. Phillips, RA, Coplan, NL, Krakoff, LR, et al: Doppler echocardiographic analysis of left ventricular filling in treated hypertensive patients. J Am Coll Cardiol 9:317–322, 1987.

55. Appleton, CP, Hatle, LK, Popp, RL: Relation of transmitral flow-velocity patterns to left ventricular diastolic function: New insights from a combined hemodynamic and Doppler echocardiographic study. J Am Coll Cardiol 12:426–440, 1988.

56. Rokey, R, Kuo, LC, Zogbi, WA, et al: Determination of parameters of left ventricular diastolic filling with pulsed Doppler echocardiography: Comparison with cineangiography. Circulation 71:543–550, 1985.

57. Spirito, P and Maron, BJ: Doppler echocardiography for assessing left ventricular diastolic function. Ann Intern Med 109:122–126, 1988.

58. Grossman, W, McLaurin, LP, Moos, SP, et al: Wall thickness and diastolic properties of the left ventricle. Circulation 49:129–135, 1974.

59. Froehlich, JP, Lakatta, EG, Beard, E, et al: Studies of sarcoplasmic reticulum function and contraction duration in young adult and aged rat myocardium. J Mol Cell Cardiol 10:427–438, 1978.

# CHAPTER 4

# Changes with Aging as Reflected in Noninvasive Cardiac Studies

*Simon Chakko, M.D.*
*Kenneth M. Kessler, M.D.*

Cardiovascular disease is the major cause of morbidity and mortality in the elderly population.[1] Noninvasive cardiac studies are commonly used to evaluate the structure and function of the heart. Aging causes anatomic and physiologic changes that are difficult to separate from pathologic changes caused by diseases of the cardiovascular system because of the high prevalence of heart disease among the elderly in Western societies.[2] In one clinical study of 500 old people living at home, there was evidence of heart disease in 50% of those aged 65 to 74 and in 60% of those aged 75 or older.[3] By definition, aging processes are usually progressive and physiologically irreversible and are considered normal in that they occur in all members of the population.[4] However, the presence of age-related changes is not uniform. For example, autopsy studies have shown that senile cardiac amyloidosis, which is commonly associated with aging, is present in only about 50% of those aged 75 or older.[5] Many changes that are present in the majority of elderly subjects, such as coronary atherosclerosis, must be regarded as diseases and not expressions of normal aging.[5]

## MORPHOLOGIC CHANGES OF AGING

To understand the changes observed in noninvasive cardiac studies, knowledge of the morphologic changes encountered in aged hearts is essential. Recent autopsy studies of large numbers of aged hearts describe these changes in detail[5-9] and are summarized in Table 4–1. Brown atrophy of the elderly heart is the result of lipofuscin deposits in the paranuclear sarcoplasm. It accumulates linearly with age and does not cause any clinical cardiac dysfunction.[9] Basophilic degeneration also is very common. It appears as solid amorphous masses that stain basophilic with hematoxylin and eosin and is found in the sarcoplasm.[5] Like lipofuscin, this substance is strongly age-associated.

Prevalence of amyloid deposits increases sharply after age 70; it is demonstra-

35

**Table 4–1.** Morphologic Changes Observed in Elderly Hearts

1. Myocardium
    Brown atrophy and basophilic degeneration
    Increased subepicardial fat
    Amyloid deposits
    Ventricular hypertrophy
2. Chambers
    Enlarged atrial cavities
    Decreased ventricular cavity
    Sigmoid-shaped ventricular septum
    Lipomatous hypertrophy of atrial septum
3. Valves
    Mitral annular calcification
    Aortic valve calcification
    Buckling of mitral leaflets toward atrium
4. Aorta
    Dilated and tortuous
    Rightward shift
    Medial atrophy, calcification
5. Coronary Arteries
    Ectatic and tortuous
    Atherosclerotic plaques, calcification

ble in 50% of patients older than age 65 although limited to fine atrial deposits in over half the cases and with ventricular involvement in only 16.5%.[5] Clinical significance of amyloid deposits depends upon its severity; small deposits are of no clinical consequence but extensive ventricular involvement results in cardiac failure. The walls of the ventricles are firm, rubbery, and noncompliant. Amyloid deposits may be found on the cardiac valves, and endocardial involvement may be associated with overlying thrombi.[10] Amyloidosis may result in systolic or diastolic dysfunction or a combination of both. The amount of subepicardial fat increases with age and is prominent over the anterior surface of the right ventricle and atrioventricular groove. Lipomatous hypertrophy of the interatrial septum is the accumulation of fatty deposits that may produce a tumor-like mass and may cause arrhythmias.[11]

Heart weight increases progressively with age. In a necropsy study of patients aged 90 years or older, the mean heart weight was increased in 67%, > 350 g in elderly women and > 400 g in elderly men.[12] Heart weight was 0.7% of body weight in elderly women and 0.6% in elderly men, compared with 0.4% and 0.45% in normal young women and men respectively. Some studies have reported a decrease in heart weight after the seventh decade.[13] The atrial cavities enlarge and the ventricular cavities become smaller (Fig. 4–1). Ventricular septal thickness is increased in the elderly, and the mean ratio of septal to left ventricular free wall ratio may exceed 1.20.[13] The ventricular septum bends leftward, bulging into the left ventricular outflow tract and is described as a "sigmoid septum."[9] These changes may be mistaken for hypertrophic cardiomyopathy. There is an increase in the subendocardial and subepicardial collagen; muscle decreases and fibrosis increases around 60 years of age.[9] These changes affect the elasticity and compliance of the heart.

Morphologic changes of aging are prominent on the aortic and mitral valves. Focal fibrous thickening at valvular margins of closure is common. Calcific deposits are often encountered at the bases of aortic cusps and margins of closure of the

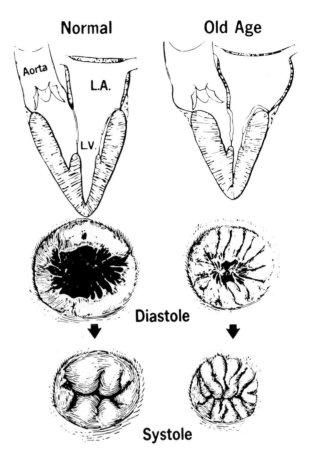

**Normal**      **Old Age**

Aorta   L.A.

L.V.

Diastole

Systole

**Figure 4–1.** Cardiac changes in the very elderly: Left atrial enlargement and left ventricular hypertrophy with small cavity are observed. The amount of space available for the mitral leaflets is decreased and consequently the number of scallops in the leaflets appears to increase. (From Waller and Roberts,[12] with permission.)

mitral valves. Mounds of calcium deposits can cause rigidity of the aortic cusps (aortic sclerosis); occasionally the deposits are heavy enough to produce aortic stenosis.[9] Calcification of the mitral annulus, considered to be the hallmark of the aged heart, is more common in women. Heavy deposits may cause mitral regurgitation, heart block, and rarely mitral stenosis. Owing to the small left ventricular cavity, the mitral leaflets protrude or "buckle" toward the left atrium in systole and may be mistaken for mitral valve prolapse (see Fig. 4–1).[13] The normal aorta of the elderly is characterized by dilation of the ascending aorta and the sinuses of Valsalva; dilation and elongation of the thoracic aorta is described as an "uncoiled aorta."

The conduction system is affected by aging. In the sinus node, the number of pacemaker cells decrease, and there is an increase in the fibrous and fatty tissue. Some fibrous infiltration of the bundle of His and bundle branches is common in the elderly.[9] More severe forms may lead to heart block due to bundle branch fibrosis. Although there is a continuous spectrum of disease, two patterns have been described. In the first (Lev's disease), fiber loss is maximal proximally, involving the branching atrioventricular bundle; whereas in the second (Lenegre's disease), fiber loss occurs in the middle and distal portions of both bundle branches.[14] Amyloid deposits and extensions of the calcific deposits of mitral annular calcification can involve the conducting system and lead to complete heart block.

The clinical significance of the aforementioned normal morphologic changes of aging depends upon their severity. Mild forms are common and are of no clinical significance; more severe forms are uncommon but can cause significant morbidity and mortality. The next section will discuss how these changes are reflected in non-invasive cardiac studies.

## NONINVASIVE CARDIAC STUDIES

### ELECTROCARDIOGRAPHY

In the past 60 years, many studies dealing with electrocardiographic (ECG) changes of aging have been published. Results of these studies are sometimes conflicting owing to the lack of uniform criteria and small sample size. Mihalick and Fisch[15] reported the ECG findings of 671 patients aged 65 or older without clinical evidence for heart disease and compared the findings with those reported in the literature.[16,17] Their findings are summarized in Table 4–2. Minor age-related increases in P-wave duration, P-R interval, and QRS duration have been reported, but these are of no clinical significance. Epidemiologic studies show that there is a decrease in S V1 and R V5 amplitude, and a leftward QRS axis shift with aging.[15,18] These changes may be secondary to changes in body habitus or the presence of heart disease. First degree AV block is more common in the elderly. Bundle branch blocks are rare in the young normal population, right bundle branch block (RBBB) occurring in 0.16% and left bundle branch block (LBBB) in 0.02%.[18] Prevalence of bundle branch block is higher in the aged; LBBB suggests the presence of heart disease, and RBBB is usually benign. Nonspecific ST-segment and T-wave changes are encountered in nearly 16% of subjects older than the age of 70[15] and are associated with heart disease. An abnormal ECG is present in half the elderly subjects. Approximately half of the patients with unequivocal infarct on ECG do not give a history of angina or myocardial infarction.[15] In the Bronx aging study, among elderly persons aged 75 or older, 6.4% had an electrocardiographic Q wave without a history of infarction; morbidity and mortality of these subjects were not different from those with clinically recognized infarction.[19] Atrial fibrillation and premature

**Table 4–2.** Prevalence of Electrocardiographic Abnormalities and Their Association with Clinically Evident Heart Disease in 671 Elderly Subjects, Compared with 5000 Normal Young Adults[16,17]

| ECG Abnormality | Elderly | | Young |
| --- | --- | --- | --- |
| | Prevalence n (%) | % with Heart Disease | Prevalence (%) |
| Atrial fibrillation | 34 (5.0) | 79 | — |
| First degree AVB | 39 (6.1) | 49 | 0.52 |
| LAD ≥ 30 | 74 (11) | — | 0.10 |
| LAHB | 51 (7.6) | 61 | — |
| RBBB | 40 (7.1) | 50 | 0.16 |
| LBBB | 28 (4.9) | 78 | 0.02 |
| RAD ≥ 120 | 6 (0.9) | 33 | 0.10 |
| ST-T changes | 106 (16) | 61 | 0.86 |

*AVB = atrioventricular block; ECG = electrocardiogram; LAD = left axis deviation; LAHB = left anterior hemiblock; LBBB = left bundle branch block; RBBB = right bundle branch block; RAD = right axis deviation.

atrial and ventricular beats are the most common arrhythmias encountered. The prevalence of ECG abnormalities increases with age, as does the prevalence of heart disease. Criteria for a normal ECG are not different in the elderly. Abnormalities that suggest the presence of heart disease include atrial fibrillation, LBBB, and ST-T changes.

The ECG is usually abnormal in cardiac amyloidosis that is severe enough to cause congestive heart failure; the most characteristic feature is diffusely diminished voltage. Myocardial infarction may be simulated by the absence of septal R waves or the presence of inferior Q waves. Arrhythmias are common; complex ventricular arrhythmias, atrioventricular conduction defects, and manifestations of sick sinus syndrome may be observed.[10] The ECG is neither sensitive nor specific in the diagnosis of left ventricular hypertrophy. In patients with severe mitral annular calcification, the conduction system may be invaded by the calcium, leading to atrioventricular or intraventricular conduction defects. These conduction defects are more common when the annular calcification is located medially, close to the conduction system.[20] In calcific aortic stenosis, the ECG is usually abnormal; a normal ECG is an important diagnostic point against significant aortic stenosis.[21]

## ECHOCARDIOGRAPHY

Echocardiography is particularly well suited for the evaluation of elderly patients, inasmuch as it provides important diagnostic information, is noninvasive, and can be used to follow patients serially for clinical or research purposes. Technically adequate echocardiograms are more difficult to obtain in the elderly because of chest-wall deformities and pulmonary hyperinflation. Most laboratories use the same normal ranges for adults of all ages. However, the echocardiographic measurements should be interpreted in light of the known morphologic changes of aging. As already discussed, mild atrial enlargement is an expected finding but ventricular enlargement is abnormal. A 20% increase in left atrial dimension is observed between the ages of 18 and 93.[22] Left ventricular wall thickness increases with age; Gerstenblith and associates[23] studied 105 male volunteers and found that the mean wall thickness was 8.7 mm between the ages of 25 and 44 years, but increased to 9.8 mm in the group aged 45 to 64 years, and 10.7 mm in the group aged 65 to 84 years. Increased amounts of subepicardial fat results in an echo-free space, especially anteriorly, but the diagnosis of pericardial effusion can be excluded if there is no echo-free space seen posteriorly. The dilated and tortuous aorta and dilated sinuses of Valsalva may be mistaken for an aortic aneurysm, especially on M-mode echocardiography. The aortic root diameter is 2 to 3 mm larger in the elderly.[23]

### Left Ventricular Function

Echocardiography can be used to evaluate systolic and diastolic function. Aging does not affect the systolic function of the ventricle. Gerstenblith and coworkers[23] studied the effects of aging on left ventricular function by performing M-mode echocardiograms on 105 healthy men between the ages of 25 and 84 years, without any evidence for cardiovascular disease or hypertension. Aging did not appear to affect the left ventricular cavity dimension or the velocity of circumferential fiber shortening. Ejection fraction at rest, the most widely used index of pump function, is not age-related in healthy volunteers.[24]

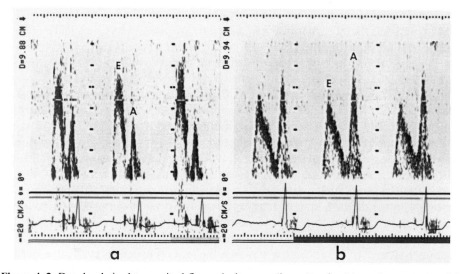

**Figure 4–2.** Doppler-derived transmitral flow velocity recordings. *Panel a:* Normal pattern. *Panel b:* Recording from an elderly hypertensive patient; atrial filling velocity (*A*) is higher than that of early filling (*E*). Deceleration slope of E wave is prolonged.

Recently, it has become apparent that diastolic dysfunction may lead to heart failure even in the presence of normal systolic function,[25] especially in the elderly. Doppler echocardiography is now used to evaluate diastolic function of ventricles.[26,27] This method is based on measurements derived from the waveform that reflects the velocity of blood flow through the mitral valve during ventricular filling. The contour of this transmitral flow-velocity waveform has an M shape. The initial peak represents the early filling phase (E) and the second peak represents atrial filling (A). Normally E is larger than A. With diastolic dysfunction, ventricular filling becomes more dependent on atrial contraction, A becomes larger, and the E/A ratio becomes reversed (Fig. 4–2). Owing to the reduced rate of early diastolic filling, the descending slope of E becomes prolonged. Diastole is a complex phenomenon, and a transmitral flow velocity profile alone cannot be used for its complete evaluation.

With advancing age, the compliance of the left ventricle is diminished and diastolic filling becomes more dependent on atrial contraction. Thus the E/A ratio is reduced in normal elderly subjects.[28] These age-related diastolic filling abnormalities alone usually are not sufficient to cause heart failure. However, the elderly may be more sensitive to the diastolic abnormalities caused by other conditions, for example, hypertension, aortic stenosis, or ischemic heart disease. Echocardiographic evaluation of patients with congestive heart failure revealed that heart failure with normal systolic function is more common in the elderly.[29] These patients may not respond or may deteriorate with vasodilator and diuretic therapy.

### Hypertrophy and Hypertrophic Cardiomyopathy

The ventricular septum may be thicker than the posterior wall in the elderly;[13] it may have a sigmoid shape[9] and project into the left ventricular outflow tract. These findings may mimic hypertrophic cardiomyopathy. However, is not unusual for the diagnosis of hypertrophic cardiomyopathy to be first made at an advanced age. Presence of left ventricular posterior wall hypertrophy, hypertrophied septum with a septal/posterior wall ratio $>$ 1.3, systolic anterior motion of the mitral leaflet, and a gradient across the outflow tract are highly suggestive of the diagnosis.

Recently the prevalence and risk factors associated with echocardiographically detected left ventricular hypertrophy were examined in the Framingham Study.[30] Prevalence of hypertrophy increased dramatically with age, and 33% of men and 49% of women older than the age of 70 were affected (Fig. 4–3). The association between age and left ventricular hypertrophy was an independent one. Echocardiographic assessment of left ventricular hypertrophy offers prognostic information beyond that provided by traditional risk factors. During a 4-year follow-up of elderly volunteers, left ventricular hypertrophy was positively correlated to the incidence of coronary events after adjusting for the traditional risk factors.[31] The ECG is neither sensitive nor specific in the diagnosis of left ventricular hypertrophy. Left

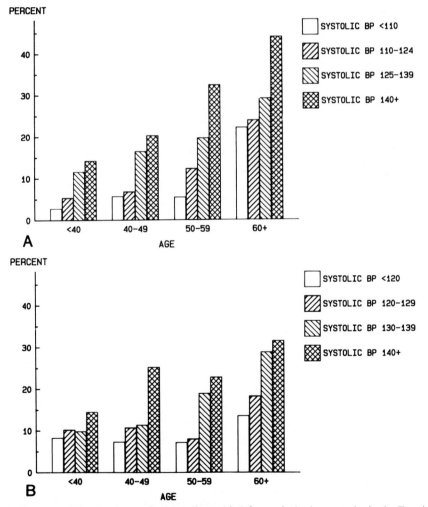

**Figure 4–3.** Age specific prevalence of echocardiographic left ventricular hypertrophy in the Framingham Heart Study according to quartiles of systolic blood pressure in women *(Panel A)* and in men *(Panel B)*. (From Levy, Anderson, and Savage,[30] with permission.)

ventricular mass estimated from the echocardiogram using geometric formulas that include wall thickness and cavity size in the calculation are very accurate.[32]

In 1985, Topol and associates[33] described the syndrome of "hypertensive hypertrophic cardiomyopathy of the elderly." The features of this syndrome included severe concentric left ventricular hypertrophy, a small left ventricular cavity, and supernormal indexes of systolic function without concurrent medical illness or ischemic heart disease. The left ventricular ejection was supernormal (mean = 0.79), but the diastolic function was abnormal. In this syndrome, Doppler echocardiography has been reported to reveal increased peak atrial velocity and reduced ratio of peak early to peak atrial velocity.[34] Patients with this syndrome may present with congestive heart failure. This is an example of heart failure due to diastolic dysfunction in the presence of normal systolic function.[25] These patients tend to do poorly when given vasodilators and diuretics and may show improvement when treated with negative inotropic agents such as beta-adrenergic blocking drugs or calcium channel blocking agents.

**Aortic Valvular Disease**

Degenerative aortic valve calcification is an age-related condition. In most cases, the degree of valve distortion is mild (aortic sclerosis) and the clinical effect is limited to an audible systolic murmur; there is no significant obstruction of the valve. Severe degenerative calcification of previously normal three-leaflet aortic valve leads to aortic stenosis, and this is the most common cause of aortic stenosis in the elderly. Calcification progresses from the base toward the edge of the valve; severity of stenosis worsens as the leaflets become more rigid.[35]

A systolic murmur originating from the aortic valve is a common finding in the elderly, and noninvasive studies can differentiate between aortic sclerosis and stenosis. Absence of dense aortic valve calcification on radiographic examination and a normal ECG are diagnostic points against severe senile aortic stenosis.[21] M-mode or two-dimensional echocardiograms may reveal a normal aortic valve and exclude the diagnosis of aortic stenosis. However, aortic valve calcification, often noted on echocardiography, does not differentiate aortic sclerosis from stenosis. Continuous-wave Doppler echocardiography has been used to estimate the severity of aortic stenosis by measuring the velocity of the aortic outflow jet. As the aortic valve orifice becomes smaller, the velocity of the aortic jet increases. The gradient across the aortic valve is calculated by the simplified Bernoulli equation, gradient = $4(\text{velocity})^2$; the aortic valve area is estimated using the continuity equation.[36,37] Many studies have validated this method by showing very good correlation between the aortic gradient and valve area estimated by Doppler echocardiography and cardiac catheterization.[37] Although Doppler echocardiography is adequate to diagnose aortic stenosis in most cases, the clinician should be aware of two pitfalls. The ultrasound beam must be almost parallel to the direction of the blood flow to accurately estimate its velocity; in some cases, this may not be feasible due to an unusual orientation of the jet; therefore, the severity of aortic stenosis may be underestimated. Rarely, a mitral regurgitation jet (which is similar to an aortic jet in direction and timing) may be mistaken for an aortic jet, and the misdiagnosis of aortic stenosis may be made.

The aorta tends to become dilated and tortuous with advancing age. These changes may be mistaken for aortic aneurysm on M-mode echocardiography, but an accurate diagnosis can be made by two-dimensional or transesophageal echocardiography. The combination of degenerative changes involving the aortic root and leaflets may result in aortic insufficiency, which is usually mild.

## Mitral Valvular Disease

Mitral annular calcification is an age-related degenerative change that is more common in women. It is accelerated by the presence of systemic hypertension, aortic stenosis, diabetes, and chronic renal failure.[38] Massive mitral annular calcification is almost exclusively a disease of elderly women.[5] While mild annular calcification is of little functional consequence, severe calcification forms a rigid curved bar of calcium that encircles the mitral orifice and may cause mitral regurgitation or stenosis. The calcification was frequently located in the angle between the posterior mitral leaflet and the left ventricular posterior wall.[39] The anterior leaflet is not attached to a true fibrous annulus as is the posterior leaflet; therefore the mitral annulus is deficient anteriorly, and the annular calcification has a C shape or U shape on radiographs. Mitral regurgitation results from the loss of sphincter action of the mitral ring.[38] The calcification may extend into the basal portion of the mitral leaflets, preventing their normal coaptation and worsening the regurgitation. Rarely, calcification protrudes into the mitral orifice, resulting in obstruction to the left ventricular inflow, a hemodynamic state similar to mitral stenosis.[40] Mitral annular calcium can be easily visualized by two-dimensional echocardiography. Presence and severity of mitral regurgitation and stenosis can be evaluated by Doppler echocardiography.

## Mitral Valve Prolapse

Mitral valve prolapse is a common valvular abnormality affecting 5% to 10% of the population. Most patients with this disorder have an uncomplicated course.[41] However, the risk for complications including severe mitral regurgitation requiring surgery, infective endocarditis, and rupture of the chordae tendineae increase with advancing age.[42,43] Mitral regurgitation due to mitral valve prolapse is a progressive disease in some patients, and symptoms may appear only around age 60, even though the prolapse has been present since a young age.[42] Infective endocarditis, cerebral ischemic events, and spontaneous rupture of the chordae tendineae are all more common in the elderly.[43] Mitral valve prolapse is diagnosed when two-dimensional echocardiography reveals prolapsing of the mitral leaflet toward the left atrium in systole. Diagnosis of mitral valve prolapse should be made cautiously when only a mild degree of prolapse is seen in a single apical view. Elderly subjects have a small hypertrophied left ventricle, and the mitral leaflets tend to protrude toward the left atrium.[12] Recent studies have shown that the mitral annulus may have a nonplanar, saddle-shaped configuration in normal subjects that results in the echocardiographic appearance of prolapse without actual leaflet displacement above the mitral annulus.[44] Thus, the diagnosis of mitral valve prolapse is more secure when seen in two different views and when accompanied by leaflet thickening and mitral regurgitation.

## Senile Amyloidosis

Echocardiographic features of cardiac amyloidosis are well described.[45,46] In advanced cases, thickened ventricular walls, dilated atria, and impaired ventricular function are seen. The thickened walls may have a granular sparkling texture, presumably due to amyloid deposits. Findings of congestive cardiomyopathy or restrictive cardiomyopathy may be seen. Cardiac valves may be thickened, but they have normal motion. Pericardial effusion is common. The combination of thickened ventricular walls on echocardiography and low voltage on electrocardiography is suggestive of the diagnosis.

## EXERCISE TESTING

The age-related physiologic changes in the cardiovascular system are described in detail in another chapter. Exercise capacity diminishes with age; cardiac output, heart rate, maximal oxygen consumption, and vital capacity decrease. Muscle atrophy, osteoarthritis, and osteoporosis also decrease the exercise capacity. The aging process explains only a portion of the functional deterioration; disease states and inactivity play a significant role.[47] Maximal heart rate that can be achieved with exercise declines with age. Standard indications and contraindications for exercise testing apply to the elderly also. It is prudent to employ an exercise protocol that has a slow treadmill speed at the beginning, making advances in small increments using, for example, Naughton or modified Bruce protocols. The physician can observe the patient's performance and ascertain if coordination and musculoskeletal strength for higher grades of exercise exist. Falls and injuries may be avoided by this approach. Bicycle ergometer may be more appropriate for patients with gait disturbances. In patients who are unable to exercise adequately, thallium scintigrams obtained after the infusion of pharmacologic agents (e.g., dipyridamole, adenosine, or dobutamine) may be helpful.

Interpretation of ST-segment changes is not influenced by age. Significance of a less than perfect diagnostic test is determined by the prevalence of disease in the population being studied. Thus, an ischemic electrocardiographic response to exercise in young healthy populations has low predictive value for future cardiac events. Coronary artery disease is common in the elderly. In a recent study of asymptomatic elderly volunteers, exercise induced silent myocardial ischemia, defined as concordant ST-segment depression and thallium perfusion defect, had good predictive value for future cardiac events; 48% of those in whom both tests were positive developed new angina pectoris, myocardial infarction, or death during a follow-up period of 4.6 years.[48] Further studies are needed to determine the usefulness of screening the elderly for coronary artery disease.

## SCINTIGRAPHY

Radionuclide methods are used to assess a variety of cardiac functions. Ejection fraction measured by radionuclide ventriculography is used to assess systolic function of the ventricle. In healthy volunteers, there is no age-related decline in the left ventricular ejection fraction.[24] Radionuclide ventriculography performed during exercise is used in the diagnosis of coronary artery disease. A 5% to 10% decrease in ejection fraction or the appearance of a segmental wall motion abnormality with exercise are abnormal findings; the former finding is very sensitive but not specific, and the latter is very specific but not sensitive in the diagnosis of ischemia. Elderly subjects without heart disease may demonstrate no increase in ejection fraction and may in fact have a decrease in ejection fraction at exercise. Port and coworkers[49] studied 77 healthy volunteers with no evidence for heart disease. At rest, the ejection fraction ranged from 47% to 80% with no significant relationship to age. In contrast, the ejection fraction at peak exercise showed a significant decline with increasing age. Of the 29 subjects older than the age of 60, 21 had a decrease in ejection fraction from rest to exercise. This appears to be an age-related change. Coronary arteriography was not performed since these patients were asymptomatic. Hitzhusen and colleagues[50] did not find an exercise-induced decrease in ejection fraction in asymptomatic elderly volunteers; however, among the 34 volunteers with a normal exercise thallium test, 35% had regional wall motion abnormalities by radionuclide ventriculography at peak exercise. Thus, in elderly patients, exercise radionuclide ventriculography will produce many false-positive results, and exercise thallium scintigraphy is the preferred approach. Exercise thallium scintigraphy has excellent sensitivity and specificity in the diagnosis of coronary artery disease. In patients who cannot exercise adequately, a stress test performed with pharmacologic agents such as dipyridamole and adenosine are good alternatives.

Radionuclide ventriculography can be used to evaluate diastolic function of the ventricle. Diastolic dysfunction causes a slower rate of rapid filling and a compensatory increase in the atrial filling due to atrial systole. An age-related decrease in peak filling rate at rest and exercise has been demonstrated.[51] These changes were more pronounced in hypertensive patients.

Scintigraphy using Tc-pyrophosphate is used for the diagnosis of myocardial infarction. This agent has been reported to be useful in the diagnosis of amyloidosis.[52] Positive scans correlate with extensive involvement, and scans are usually negative when the echocardiogram does not demonstrate abnormalities. Scintigraphy does not appear to be of value for the early detection of cardiac amyloidosis without echocardiographic abnormalities.[10]

## NEWER IMAGING TECHNIQUES

Computerized tomography (CT) of the heart is useful in diagnosing cardiac masses, pericardial effusion, constrictive pericarditis, and dissecting aneurysm. In the elderly, cardiac CT may be helpful in differentiating subepicardial fat from pericardial effusion.[53] A major drawback of this procedure is the need for the injection of iodinated contrast media. Magnetic resonance imaging can be used to evaluate cardiac anatomy, and ventricular function can be assessed by gating the image acquisition; because of its high cost, its use is limited to cases where adequate echocardiography cannot be obtained.

## REFERENCES

1. Fleg, JL, Lakatta, E: Cardiovascular disease in old age. In Rossman, I (ed): Clinical Geriatrics. JB Lippincott, Philadelphia, 1986, pp 169–196.
2. Kennedy, RD and Caird, FI: Physiology of the aging heart. In Brest, AN (ed): Geriatric Cardiology. Philadelphia, FA Davis, 1982, pp 1–8.
3. Kennedy, RD, Andrews, GR, Caird, FI: Ischemic heart disease in the elderly. Br Heart J 39:1121, 1977.
4. Waller, BF: Hearts of the "oldest old." Mayo Clin Proc 63:625, 1988.
5. Pomerance, A: Cardiac pathology in the elderly. In Brest, AN (ed): Geriatric Cardiology. Philadelphia, FA Davis, 1982, pp 9–53.
6. Lie, JT and Hammond, PI: Pathology of the senescent heart: Anatomic observations on 237 autopsy studies of patients 90 to 105 years old. Mayo Clin Proc 63:552, 1988.
7. Kitzman, DW, Scholz DG, Hagen PT, et al: Age-related changes in normal human hearts during

the first 10 decades of life. Part II (maturity): A quantitative anatomic study of 765 specimens from subjects 20 to 99 years old. Mayo Clin Proc 63:137, 1988.

8. Gross, JS, Neufeld, RR, Libow, LS, et al: Autopsy study of the elderly institutionalized patient. Review of 234 autopsies. Arch Intern Med 148:173, 1988.

9. Waller, BF and Morgan, BS: The very elderly heart. In Brest AN (ed): Contemporary Issues in Cardiovascular Pathology. Philadelphia, FA Davis, 1982, pp 361–410.

10. Wynne, J and Braunwald, E: The cardiomyopathies and myocarditis. In Braunwald, E (ed): Heart Disease. Philadelphia, WB Saunders, 1988.

11. Reyes, CV and Jablokow, VR: Lipomatous hypertrophy of the interatrial septum. Am J Clin Pathol 72:785, 1979.

12. Waller, BF and Roberts, WC: Cardiovascular disease in the very elderly. Analysis of 40 necropsy patients aged 90 years or over. Am J Cardiol 51:403, 1983.

13. Kitzman, DW, Scholz, DG, Hagen, PT, et al: Age related changes in normal human hearts during first 10 decades of life. Part II (maturity): A quantitative anatomic study of 765 specimens from subjects 20 to 99 years old. Mayo Clin Proc 63:137, 1988.

14. Smith, WM: Mechanisms of cardiac arrhythmias and conduction disturbances. In Hurst, JW (ed): The Heart. New York, McGraw-Hill, 1990, pp 473–488.

15. Mihalick, MJ and Fisch, C: Electrocardiographic findings in the aged. Am Heart J 87:117, 1974.

16. Johnson, RL, Averill, KH, Lamb, LE: Electrocardiographic findings in 67,375 asymptomatic individuals. Am J Cardiol 6:153, 1960.

17. Manning, GW: Electrocardiography in the selection of Royal Canadian airforce aircrew. Circulation 10:401, 1954.

18. Levy, D, Bailey, JJ, Garrison RJ, et al: Electrocardiographic changes with advancing age. A cross-sectional study of the association of age with QRS axis, duration and voltage. J Electrocardiol 20:44, 1987.

19. Nadelmann, J, Frishman, WH, Ooi, WL, et al: Prevalence, incidence and prognosis of recognized and unrecognized myocardial infarction in persons aged 75 years or older: The Bronx aging study. Am J Cardiol 66:533, 1990.

20. Takamato, T and Popp, RL: Conduction disturbances related to the site and severity of mitral annular calcification: A 2-dimensional echocardiographic and electrocardiographic correlative study. Am J Cardiol 51:1644, 1983.

21. Lombard, JT and Selzer, A: Valvular aortic stenosis. A clinical and hemodynamic profile of patients. Ann Intern Med 106:292, 1987.

22. Gardin, JM, Henry WL, Savage DD, et al: Echocardiographic measurements in normal subjects: Evaluation of an adult population without clinically apparent heart disease. Journal of Clinical Ultrasound 7:439, 1979.

23. Gerstenblith, G, Frederikson, J, Yin, FCP, et al: Echocardiographic assessment of a normal aging population. Circulation 56:273, 1977.

24. Fleg, JL: Alterations in cardiovascular structure and function with advancing age. Am J Cardiol 57:33C, 1986.

25. Kessler, KM: Heart failure with normal systolic function. Arch Intern Med 148:2109, 1988.

26. Spirito, P and Maron, BJ: Doppler echocardiography for assessing left ventricular diastolic function. Ann Intern Med 109:122, 1988.

27. Chakko, S, de Marchena, E, Kessler, KM, et al: Right ventricular diastolic function in systemic hypertension. Am J Cardiol 65:1117, 1989.

28. Bryg, RJ, Williams GA, Labovitz, AJ: Effect of aging on left ventricular diastolic filling in normal subjects. Am J Cardiol 59:971, 1987.

29. Wong, WF, Gold, S, Fukuyama, O, et al: Diastolic dysfunction in elderly patients with congestive heart failure. Am J Cardiol 63:1526, 1989.

30. Levy, D, Anderson, KM, Savage DD, et al: Echocardiographically detected left ventricular hypertrophy: Prevalence and risk factors. The Framingham study. Ann Intern Med 108:7, 1988.

31. Levy, D, Garrison, RJ, Savage, DD, et al: Left ventricular mass and incidence of coronary heart disease in an elderly cohort. The Framingham Study. Ann Intern Med 110:101, 1989.

32. Devereux, RB, Alonso, DR, Lutas EM, et al: Echocardiographic assessment of left ventricular hypertrophy: Comparison to necropsy findings. Am J Cardiol 57:450, 1986.

33. Topol, EJ, Traill, TA, Fortuin, NJ: Hypertensive hypertrophic cardiomyopathy of the elderly. N Engl J Med 31:227, 1985.

34. Pearson, AC, Gudipati, CV, Labovitz, AJ: Systolic and diastolic flow abnormalities in elderly patients with hypertensive hypertrophic cardiomyopathy. J Am Coll Cardiol 12:989, 1988.

35. Selzer, A: Changing aspects of the natural history of valvular aortic stenosis. N Engl J Med 317:91, 1987.
36. Saini, VD, Nanda, NC, Maalik, D: Physics of blood flow. In Nanda, NC (ed): Doppler Echocardiography, ed 1. New York, Igaku-Shoin, 1985, pp 42–50.
37. Miller, FA: Aortic stenosis: Most cases no longer require invasive hemodynamic study. J Am Coll Cardiol 13:551, 1989.
38. Braunwald, E: Valvular heart disease. In Braunwald, E (ed): Heart Disease. Philadelphia, WB Saunders, 1988, pp 1023–1092.
39. D'Cruz, I, Panetta, F, Cohen, H, et al: Submitral calcification or sclerosis in elderly patients: M-mode and two dimensional echocardiography in "mitral annulus calcification." Am J Cardiol 44:31, 1979.
40. Labovitz, AJ, Nelson, JG, Windhorst, DM, et al: Frequency of mitral valve dysfunction from mitral annular calcium as detected by Doppler echocardiography. Am J Cardiol 55:133, 1985.
41. Kessler, KM: Prolapse paranoia. J Am Coll Cardiol 11:48, 1988.
42. Kolibash, AJ, Kilman, JW, Bush, CA, et al: Evidence for progression from mild to severe mitral regurgitation in mitral valve prolapse. Am J Cardiol 58:762, 1986.
43. Naggar, CZ and Pearson, WN: Frequency of complications of mitral valve prolapse in subjects aged 60 years and older. Am J Cardiol 58:1209, 1986.
44. Levine, RA, Triulzi, MO, Harrigan, P, et al: The relationship of mitral annular shape to the diagnosis of mitral valve prolapse. Circulation 75:756, 1987.
45. Nicolosi GL, Pavan, D, Lestuzzi, C, et al: Prospective identification of patients with amyloid heart disease by two-dimensional echocardiography. Circulation 70:432, 1984.
46. Siqueira-Filho, AG, Cunha, CLP, Tajik, AJ, et al: M-mode and two-dimensional echocardiographic features in cardiac amyloidosis. Circulation 63:188, 1981.
47. Landin, RJ, Linnemeier, TJ, Rothbaum, DA, et al: Exercise testing and training of the elderly patient. In Wenger, NK (ed): Exercise and the Heart, ed 2. Philadelphia, FA Davis, 1985, pp 201–218.
48. Fleg, JL, Gerstenblith, G, Zonderman, AB, et al: Prevalence and prognostic significance of exercise induced silent myocardial ischemia detected by thallium scintigraphy and electrocardiography in asymptomatic volunteers. Circulation 81:428–436, 1990.
49. Port, S, Cobb, FR, Coleman, E, et al: Effect of age on the response of the left ventricular ejection fraction to exercise. N Engl J Med 303:1133, 1980.
50. Hitzhusen, JC, Hickler, RB, Alpert, JS, et al: Exercise testing and hemodynamic performance in healthy elderly persons. Am J Cardiol 54:1082, 1984.
51. Iskandrian, AS and Hakki, A-H: Age-related changes in left ventricular diastolic performance. Am Heart J 112:75, 1986.
52. Falk, RH, Lee, VW, Rubinow, A, et al: Sensitivity of technetium-99m-pyrophosphate scintigraphy in diagnosing cardiac amyloidosis. Am J Cardiol 51:826, 1983.
53. Baron, MG: Computed tomography of the heart. In Hurst, JW (ed): The Heart. New York, McGraw-Hill, 1985, pp 1950–1961.

# CHAPTER 5

# Hypertension in the Elderly

*Leonard Williams, M.D.*
*David T. Lowenthal, M.D., Ph.D.*

In the United States and in most of the other industrialized countries, the elderly (i.e., those older than the age of 65) represent the most rapidly growing portion of the population. Currently, the elderly represent about 12% of the U.S. population; however, they consume over one-third of all the healthcare dollars spent in this country. This demographic shift has focused attention on hypertension in the elderly because this condition has a high prevalence in this population and is responsible for much mortality and morbidity, with loss of functional capacity and resulting decline in quality of life. The major goals of therapy in geriatrics are the prevention of premature mortality and disability, and the maintenance of functions and independence and improvement in quality of life.[1]

In recent years, there has been a re-assessment of knowledge regarding the epidemiology, pathophysiology, and treatment of hypertension in the elderly.[2] In the elderly, hypertension is considered the single most potent, common, and remediable risk factor for cerebrovascular disease, congestive heart failure, and coronary artery disease, which are the major causes of cardiovascular morbidity and mortality in this age group.[3] Cardiovascular disease does not seem to be an inevitable result of aging, and its prevention would help decrease disability and premature mortality as well as improve the quality of life in the elderly.

## DEFINITION

The risk of cardiovascular morbidity and mortality is independently related to rises in both the systolic (SBP) and diastolic (DBP) blood pressure. This risk increases in a continuous fashion as the SBP or the DBP rises, but the increase in risk for each increment in blood pressure becomes more pronounced with advancing age.[4] Generically, hypertension can best be defined as that level of blood pressure at which the benefits of therapy exceed the risks and costs of withholding treatment. Various investigational studies have used different levels of SBP and DBP to define hypertensive patients. This variance makes analyzing the data somewhat more difficult.

**Table 5–1.** Classification of Arterial Hypertension by Arterial
Pressure Levels

|  | Pressure (mmHg) | Class |
|---|---|---|
| Systolic (when diastolic pressure < 90) | < 140 | Normal BP |
|  | 140–159 | Borderline isolated systolic hypertension |
|  | ≥ 160 | Isolated systolic hypertension |
| Diastolic | < 85 | Normal BP |
|  | 85–89 | High normal BP |
|  | 90–104 | Mild hypertension |
|  | 105–114 | Moderate hypertension |
|  | ≥ 115 | Severe hypertension |

The Joint National Committee on Detection, Evaluation, and Treatment of
High Blood Pressure has developed a useful classification of blood pressure in
adults based on the average of two or more readings on two or more occasions
(Table 5–1). This categorization is based on risk level for the various determinations of SBP and DBP. High-normal blood pressure is a category included because
these patients need closer monitoring. In addition, the term *mild* is relative to other
categories and does not imply that these patients are unimportant, inasmuch as
data from clinical trials indicate that these patients require medical attention.[5]

The Working Group on Hypertension in the Elderly defines hypertension as
an average SBP > 160 mmHg and/or an average DBP ≥ 90 mmHg on three consecutive visits. A SBP of 140 to 160 mmHg with a DBP < 90 represents *borderline
isolated systolic hypertension.*[6]

A subclassification of hypertension devised in relation to risk and applicable
to the elderly has been proposed[1] (Table 5–2). According to this profile, elderly
patients with *combined hypertension* (blood pressure > 160/90 mmHg) should be
treated. Those with *borderline hypertension* (blood pressure 140 to 159/90 mmHg
or more) should be observed closely and many could be treated empirically with
nonpharmacologic measures. Other patients in this category (e.g., those with a mild
elevation of SBP and evidence of cardiovascular disease) should be treated. The
significance of the *predominant systolic hypertension* group (SBP > (DBP − 15)
× 2) is still being debated. It is established, however, that patients with isolated

**Table 5–2.** Classification of Hypertension in the
Elderly Based Upon the Level of Systolic and
Diastolic Blood Pressure

| Classification | Blood Pressure (mmHg) | |
|---|---|---|
|  | Systolic | Diastolic |
| Combined hypertension | > 160 | > 90 |
| Borderline hypertension | 140–159 | > 90 |
| Predominant systolic hypertension | > (DBP − 15) × 2 | > 90 |
| Isolated systolic hypertension | > 160 | < 90 |

*DBP = diastolic blood pressure

systolic hypertension are at an increased risk of cardiovascular morbidity and mortality even though DBP is normal.[1]

# EPIDEMIOLOGY

## GENERAL OBSERVATIONS

Both the SBP and DBP increase with age in the industrialized world; SBPs continue to rise until the age of 70 or 80 whereas DBPs rise up to the age of 50 or 60 and then show a tendency to level off or even decrease slightly. In the U.S. population, from age 40 to 70 the SBP tends to rise 5 to 10 mmHg whereas the DBP shows an increase of 5 to 6 mmHg. Peak blood pressure recordings occur at a slightly younger age in men than in women. In relation to racial influences, in blacks both the SBP and DBP are higher than in whites during each decade after the age of 30. Persons with higher blood pressures at younger ages show the greatest increase in blood pressure as they grow older.

An increase in blood pressure is not inevitable, however, as demonstrated by studies with primitive populations in parts of South America and the South Pacific where blood pressure does not increase with age.[7-10] It seems likely that environmental factors as well as social and cultural habits play an important role. In many elderly individuals, blood pressure remains normal or even low with aging, and these individuals actually have lower cardiovascular mortality and morbidity rates.

## PREVALENCE

The overall prevalence of hypertension and, in particular, isolated systolic hypertension (ISH) is considerable in the geriatric population. As pointed out, the average DBP tends to level off between the ages of 50 and 60, and therefore the prevalence of hypertension tends to level off somewhere between the ages of 55 to 60.[3] It is actually the rise in ISH that is responsible for the overall increase in the prevalence of "hypertension" with age. There are other factors that affect prevalence estimates of either hypertension or ISH. As the *number of measurements* taken increases, prevalence tends to decrease. Naturally, the *levels of DBP and SBP* used for making the diagnosis will affect prevalence as well as the choice of population that is studied.

When blood pressure measurements on more than one occasion are used to estimate prevalence, as in the Hypertension Detection and Follow-up Program (HDFP)[11] and the Systolic Hypertension in the Elderly Program (SHEP),[12] the prevalence of hypertension in the elderly is about 15% in whites and 25% in blacks, and the prevalence of ISH ranges from 10% to 20%.[13]

The actual total prevalence of hypertension in the elderly does not seem to be as high as the figures of 50% to 60% frequently reported.[6,14]

## RISKS

Analysis of hypertensive prevalence data indicates that blood pressure is a particularly important risk factor for cerebrovascular accidents (CVA) and congestive heart failure (CHF). Blood pressure is also an impressive risk factor for the most frequent cardiovascular complication, coronary artery disease (CAD), even though this risk relationship is somewhat less important than that between blood pressure and cerebrovascular disease.[15]

The Framingham Study showed that the *overall mortality* rates were more than doubled and *cardiovascular mortality* was basically tripled in hypertensives as compared with normotensives, and this persists with age and is more significant for women especially after the age of 65.[3]

When assessing *cardiovascular morbidity,* the rise of CHF is particularly impressive. Analysis of Framingham data once again shows that the risk of developing CHF in hypertensives is six times the risk for normotensives and that there is evidence of a stronger level of risk with SBP when compared with DBP for both men and women.[16]

The Framingham data indicate that DBP is more closely linked to the development of CAD in persons younger than the age of 45. In individuals older than the age of 45, the DBP declines somewhat as a predictor of CAD whereas SBP increases as a predictor. In fact, older than the age of 60, SBP is more predictive of CAD. In the elderly, SBP by itself is as predictive as SBP and DBP combined.[17]

Data from the Framingham Study also have been used to examine the role of hypertension in regards to CVAs or stroke. These analyses show that there is no more important factor in the development of stroke than hypertension, and the relationship between blood pressure and stroke was stronger than for any other cardiovascular disease outcome except CHF. A person with a blood pressure $\geq$ 160/95 mmHg has three times the risk for stroke than a normotensive. Both SBP and DBP were shown to have similar gradients of risk for stroke, as with CHF, with no evidence of declining importance for SBP with age.[18,19]

The Chicago Stroke Study was an epidemiologic investigation that was designed to examine the precursors of stroke in an elderly population. The results of this study were in accordance with the Framingham data in that the incidence of stroke was significantly increased by hypertension. The gradient of risk for both SBP and DBP was examined, and it was found that the SBP had a stronger effect. For persons with a SBP > 179 mmHg, the 3-year incidence of stroke was approximately three times greater than persons with a SBP < 130 mmHg.[20]

Isolated systolic hypertension also has been associated with an increased risk of cardiovascular morbidity; however there have been few studies designed to examine exclusively this form of hypertension. Data from the Framingham Study showed that in a 20-year follow-up of men aged 55 to 74 years, overall mortality was twice that in persons with ISH when compared with normotensive controls. Cardiovascular mortality was 1.8 times greater for men with ISH and 4.7 times greater for women with ISH compared with their respective normotensive controls. Risk was shown to increase with a rise in SBP at all ages. In elderly persons with a DBP < 95 mmHg, the rise in the mortality rate with SBP was as steep as the mortality rate noted in middle-aged individuals.[21] Colandrea and associates[22] conducted a small study in a retirement community in which 72 persons with ISH were identified. The investigators found that the cardiovascular mortality in the study group (seven deaths) was significantly greater than in the control group (one death). Garland and coworkers[23] studied 2636 persons aged 60 and older an average of 6.4 years. Of these subjects, 6.3% were determined to have ISH based on a single-day reading. The subjects who had untreated ISH had a one and a half times elevated risk for overall mortality compared with normotensive subjects. Data from HDFP were analyzed by Curb and associates[24] to examine the effect of ISH in overall mortality. The sex-race–adjusted mortality rate for persons in the 60 to 69 years old age group at baseline was higher in persons with ISH, and increasing SBP in this group was found to have a significant association with mortality—for every 1 mmHg increase in SBP there was a 1% increase in mortality.

Regarding stroke, the Framingham Study showed that in 24 years of follow-up for incidence of stroke, the subjects with ISH had a two to four times increase in stroke when compared with normotensives.[25] In the Chicago Stroke Study, elderly persons with ISH were found to have a two and a half times higher 3-year incidence of stroke than persons with a SBP < 140 mmHg.[20] Hopefully the forthcoming SHEP results will indicate whether treatment of ISH will prevent stroke.

## PATHOPHYSIOLOGY

An increase in blood pressure is not a normal part of aging despite the fact that there is a high incidence of hypertension in the elderly. The mechanisms responsible for hypertension in the elderly are as multifactorial and complex as in the young hypertensive.

There is an increase in aortic impedance and peripheral vascular resistance with age due to a decrease in connective tissue elasticity and an increase in the prevalence of atherosclerosis. Inasmuch as much of the rise in prevalence of hypertension in the elderly seems attributable to a rise in ISH, it has been proposed that *structural changes* in the *large vessels* may play a predominant role in the rise in SBP found with advancing age.[13] In the walls of the aorta and other large vessels, there is a continuous fracturing and unrolling of the elastic fibers with deposition of calcium and collagenous matrix with age. These changes lead to an increase in the rigidity and a decrease in elasticity of the aorta and large vessels with age. Because of this reduced compliance in the aorta and large vessels, the pulse generated during systole results in a steeper rise in pressure per unit of stroke volume into the large arteries. Owing to the loss of elasticity in the aorta and large vessels, the left ventricle is required to pump against increased impedance. Echocardiographically, elderly hypertensives have been shown to have increased left ventricular wall and septal thickening with higher left ventricular mass when compared with young hypertensives.[26] Unfortunately there are few data comparing elderly hypertensives to elderly normotensives and therefore it is difficult to determine whether the aforementioned findings are related to the effects of age or hypertension or both.

There are also structural changes in *small vessels* with aging. Aging small arteries and arterioles demonstrate hyaline degeneration within the media with a resulting decrease in the lumen to wall ratio and the overall cross-sectional area of the lumen.[27] The structural changes that occur with aging in the vasculature are qualitatively similar to but not as extreme as those encountered in hypertension. In hypertension, vascular morphologic changes include the changes in collagen and elastin in the vessel walls found with aging but there is also hypertrophy and hyperplasia of smooth muscle cells and possibly hyperplasia of the cells in the vascular endothelium.[13] These changes in small arteries and arterioles result in thickening and a decrease in cross-sectional area. This results in an increase in total vascular resistance.[28]

The increase in aortic and large vessel impedance and the increase in peripheral vascular resistance result in an increased SBP. The increase in arterial impedance, however, is responsible for about twice the increment in SBP when compared with the rise in peripheral vascular resistance. The natural history of hypertension is not that of further increases in peripheral resistance but is characterized by accelerated arterial impedance that further increases the SBP more than the DBP.[29]

There are also *functional changes* that may have significance in hypertension and aging. There seems to be no change in *alpha-adrenoreceptor*-mediated responses[30] but there is a decrease in *beta-adrenergic* function due to a decrease in $\beta$-adrenergic receptor affinity for agonist[31] and to defects in postreceptor activity[32] with aging. This adrenergic imbalance between the preserved vasoconstricting $\alpha$-receptor activity and decreased vasodilation $\beta$-receptor activity may contribute to the development of hypertension in the elderly.

Baroreceptor sensitivity is reduced in the elderly.[33] This too may play a role in the development of hypertension. A rise in blood pressure should activate baroreceptor mechanisms to inhibit sympathetic nervous system outflow, which would lead to a decrease in norepinephrine release and a lowering of blood pressure. The failure of this system to function properly could sustain an increased blood pressure.

*Plasma norepinephrine* levels increase with age. It is not known whether this is the cause or a result of diminished $\beta$-receptor activity and/or baroreceptor reflex dysfunctions, or whether this is a primary event related to age. It is thought, however, that the rise in norepinephrine levels is probably not a cause of hypertension but rather an epiphenomenon. Plasma epinephrine levels increase with age in both hypertensive and normotensive elderly subjects but the increase actually is greater in the normotensive group.[34]

It is uncertain whether the *renin-angiotensin system* plays a significant role in the development of hypertension in the elderly. Most studies describe a decrease in plasma renin activity with age. The plasma renin activity is low in most elderly patients in the basal state, in response to sodium depletion,[35] after diuretic administration,[36] or with upright posture.[37] Although plasma renin activity is usually low in elderly hypertensives, the response to angiotensin converting enzyme (ACE) inhibitor in this population suggests either some role for the renin-angiotensin system or a different (bradykinin) mechanism in the pathogenesis of hypertension in the elderly.[38]

Although the glomerular filtration rate[39] and renal blood flow[40] decline with age and elderly persons take longer to excrete excess sodium and are slow in retaining needed sodium,[36] the relationship between these *renal factors* and hypertension in the elderly has not been defined and requires further investigation.

It has been postulated that changes in vascular responsiveness to vasoactive agents with age might be related to alterations in the handling of the calcium cation with age. There have been conflicting reports concerning vascular smooth muscle response to $Ca^{++}$ in aging rats.[13] However, the clinical effectiveness of calcium channel blockers in treating elderly hypertensives suggests a possible relationship between calcium and hypertension in the aged.[41]

## EVIDENCE OF EFFICACY OF ANTIHYPERTENSIVE THERAPY

Although there remains concern about the potential risks from antihypertensive medications in the elderly, it now appears that the benefits of treating hypertension in patients between the ages of 60 and 80 outweighs potential adverse effects.[1,2,42]

The *Veterans Administration Cooperative Study on Antihypertensive Agents* was a multicenter double-blind, placebo-controlled trial in men younger than the age of 75. Although only 81 patients were older than 60 years, they accounted for half of the "morbid events" that were assessed. These patients were treated with thiazides, reserpine, and hydralazine in sequence and the follow-up was for 3.3 years. This study found positive treatment effects for the prevention of CVAs and CHF in the older age group whereas CAD was not prevented. Of those aged 60 and older, morbid cardiovascular events occurred in 28.9% of the treatment group and 62.8% of the control group. Hypokalemia occurred in 15% of patients.[43] Isolated systolic hypertension was not addressed in this study.

In the *Australian National Trial* there were 582 patients aged 60 to 69 years with a DBP of 95 to 110 mmHg and a SBP < 200 mmHg. These patients were randomized to single-blind treatment with thiazide, methyldopa, beta-blockers, vasodilators, and placebo. There was a 39% reduction in trial end points of death or a specific cardiovascular event (stroke, myocardial infection, CAD, or CHF) in the treated group.[44] This study did not examine ISH.

The *Hypertension Detection and Follow-up Program (HDFP)* was a randomized, cooperative, clinical trial of 5-years duration that assessed the efficiency of rigorous, systematic, antihypertensive therapy in special program centers (stepped care) compared with the existing patterns of care in the community (referred care) in 2376 patients between the ages of 60 and 69 years. Stepped-care patients were treated with thiazides followed by reserpine and hydralazine. Of the referred care patients, 54% received antihypertensive medication. In the population with mild hypertension, the stepped-care group had a 17.2% reduction in overall mortality, which was due primarily to a reduction in cardiovascular deaths.[45] Isolated systolic hypertension was not specifically addressed.

The *European Working Party on High Blood Pressure in the Elderly (EWPHE)* was a trial with 840 patients older than 60 years (average age = 72 years) with a casual sitting blood pressure of 160 to 239/90 to 119 mmHg. Patients were randomized to placebo and treatment groups (thiazide and triamterene with methyldopa added if needed). After an 8-year follow-up period, there was no effect found on overall mortality but there was a 27% reduction in cardiovascular mortality rate, which was significant. There was also a statistically significant 38% reduction in cardiac mortality and a nonstatistically significant 32% reduction in cerebrovascular mortality.[46] The beneficial effects of treatment on cardiovascular mortality was limited to patients younger than the age of 80 years.[47] Isolated systolic hypertension was not assessed.

An overall view of the aforementioned trials show that in general patients older than the age of 60 had relative reductions in mortality and morbidity similar to patients younger than 50 years of age. It is also apparent that more total "morbid events" are prevented in patients older than the age of 60. Lower levels of absolute benefit from treatment of mild hypertension in elderly individuals was found. Although there is uncertainty in the prevention of CAD and overall mortality, it is evident that treating the elderly hypertensive population will prevent strokes. These studies also showed that there is no evidence that the elderly have more frequent side effects to antihypertensive medications than do younger patients.[1,13,42,48] However, it must be remembered that the patients treated in these studies were usually relatively healthy, which does not reflect the general clinical practice of geriatrics.

Regarding ISH, there are limited data available on the potential benefits of treatment. The Systolic Hypertension in the Elderly Program (SHEP)[12,49] pilot study was a randomized, double-blind, placebo-controlled clinical trial that was undertaken to assess the feasibility of a larger study planned to assess the safety and efficiency of drug treatment of ISH in persons 60 years or older. A total of 2365 patients with SBP > 160 mmHg and DBP < 90 mmHg were randomized to treatment with chlorthalidone (with reserpine or atenolol as additional drugs if necessary) and to placebo (2371). Of the patients in the active treatment group, 65% to 72% had their blood pressure lowered to goal value. The primary outcome of this trial related to the lowering of SBP was the reduction in incidence of nonfatal and fatal (total) stroke. Secondarily, cardiovascular and coronary morbidity and mortality, all-cause mortality, and quality of life measures were assessed.

The data show that in persons aged 60 years and older with ISH, drug therapy for 5 years reduced the incidence of total stroke by 36%. The reduction in secondary or coronary events was 27%.

Another trial in its pilot stage, the *Syst-Eur* trial, is under way. This study enters patients older than the age of 60 years with a DBP < 95 mmHg and a SBP ≥ 160 mmHg. It is a double-blind, placebo-controlled trial with the main purpose of examining the influence of ISH on morbidity, mortality, and general well-being.[50]

In conclusion, the results of the aforementioned trials suggest that the benefits of treatment outweigh the risks and side effects for the majority of patients between 60 and 79 years of age with mild-to-moderate hypertension (SBP > 160 mmHg and DBP > 90 mmHg). For patients older than the age of 80, those with other risk factors or cardiovascular, renal, or other disease processes due to or worsened by hypertension should probably be treated. For the patients who fall in the borderline group (SBP 140 to 160 mmHg and DBP 90 to 95 mmHg), the same recommendations would apply as for those older than 80 years of age.[1]

## DIAGNOSIS AND CLINICAL ASSESSMENT

In the evaluation of the elderly patient with hypertension, there are three factors to be considered carefully: the accuracy for determining the baseline blood pressure; the assessment for possible end-organ damage; and, under certain situations, further evaluation to rule out underlying conditions that may be responsible for blood pressure elevations.[2]

When measuring blood pressure, the average of two or more readings should be obtained with the patient seated comfortably with their arm bare. The first systolic sound (phase I) represents the SBP, whereas the disappearance of the sound (phase V) represents the DBP. For persons with an arm circumference of 32 cm (12½ in.), a large cuff should be used. These measurements should be repeated with the patient supine, and after 1 minute and 5 minutes standing. The diagnosis of hypertension is made when on three consecutive subsequent visits the average blood pressure is ≥ 160/90 mmHg.[1,51]

In pseudohypertension, there may be an overestimation of the real blood pressure because thickened or calcified arteries may not be easily compressed by the standard blood pressure cuff. The Osler maneuver can help determine this. In this maneuver, the cuff is inflated above the SBP. If the brachial or radial arteries are still palpable, pseudohypertension may be present.[52]

Certain laboratory tests should be performed to detect target organ damage and to help guide therapeutic decisions. These include a hemogram; blood chemistry profile with a serum creatinine, plasma glucose, serum potassium, uric acid, and cholesterol; and an electrocardiogram.

Under certain circumstances, patients should be evaluated for secondary causes of hypertension. One should be concerned when the following occur: 1) when, at the onset, the DBP is $\geq$ 105 mmHg in a male after the age of 55; 2) when the DBP continues to be > 100 mmHg despite a triple-drug therapy regimen; 3) if accelerated hypertension occurs in the elderly; 4) when spontaneous hypokalemia (not related to drug therapy) exists; 5) when signs and symptoms related to pheochromocytoma are present; 6) when signs of renovascular disease are found; and 7) when a rise in serum creatinine occurs when ACE inhibitor therapy is instituted, which could suggest bilateral renal artery stenosis (RAS) in a solitary kidney.[6]

## PHYSIOLOGIC CHANGES WITH AGING

Certain physiologic changes occur with age that involve the cardiovascular system, central nervous system, renal and hepatic function, and body composition. These changes are also discussed elsewhere in this book but will be briefly addressed in this chapter in relation to antihypertensive medications.

With aging, there is a reduction in body size with a decrease in lean body mass (mostly muscle mass) and body water with an increase in fat per unit of body weight (Table 5–3). There is a decrease in hepatic albumin synthesis with lower albumin serum levels, which could yield more free drug for entry into tissues for elimination. With aging, there is a gradual decrease in blood flow through the liver and the kidney, which reduces drug clearance. Because of these changes, water soluble drugs (atenolol, nadolol, ACE inhibitors) may result in higher blood concentrations with increased pharmacologic activity, and, conversely, a highly lipid-soluble drug (propranolol, timolol, central alpha-agonists, calcium channel blockers) could have longer pharmacologic activity because of increased volume of distribution and delayed elimination.

Symptomatic or asymptomatic CAD can reduce ventricular function in the elderly. Diuretic therapy causes volume contraction and if superimposed on impaired ventricular function could result in orthostatic hypotension. Orthostatic hypotension also could be caused by alpha-adrenergic blockers such as prazosin or terazosin. Beta-blockers and verapamil can produce significant negative inotropic effects, especially when given in combination, and may precipitate heart failure.

**Table 5–3.** Age-Related Changes
Affecting Pharmacokinetics

| Body Component of Function | Direction of Change |
|---|---|
| Renal function | ↓ |
| Hepatic blood flow | ↓ |
| Serum albumin | ↓ |
| $\alpha_1$-acid glycoprotein | ↑ |
| Body fat | ↑ |
| Lean muscle mass | ↓ |
| Total body water | ↓ |

As a result of a decrease in responsiveness and sensitivity of the baroreceptor reflex, elderly hypertensives may develop postural hypotension when treated with diuretics and/or peripheral alpha-blocking antihypertensive agents.

Owing to the possibility of neuron loss in the brain due to atherosclerosis, there is an altered sensitivity to many centrally acting drugs. Highly lipid-soluble drugs like beta-blockers and calcium channel blockers penetrate the central nervous system and may cause central nervous system side effects. Central alpha-agonists (e.g., methyldopa, clonidine, guanfacine, and guanabenz) can have similar effects.

Because of the decline in plasma renin activity with age, drugs that further depress the renin-angiotensin system (such as beta-blockers and ACE inhibitors) can potentiate potassium retention.

Because of the kidneys' slowed response in correcting salt and water imbalance with aging, the use of diuretics can give rise to hyponatremia, hypomagnesemia, hypokalemia, and hypercalcemia. These diuretic-induced changes can then propagate additional cerebral and cardiac complications.

Because of changes in hepatic function with age, there is a decrease in hepatic clearance of some drugs such as metoprolol and propranolol. Calcium channel blockers are extensively metabolized by the liver, but no data confirm any untoward pharmacodynamic events as a result of possible drug accumulation.

## THERAPY

### NONPHARMACOLOGIC THERAPY

Although nonpharmacologic treatment of hypertension in the elderly has not been conclusively evaluated, the low risk and cost of a short trial of these measures seem warranted in most elderly persons with mild hypertension. These measures include salt restriction, weight loss, exercise conditioning, reduction of excessive alcohol intake, and calcium supplementation.

### DIURETIC THERAPY

Initial therapy of hypertension in the elderly should include a thiazide diuretic in small doses (hydrochlorothiazide, 12.5 to 25 mg/d). This approach has been shown to be effective with minimal side effects in both the EWPHE trial and SHEP pilot study. The drugs do tend to lower serum potassium and raise serum creatinine levels slightly and may have an adverse effect on serum lipids. Decreased plasma volume may lead to orthostatic hypotension. The use of small doses of hydrochlorothiazide, which can be combined with a potassium-sparing diuretic, may minimize the adverse effects.

### BETA-BLOCKERS

Although the physiologic changes with aging as described seem to suggest that beta-blockers theoretically might not be very effective in lowering blood pressure, there is evidence that this class of drugs can be used effectively and safely in the elderly. Using a less lipid-soluble agent such as atenolol *may* reduce central nervous system side effects such as depression or sleep disorders.

## Calcium Channel Blockers

Calcium channel blockers seem to be an ideal class of antihypertensive drugs for the elderly. They are effective in lowering blood pressure, and they tend not to cause fluid retention, postural hypotension, sedation, depression, or metabolic abnormalities. The major side effects are constipation, dizziness, and tachycardia.[1]

## Angiotensin Converting Enzyme Inhibitors

The ACE inhibitors theoretically would seem less than ideal in the elderly for the reasons already described; however, their efficacy has been demonstrated in the treatment of elderly hypertensives.[53] Although there is a potential problem with hyperkalemia, they do not produce metabolic changes and central nervous system side effects.

## Central Alpha-adrenergic Agents

Central alpha-adrenergic agents appear to be effective in elderly hypertensives and are usually well-tolerated. Common side effects include dry mouth, drowsiness, and constipation. The transdermal delivery of clonidine has been shown to be effective in the elderly and is associated with a lower and smoother plasma curve, absence of peaks and valleys, and fewer side effects.[54,55]

## Overall Approach

We consider the diuretics to be the drugs of first choice for most elderly hypertensives. The choice of a second-step drug depends mostly on the individual patient inasmuch as there are not data available on the relative benefits of the various second-step regimens. In general, one half of the usual middle-aged adult dose should be the initial dose at each step.[56]

# REFERENCES

1. Byyny, RL: Hypertension in the elderly. In Laragh, JH and Brenner, BM (ed): Hypertension: Pathophysiology, Diagnosis, and Management. Raven Press, New York, 1990, pp 1869–1887.
2. Applegate, WB: Hypertension in elderly patients. Ann Intern Med 110:901–915, 1989.
3. Kannel, WB and Gordon, T: Evaluation of cardiovascular risk in the elderly: The Framingham Study. Bull NY Acad Med 54:573–591, 1978.
4. Kannel, WB: Some lessons in cardiovascular epidemiology from Framingham. Am J Cardiol 37:269–274, 1976.
5. Joint National Committee: The 1988 report of the Joint National Committee on detection, evaluation, and treatment of high blood pressure. Arch Intern Med 148:1023–1038, 1988.
6. Working Group on Hypertension in the Elderly: Statement on hypertension in the elderly. JAMA 256:70–74, 1986.
7. Maddocks, I: Possible absence of hypertension in two complete Pacific Island populations. Lancet 2:396–399, 1961.
8. Prior, IAM, Grimley, EJ, Harvey HPB, et al: Sodium intake and blood pressure in two Polynesian populations. N Engl J Med 279:515, 1968.
9. Page, LB, Damon, A, Moellering, RC: Antecedents of cardiovascular disease in six Solomon Islands societies. Circulation 49:1132–1146, 1974.
10. Lowenstein, FW: Blood pressure in relation to age and sex in the tropics and subtropics. A review of the literature and an investigation in two tribes of Brazil Indians. Lancet 1:389, 1961.

11. Hypertension Detection and Follow-up Program Cooperative Group: Blood pressure studies in 14 communities. JAMA 237:2385, 1977.

12. Hulley, S, Feigal, D, Ireland, C et al: Systolic hypertension in the elderly program (SHEP): The first three months. J Am Geriatr Soc 34(2):101–105, 1986.

13. Applegate, WB: Hypertension. Hazard, WR, Andres, R, Bierman, EL, et al (eds): In Principles of Geriatric Medicine and Gerontology, ed 2. New York, McGraw-Hill, 1990, pp 485–498.

14. Joint National Committee: Hypertension prevention and the status of awareness, treatment and control in the United States: Final report of the subcommittee on definition and prevalence of the 1984 Joint National Committee. Hypertension 7:457–468, 1985.

15. Whelton, PK and Klag MJ: Epidemiology of high blood pressure. Clinics in Geriatric Medicine: Hypertension 5(4):639–655, 1989.

16. Kannel, WB, Castelli, WP, McNamara, PM et al: Role of blood pressure in the development of congestive heart failure: The Framingham Study. N Engl J Med 287(16):781–787, 1972.

17. Kannel, WB and Gordon, T: Systolic vs diastolic blood pressure and risk of coronary artery disease. Am J Cardiol 27:335, 1971.

18. Kannel, WB, Wolf, PA, Verter, J et al: Epidemiologic assessment of the role of blood pressure in stroke: The Framingham Study. JAMA 214(2):301–310, 1970.

19. Kannel, WB, Dawber, TR, Sorlie, P et al: Components of blood pressure and risk of atherothrombotic brain infarction: The Framingham Study. Stroke 7(4):327–331, 1976.

20. Shekelle, R and Ostfeld, A: Hypertension and risk of stroke in an elderly population. Stroke 5:71–75, 1974.

21. Kannel, WB and Dawber, T: Perspectives on systolic hypertension: The Framingham Study. Circulation 61(6):1179–1182, 1980.

22. Colandrea, M, Friedman, GD, Nichaman MZ et al: Systolic hypertension in the elderly: An epidemiologic assessment. Circulation 41:239–245, 1970.

23. Garland, C, Barrett-Connor, E, Suarez, L et al: Isolated systolic hypertension and mortality after age 60 years. Am J Epidemiol 118(3):365–476, 1983.

24. Curb, J, Curb, JD, Borhani, NO, Entwisle, G et al: Isolated systolic hypertension in 14 communities. Am J Epidemiol 121(3):362–370, 1985.

25. Kannel, WB, Wolff, PA, McGee DL et al: Systolic blood pressure, arterial rigidity and risk of stroke: The Framingham Study. JAMA 245(12):1225–1229, 1981.

26. Messerli, FH and Ventura, HO: Essential hypertension in the elderly: Hemodynamics, intravascular volume, plasma renin activity and circulating catecholamine levels. Lancet 2:983–986, 1983.

27. Weller, RO: Vascular pathology in hypertension. Age Aging 8:99–103, 1979.

28. Guyton, AC: Textbook of medical physiology, ed 7. Philadelphia, WB Saunders, 1986, p 219.

29. Hickler, RB: Aging and hypertension. J Am Geriatr Soc 3:421–425, 1983.

30. Abrass, IB, Ko, T, Scarpace, PJ: Platelet alpha-adrenergic function in aging. (Abstract) Clin Res 32:479a, 1984.

31. Feldman, RD and Linbird, LE: Alteration in leukocyte beta-receptor affinity with aging: A potential explanation for altered beta adrenergic sensitivity in the elderly. N Engl J Med 310:815–819, 1984.

32. Abrass, IB, Scarpace, PJ: Catalytic unit of adenylate cyclase: Reduced activity in aged-human lymphocytes. J Clin Endocrinol Metab 55:1026–1028, 1982.

33. McGarry, K, Laher, M, Fitzgerald, D et al: Baroreflex function in elderly hypertensives. Hypertension 5:763–766, 1983.

34. Goldstein, DS, Lake, CR, et al: Age dependence of hypertensive-normotensive differences in plasma norepinephrine. Hypertension 5:100–107, 1982.

35. Noth, RH, Lassman, MN, Tan SY et al: Age and the renin-aldosterone system. Arch Intern Med 137:1414–1417, 1977.

36. Luft, FC, Grim, CE, Fineberg, N et al: Effects of volume expansion and contraction in normotensive whites, blacks, and subjects of different ages. Circulation 59:643, 1979.

37. Wiedman, P and Beretta-Piccoli, C: Age versus urinary sodium for judging renin, aldosterone and catecholamine levels. Kidney Int 14:619, 1978.

38. Jenkins, AC and Knill, JR: Captopril in the treatment of elderly hypertensive patients. Arch Intern Med 145:2029, 1985.

39. Lindeman, RD and Tubin, J: Longitudinal studies on the rate of decline in renal function with age. J Am Geriatr Soc 33:178–185, 1985.

40. Hollenberg, NA and Adams, DR: Senescence and the renal vasculature in normal man. Cir Res 34:309–316, 1974.

41. Pool, PE and Massie, BM : Diltiazem as a model therapy for systemic hypertension. Am J Cardiol 57:212, 1986.
42. Davidson, DA and Caranasos, GJ: Should the elderly hypertensive be treated? Evidence from clinical trials. Arch Intern Med 147:1933–1937, 1987.
43. Veterans Administration Co-operative Study on Antihypertensive Agents: Effects of treatment on morbidity in hypertension: III. Influence of age, diastolic pressure and prior cardiovascular disease. Circulation 45:991–1004, 1972.
44. Report by the Management Committee: Treatment of mild hypertension in the elderly. Med J Aust 68:398–402, 1981.
45. Hypertension Detection and Follow-up Program: Detection and treatment of hypertension in older individuals. Am J Epidemiol 121:371–376, 1985.
46. Amery, A and Birkenhager, W: Mortality and morbidity result from the European Working Party on high blood pressure in the elderly trial. Lancet 2:1349, 1985.
47. Amery, A, Birkenhäger, W, Brixko, R et al: Efficiency of antihypertensive drug treatment according to age, sex, blood pressure and previous cardiovascular disease in patients over the age of 60. Lancet 2:589, 1986.
48. Viscoli CM and Ostfeld, A: Epidemiology of hypertension in the elderly. In Laragh, JH and Brenner, BM (eds): Hypertension: Pathophysiology, Diagnosis and Management. New York, Raven Press, 1990, pp 191–202.
49. The Systolic Hypertension in the Elderly Program (SHEP) Cooperative Research Group: Prevention of stroke by antihypertensive drug treatment in older persons with isolated systolic hypertension. Final results of the SHEP. JAMA 265:3255–3264, 1991.
50. Amery, A, Fagard, J, Staessen, J et al: Isolated systolic blood pressure elevation in the elderly: Mechanisms, risks and the need for further studies. J Card Pharm 14(Suppl 10):S:14–520, 1989.
51. Joint National Committee: The 1984 report of the Joint National Committee on detection, evaluation and treatment of high blood pressure. Arch Intern Med 144:1045–1057, 1984.
52. Messerli, FH and Ventura, HO: Osler's maneuver and pseudohypertension. N Engl J Med 312:1548, 1985.
53. Jenkins, AC, Knill, JR, Dreslinski, GR et al: Captopril in the treatment of the elderly hypertensive patient. Arch Intern Med 145:2029–2031, 1985.
54. Jeunemaitre, X, Ged E, Ducrocq, MB et al: Effects of transdermal clonidine in young and elderly patients with mild hypertension: Evaluation by three noninvasive methods of blood pressure measurements. J Cardiovasc Pharmacol 10:162–167, 1987.
55. Thananopavarn, C, Golub, MS, Sambhi, MP et al: Clonidine in the elderly hypertensive: Monotherapy and therapy with a diuretic. Chest 83:410–411, 1983.
56. Applegate, WB and Miller ST: Choice of antihypertensive medication regimen. Clinics in Geriatric Medicine: Hypertension 5(4):803–812, 1989.

# CHAPTER 6

# Clinical Features of Coronary Heart Disease in the Elderly

*Marian C. Limacher, M.D.*

The clinical spectrum of coronary heart disease (CHD) ranges from silent ischemia to fulminant congestive heart failure, with chest symptoms, typical exertional angina, acute myocardial infarction (MI) and its complications, arrhythmias, and sudden death completing the array of possible manifestations. The components of the spectrum do not differ with patient age, but the frequency distribution of these clinical signs does appear to shift in the elderly. Numerous reports have identified variable appearances in the clinical signs and symptoms in older compared with younger patients. In addition, as the incidence and prevalence of CHD increases with age, so too do most other conditions likely to produce clinical manifestations easily confused with ischemic disease. Therefore, this chapter will attempt to review information on the signs and symptoms of CHD in the elderly as well as to remind the reader of the differential diagnosis for such features.

## SILENT ISCHEMIA

It is difficult to assign a position for silent ischemia in the clinical spectrum of heart disease. Is it a more or less severe warning than the various symptomatic syndromes? When considering the role of silent ischemia in the elderly, more questions arise and few answers are available. Does asymptomatic, but detectable, ischemia necessarily develop into a symptomatic phase? What is the true prevalence of painless ischemia? What can be inferred about prognosis and outcome once detected? If the elderly are less likely to develop classic symptoms of angina, are they more likely to have asymptomatic episodes of ischemia? Can silent ischemia be distinguished from "unexpressed" symptoms, because a patient is unable or afraid to verbalize discomfort or because one is unable or unwilling to put forth enough exertion to reach an anginal threshold?

Nonetheless, with reports that the magnitude of the problem of asymptomatic ischemia approaches 85% to 90% of all episodes of ischemia,[1] the issue is far from trivial. It has been suggested also that patients who exceed 60 minutes of recorded ST-segment depression per 24-hour electrocardiogram (ECG) recording have an increase in cardiovascular events.[1] In one study, 34% of 626 elderly patients, mean age 82 ± 8 years, with known coronary artery disease (CAD) were found to have ECG recording evidence of silent ischemia. Patients with silent ischemia had a higher incidence of cardiac events in follow-up than patients without, regardless of preexisting diagnosis of CAD, hypertension, or no heart disease. Of patients with CAD and silent ischemia, 65% had new events during 26 months compared with 32% of CAD patients without silent ischemia. In comparison, among patients with other cardiac diagnoses the detection of silent ischemia was associated with a 33% incidence of subsequent events compared with an 18% occurrence in patients with the same conditions but no evidence of silent ischemia.[2] In this same study, cardiac events were quite uncommon (5%) in patients without a preexisting cardiovascular disease.[2] These figures are higher than those reported for younger patients. Stern and associates[3] reported a 30% cardiac event recurrence rate during 2 years for patients with prior MI and evidence of silent ischemia, compared with an 11% recurrence without silent ischemia.[3] In a high risk, younger, postinfarction population, silent ischemia was associated with a 37% event rate at 1 year compared with an 11% recurrence in patients without silent ischemia.[4]

Why the elderly might have a higher incidence of asymptomatic versus symptomatic ischemia could be postulated as a physiologic impairment of pain perception related to aging that would reduce the incidence of painful episodes. One study in a small number of subjects supports such a contention. Miller and coworkers[5] examined the time delay between exercise-induced ST changes and onset of pain in patients with ages ranging from 35 to 75 years and found that the duration of silent ischemia increased with age.

Another extension of the impaired sensitivity to pain theory is examined by the rates of unrecognized or silent MIs by age. The Framingham Study reported that 25% of MIs were discovered only by new ECG changes without clinically recognizable associated events. Moreover, both women and older men had higher frequencies of unrecognized infarcts than other groups.[6] Aronow and colleagues[7] reported that the prevalence of unrecognized MIs in this very elderly population (mean age 82) was 68%. This exceptionally high percentage was thought to demonstrate that the likelihood of unrecognized or asymptomatic infarction increases markedly with age, although it should be pointed out that the definition of MI was by the appearance of new Q waves only. In addition, these data may not be generalizable because a prerequisite for inclusion of patients in the study by Aronow and coworkers[7] was residency in a long-term care facility. A 4-year follow-up study of this population demonstrated that new coronary events were just as common among patients with symptomatic as silent MI, at a rate of 59%.[8] This contrasts with the Framingham findings that suggest a reduced risk of recurrent events among patients with unrecognized compared with symptomatic MIs.[6] The discrepancy may lie in differences in population, ages included, or with the criteria for diagnosis. Kannel and Abbott[6] suggest that denial, the lack of healthcare-seeking behavior, a sensory neuropathy, and/or defective anginal "warning system" are mechanisms that may explain the consistent finding of more silent episodes, both of ischemia and infarction, among the elderly.

## ANGINA PECTORIS

The frequency with which chest pain typical of angina (as defined by the classic description of midsternal or left-sided chest pain provoked by exertion and relieved by rest) is present and how it portends prognosis has been recently investigated among the elderly. In an epidemiologic study of men and women older than age 65 in three American communities, histories of symptoms of chest pain as delineated by the six questions of the Rose questionnaire were carefully obtained.[9] The prevalence rates, adjusted for age, of nonexertional chest pain, chest pain on exertion, and "Rose angina" (positive responses to all six Rose questionnaire items) were 16%, 7.5%, and 4.6% respectively for the 8,359 patients surveyed. Reports of exertional chest discomfort, with or without positive responses to ability to relieve the pain with rest or nitroglycerin, and regardless of localization, were associated with a substantial increase in risk for CHD mortality (relative risk 2.4 for men and 2.7 for women) during the 3-year follow-up.[10]

Among patients with known underlying CHD, chest pain of an anginal quality is reported in 25% to 43% of persons older than age 65. Dyspnea only is reported by 8% to 25% of the patients and both chest pain plus dyspnea by nearly 50%.[11] Other researchers[12] have found that 80% of elderly patients have angina as a presenting symptom in chronic CHD. The Coronary Artery Surgery Study (CASS) report indicated that older patients were more likely to have severe unstable angina than younger patients who were more likely to have stable exertional symptoms,[13,14] Thus, angina is common among the elderly as a symptom of CAD, and among patients brought to consideration for revascularizing surgery, the elderly may have more severe symptoms than younger patients. It is also relevant to learn that the prevalence of prior angina in the group of patients presenting with MI is approximately 50% and does not differ between patients younger than age 70 compared with those who are older.[15]

## MYOCARDIAL INFARCTION

### PRESENTING SYMPTOMS

The admonition that MI may present in variable and "unobtrusive" ways in elderly patients has been offered for several decades.[15–19] Pathy[17] provided an early and carefully documented case series of 387 patients with only ECG evidence of MI. He established that sudden shortness of breath was more common than a "classic" syndrome of substernal chest pain as the single presenting feature of patients older than age 65 with MI (Fig. 6–1). Even so, dyspnea and chest pain were the two most common single manifestations accounting for 19.9% and 19.4% of cases respectively.[17] By presenting only the single dominant symptom for each patient, combinations of features and total numbers of patients with each were not detailed. Some of the more uncommon symptoms (each present in 4% or less of patients) demonstrated in this report as indications of MI were palpitations, renal failure, recurrent vomiting, weakness, pulmonary embolus, restlessness, and sweating. In a follow-up study from the same institution, chest pain was, in fact, the most frequently documented complaint among 777 patients with ECG and enzyme evidence for acute MI. However, the frequency declined with age and shortness of breath increased slightly with age (Fig. 6–2).[19] Syncope, stroke, and confusion were

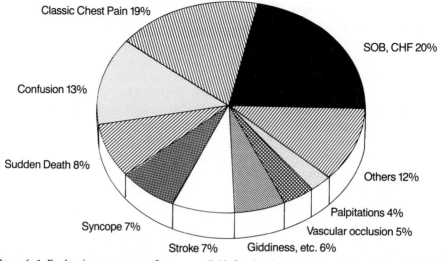

**Figure 6–1.** Predominant symptom for myocardial infarction in the elderly. (Adapted from Pathy.[17])

all more common among the older individuals. Sweating, however, declined as a presentation, from 36% among patients younger than age 70 to 13.6% of patients $\geq$ 85 years of age.[19] A smaller series examined retrospectively also confirms that substernal chest pain is the most prevalent symptom of MI patients aged 65 or older, and like in younger patients, it is commonly described as severe, dull, or pressure-like, although 62% of younger patients compared with only 29% of older patients used these descriptors.[18]

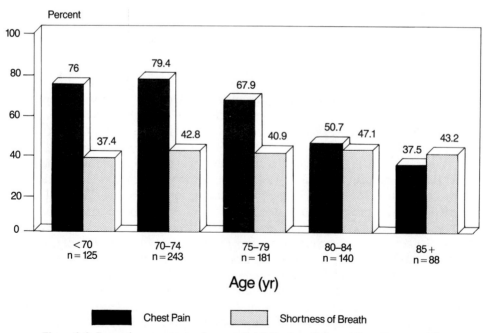

**Figure 6–2.** Presenting symptoms of myocardial infarction. (Adapted from Bayer et al.[19])

The onset of symptoms was documented by Williams and associates[15] as primarily occurring at rest in patients with acute MI, whether they were younger or older than age 70. This study also confirmed that symptoms in patients admitted to the coronary care unit were predominantly cardiovascular in orientation (chest pain and shortness of breath, alone or in combination) in 96% of patients aged 70 and older and in 99% of patients younger than age 70.[15] It is likely that the differences in frequency of reported symptoms between the cited reports reflect methodologic differences rather than true changes in clinical presentation over the years. For example, Pathy[17] reported only one single symptom in patients requiring hospitalization who were subsequently found to have ECG evidence consistent with MI. The other three studies reported the presence of any symptom (not mutually exclusive) in patients admitted to coronary care units who were diagnosed by current standard criteria of ECG changes and enzyme elevations as having MI.[15,18,19] The importance of atypical clinical presentations for elderly patients with MI should not be minimized because of bias in patient selection for the later studies.

Although it is important to remember that mild complaints of pain and dyspnea in elderly patients should be regarded with as great a concern as more severe complaints in younger people,[20] it is also mandatory to consider the multiple potential etiologies of chest discomfort. Just as atypical symptoms may actually result from an acute MI, similar, if not typical, descriptions of chest pain may be secondary to a variety of nonischemic etiologies (Table 6–1). Cardiopulmonary causes of anterior chest discomfort include critical aortic stenosis, aortic dissection, pulmonary embolism, pericarditis, pneumonia, and pleurisy. In addition, the prodrome phase of herpes zoster may be severe enough to masquerade as an acute MI.[20,21] Other organ system involvement also must be considered, including many abdominal etiologies (Table 6–2).[20,21] Cholecystitis, peptic ulcer, esophageal disease, gastritis, pancreatitis, splenic infarction, and congested hepatomegaly have all simulated the acute presentation of infarction. Finally, the numerous musculoskeletal and neurologic syndromes listed in Table 6–3 may be mistaken for cardiac syndromes.[20,21]

Careful attention to historic and physical features is imperative in making a diagnosis of CAD in the elderly. Appropriate use of laboratory and diagnostic testing usually must be undertaken. It also should be remembered that the cardiac etiologies, especially ischemic heart disease, remain the most prevalent underlying

**Table 6–1.**
Differential
Diagnosis of
Chest Pain

Coronary artery disease
Aortic stenosis
Aortic dissection
Pulmonary embolus
Pericarditis
Pneumonia
Pleurisy
Trauma/Falls
Cervical/Thoracic spine disease
Herpes zoster

**Table 6–2.**
Abdominal
Sources of Chest
Pain

Cholecystitis
Peptic ulcer
Esophageal spasm
Esophageal cancer
Hiatal hernia
Esophagitis
Gastritis
Pancreatitis
Splenic infarction
Liver congestion in CHF

CHF = congestive heart failure

conditions in the elderly, and interpretation of testing procedures must take into account the pretest likelihood of disease.[22] Analysis of the Multicenter Chest Pain Study has demonstrated that emergency room triage practices for the elderly with chest pain are more cautious than in younger patients, with 56% of patients older than 65 versus 35% of patients between age 30 and 64 admitted to the hospital and 37% versus 23% of patients admitted to the coronary care unit.[23] Additionally, the possibility of more than one condition being present in the same individual must not be discounted.

## COMPLICATIONS

Most of the described complications from acute MI are generally felt to occur more commonly in the elderly patient (Table 6–4).[12,24] Pericarditis and Dressler's syndrome do not appear to have an age-related predisposition.[12,15] Likewise, the incidence of ventricular fibrillation is not increased in the elderly.[12] The incidence of atrial flutter and atrial fibrillation may be more common, although the reports are variable.[15,25,26] Heart block, conduction defects, and asystole are all more common in the elderly.[15,27,28] Heart failure, pulmonary edema, and cardiogenic shock are also seen with increasing frequency in the elderly.[15,27,29] These factors might be assumed to be the result of prior multiple infarctions in patients surviving to have

**Table 6–3.** Musculoskeletal Causes of Chest Pain

| | |
|---|---|
| Osteoarthritis | Osteoporosis |
| Spondylosis | Kyphoscoliosis |
| Fibromyositis, myofasciitis | Tietze's syndrome |
| Costochondritis | Xiphodynia |
| Thoracic outlet syndrome | Faulty posture |
| Herniated disc | Rib fracture |
| Collagen disease | Infection/abscess |
| Muscle injury | |

**Table 6–4.** Complications of
Acute Myocardial Infarction

| Increased in Elderly | Equal Frequency |
| --- | --- |
| Atrial fib or flutter | Ventricular arrhythmias |
| AV block | Pericarditis |
| VSD | Valve disruption |
| Myocardial rupture | Aneurysm |
| Embolus | Pseudoaneurysm |
| CHF | Thrombus |
| Cardiogenic shock | |

AV = atrioventricular; CHF = congestive heart
failure; VSD = ventricular septal defect

another event at older age. However, heart failure and cardiogenic shock increase
in frequency in patients older than age 60, even among those with their first heart
attack.[27] Although the formation and detection of left ventricular thrombus does
not appear to be influenced by the patient's age, Johannessen and coworkers[30]
determined that age greater than 68, in addition to pendulous appearance and
thrombus mobility, were the best predictors of thrombus embolization. Myocardial
rupture is reported to complicate MI three times as often in patients older than age
70 compared with younger patients.[31]

Despite the increased frequency of most serious complications of MI in the
elderly, the medical care of the elderly infarction patient is no different from that
for a younger victim.[32] Future directed research would seem warranted if progress
is to be made. Meanwhile, practitioners must anticipate the more frequent complications among elderly infarction patients and react promptly and possibly
preemptively in their management strategy.

## SURVIVAL

The outcome for a group of patients who are more likely to experience serious
complications from an infarction by virtue of increasing age could easily be inferred
to be more unsatisfactory than for a comparable group at a younger age. This,
unfortunately, has been established by essentially every study addressing the topic.
Williams and colleagues reported[15] in 1976 that there was a 17% in-hospital mortality rate for patients younger than age 70 compared with a 37.5% mortality for
patients older than 70. Studies from the 1980s reflect an improvement in acute
survival, but a reproducible increase in death rate with increasing age. The in-hospital mortality rates in Robinson and associates' study[28] were 3.1% for patients
younger than 60, 8.6% for age 60 to 69, and 20.1% for those 70 and older. Hoit
and colleagues[29] reported on a wider range of patient ages but found a 2.5% mortality rate for patients younger than 45 years old during their hospitalization compared with 9.0% for patients aged 46 to 70 and 21.3% for patients older than age
70. The results of the Multicenter Investigation of the Limitation of Infarct Size
(MILIS) revealed a 7% in-hospital mortality rate for patients younger than 65 and
a 14% rate for patients 65 through 75.[33] Analysis of multiple variables demonstrated
that a number of features predicted increased mortality, including Karnofsky
score $\leq 7$, cardiomegaly or rales on admission, infarct size, left ventricular ejection

fraction ≤ 40%, atrioventricular (AV) block, intraventricular conduction defect, congestive heart failure (CHF), and infarct extension. However, these variables predicted decreased survival for both age groups. In fact, elderly patients without CHF did not have a different death rate compared with younger patients.[33] In contrast to in-hospital mortality, only a low Karnofsky score was useful in predicting the significantly higher long-term mortality rates in elderly patients whereas a predischarge left ventricular ejection fraction ≤ 40% was a strong predictor of later mortality in younger patients.[33] In another study, clinical classification by Killip class, was the only independent predictor of survival among patients age 70 or older surviving acute MI.[34] Late mortality for hospital survivors at 1- and 4-years follow-up was more than double in older compared with younger patients. The 1-year mortality rate was 5% for those younger than 65 and 19% for patients 65 to 75. The 4-year mortality rates were 13% and 35%, respectively.[33]

How specific measurable characteristics of MI influence outcome has been examined in several studies. In one series, no difference was found in the ages of patients who had Q–wave versus non-Q–wave infarctions.[35] A larger survey, the Worcester Heart Attack Study, demonstrated that older patients were more likely to have a non-Q–wave infarction.[36] Older patients were actually likely to have smaller infarcts as measured by peak creatine kinase levels, despite being at greater risk for CHF and cardiogenic shock.[36] The ECG location of MI does not appear to be more prevalent in younger or older patients and also does not predict mortality.[34,36]

Myocardial infarction can be considered the major identifiable clinical entity of CAD and has been shown to be highly associated with poor outcome both in the acute and long-term setting. Awareness of the propensity for atypical presentations, serious complications, and reduced survival in elderly patients mandates prompt diagnosis and careful management decisions. Guidelines for the role of coronary angiography have been proposed for those younger than age 75 with individual consideration suggested for those older than age 75. Ross and associates[37] recommend diagnostic catheterization in patients surviving MI with a history of previous infarction, clinical or radiographic signs of left ventricular failure, ischemic exercise response, poor workload capability, or resting ejection fraction between 20% and 44%.

## ARRHYTHMIAS AND SUDDEN DEATH DUE TO CORONARY HEART DISEASE

Atrial dysrhythmias, notably atrial fibrillation and flutter, are common problems encountered in elderly patients following MI and have been associated with increased mortality during the first year.[35] The atrial rhythms associated with sick sinus syndrome may also have CAD as an underlying condition.[38] The frequency with which supraventricular dysrhythmias present as the initial or major feature of ischemia in the chronic setting is not defined nor is it known how prognosis is affected. Supraventricular ectopic beats and nonsustained tachycardias, however, are common in apparently healthy elderly individuals.[39] Chronic AV block has been associated with severe CAD in 43% of younger patients (age 45 to 65).[40] However, in elderly patients (mean age 70), a necropsy study found that severe CAD could be attributed in only 15% as the etiology of chronic heart block.[41] Although the methodology of the two studies does not permit direct comparisons, it would seem prudent to consider that CAD may be present in most elderly patients with chronic supraventricular abnormalities or heart block, but that it is unlikely to be the primary correctable etiology of the disturbance.

Ventricular ectopic beats and ventricular tachycardia are also encountered more commonly with increasing age.[39,42] The prognostic significance of such findings on ambulatory ECG monitoring, in the absence of other known markers of CAD, remains controversial.[43] One study found that patients age 75 and older, with 10 ventricular ectopic beats (VEBs) per hour on 24-hour ambulatory ECG monitoring had an increased crude mortality rate during 5 years compared with patients who had less ectopy and that 92% of patients free of VEBs at baseline remained free on repeat study 5 years later.[44] However, without baseline comprehensive evaluation of the extent of CAD, it is not possible to directly link VEBs or asymptomatic nonsustained ventricular tachycardia with future CAD events.

Sudden cardiac death increases with age, is most frequently due to underlying atherosclerotic CHD, and is caused immediately by ventricular arrhythmias with or without acute MI.[45] In a study of elderly patients in a long-term care facility who were known to have CAD or hypertension, 24-hour ambulatory monitoring evidence of complex ventricular ectopy, nonsustained ventricular tachycardia or, interestingly, silent ischemia, was associated with a very high frequency of serious cardiac events including sudden death during 37 months of follow-up.[46] Madsen's[45] analysis of 166 patients with sudden death demonstrates the majority had some prodromal symptoms, usually cardiac, and 57% had seen a doctor within the preceding 2 months. Whether more specific markers can be identified and whether any therapy can be administered to moderate the risk of sudden death in the elderly with ischemic heart disease (the highest risk group) remains to be determined.[47]

## CONGESTIVE HEART FAILURE

Congestive heart failure is the most common principal diagnosis in geriatric patients admitted to many hospitals.[48] The incidence and prevalence of CHF is increasing and the rate of rise is greater for the elderly.[49] The major etiology for CHF, for both men and women, is CAD.[50] When complicating acute MI, heart failure is a powerful predictor of early and late mortality.[33,34] When acute pulmonary edema is the presenting symptom, Plotnick and associates[51] found that the majority of historic, physical, and laboratory findings did not predict 1-year survival. Peak creatine kinase level ($> 1000$ IU/L), admission systolic blood pressure $\leq 150$ mmHg, and response to therapy within 4 hours were the only features predictive of mortality.[51] In this group, 49% had evidence of acute MI and most also had chest pain. During the hospital admission, 16% of the population died and 36% died within 1 year (overall mortality at 1 year = 52%).[51] Thus, CHF is highly associated with CAD in the elderly in both acute and chronic presentations.

## SUMMARY

Care of the elderly patient with CHD requires an understanding of the prevalence of disease and its variability of presentation. Sound application of the diagnostic and therapeutic maneuvers developed for younger patients remains the predominant basis for the clinical approach to older individuals with heart disease. As more research is directed toward age-related issues in cardiac disease, the approach may be refined with more specific guidelines than are currently available.

## REFERENCES

1. Nademanee, K, Intarachot, V, Josephson, M, et al: Prognostic significance of silent myocardial ischemia in patients with unstable angina. J Am Coll Cardiol 10:1–9, 1987.
2. Aronow, WS and Epstein, S: Usefulness of silent myocardial ischemia detected by ambulatory electrocardiographic monitoring in predicting new coronary events in elderly patients. Am J Cardiol 62:1295–1296, 1988.
3. Stern, S, Gavish, A, Zin, D, et al: Clinical outcome of silent myocardial ischemia. Am J Cardiol 62:16F–18F, 1988.
4. Gottlieb, SO, Gottlieb, SH, Achuff, SC, et al: Silent ischemia on Holter monitoring predicts mortality in high-risk post infarction patients. JAMA 259:1030–1035, 1988.
5. Miller, PF, Sheps, DS, Bragdon, EE, et al: Aging and pain perception in ischemic heart disease. Am Heart J 120:22–30, 1990.
6. Kannel, WB and Abbott, RD: Incidence and prognosis of unrecognized myocardial infarction: An update on the Framingham Study. N Engl J Med 311:1144–1147, 1984.
7. Aronow, WS, Starling, L, Etienne, R, et al: Unrecognized Q-wave myocardial infarction in patients older than 64 years in a long-term healthcare facility. Am J Cardiol 56:483, 1985.
8. Aronow, WS: New coronary events at four-year follow-up in elderly patients with recognized or unrecognized myocardial infarction. Am J Cardiol 63:621–622, 1989.
9. Rose, G, Blackburn, H, Gillum, R, et al: Cardiovascular survey methods. World Health Organization, Geneva, pp. 162–165, 1982.
10. LaCroix, AZ, Guralnik, JM, Curb, JD, et al: Chest pain and coronary heart disease mortality among older men and women in three communities. Circulation 81:437–446, 1990.
11. Coodley, EL: Coronary artery disease in the elderly. Postgrad Med 87:223–227, 1990.
12. O'Rourke, RA, Chatterjee, K, Wei, JY: Coronary heart disease. In 18th Bethesda Conference: Cardiovascular Disease in the Elderly. J Am Coll Cardiol 10:52A–56A, 1987.
13. Mock, MD, Fisher, LD, Gersh, BJ, et al: Prognosis of coronary heart disease in the elderly patient: The CASS experience. In Coodley, EL (ed): Geriatric Heart Disease. Littleton, MA, PSG Publishing Co., pp 358–363, 1985.
14. Gersh, BJ, Kronmal, RA, Schaff, HV, et al: Comparison of coronary artery bypass surgery and medical therapy in patients 65 years of age or older. A nonrandomized study from the Coronary Artery Surgery (CASS) registry. N Engl J Med 313:217–224, 1985.
15. Williams, BO, Begg, TB, Semple, T, et al: The elderly in a coronary unit. Br Med J 2:451–453, 1976.
16. Thould, AK: Coronary heart disease in the aged. Br Med J 2:1089–1093, 1965.
17. Pathy, MS: Clinical presentation of myocardial infarction in the elderly. Br Heart J 29:190–199, 1967.
18. Applegate, WB, Graves, S, Collins, T, et al: Acute myocardial infarction in elderly patients. South Med J 77:1127–1129, 1984.
19. Bayer, AJ, Chadha, JS, Farag, RR, et al: Changing presentation of myocardial infarction with increasing old age. J Am Geriatr Soc 34:263–266, 1986.
20. Harris, R: Cardiovascular diseases in the elderly. In Symposium on clinical geriatric medicine. Med Clin N Am 67:379–394, 1983.
21. Zoob, M: Differentiating the causes of chest pain. Geriatrics 33:95–101, 1978.
22. Iskandrian, AS, Heo, J, Hakki, A: Angina: DDx of atypical presentations in the elderly. Geriatrics 10:51–60, 1986.
23. Solomon, CG, Lee, TH, Cook, EF, et al: Comparison of clinical presentation of acute myocardial infarction in patients older than 65 years of age to younger patients: The Multicenter Chest Pain Study Experience. Am J Cardiol 63:772–776, 1989.
24. Morley, JE and Reese, SS: Clinical implications of the aging heart. Am J Med 86:77–86, 1987.
25. Helmers, C, Lundman, T, Mogensen, L, Orinius, E, et al: Atrial fibrillation in acute myocardial infarction. Acta Med Scand 193:38–44, 1973.
26. Kannel, WB, Sorlie, P, McNamara, PM: Prognosis after initial myocardial infarction: The Framingham Study. Am J Cardiol 44:53–59, 1979.

27. Hunt, D and Sloman, G: Prognosis in elderly patients following myocardial infarction. In Coodley, EL (ed): Geriatric Heart Disease. Littleton, MA, PSG Publishing Co., pp 372–375, 1985.

28. Robinson, K, Conroy, RM, Mulcahy, R: Risk factors and in-hospital course of first myocardial infarction in the elderly. Clin Cardiol 11:519–523, 1988.

29. Hoit, BD, Gilpin, EA, Henning, H, et al: Myocardial infarction in young patients: An analysis by age subsets. Circulation 74:712–721, 1986.

30. Johannessen, K-A, Nordrehaug, JE, von der Lippe, G, et al: Risk factors for embolization in patients with left ventricular thrombi and acute myocardial infarction. Br Heart J 60:104–110, 1988.

31. Latting, CA and Silverman, MD: Acute myocardial infarction in hospitalized patients over age 70. Am Heart J 100:311–318, 1980.

32. Wenger, NK, Marcus, RI, O'Rourke, RA: Cardiovascular disease in the elderly. In the 18th Bethesda Conference: Cardiovascular Disease in the Elderly. J Am Coll Cardiol 10:80A–87A, 1987.

33. Tofler, GH, Muller, JE, Stone, PH, et al: Factors leading to shorter survival after acute myocardial infarction in patients ages 65 to 75 years compared with younger patients. Am J Cardiol 62:860–867, 1988.

34. Olmsted, WL, Groden, DL, Silverman, ME: Prognosis in survivors of acute myocardial infarction occurring at age 70 years or older. Am J Cardiol 60:971–975, 1987.

35. Krone, RJ, Friedman, E, Thanavaro, S, et al: Long-term prognosis after first Q-wave (transmural) or non-Q-wave (nontransmural) myocardial infarction: Analysis of 593 patients. Am J Cardiol 52:234–239, 1983.

36. Goldberg, RJ, Gore, JM, Gurwitz, JH, et al: The impact of age on the incidence and prognosis of initial acute myocardial infarction: The Worcester Heart Attack Study. Am Heart J 117:543–549, 1989.

37. Ross, J, Gilpin, EA, Madsen, EB, et al: A decision scheme for coronary angiography after acute myocardial infarction. Circulation 79:292–303, 1989.

38. Rodriguez, RD and Schocken, DD: Update on sick sinus syndrome, a cardiac disorder of aging. Geriatrics 45:26–36, 1990.

39. Kantelip, J-P, Sage, E, Duchene-Marullaz, P: Findings on ambulatory electrocardiographic monitoring in subjects older than 80 years. Am J Cardiol 57:398–401, 1986.

40. Ginks, W, Sutton, R, Siddons, H, et al: Unsuspected coronary artery disease as cause of chronic atrioventricular block in middle age. Br Heart J 40:699–702, 1980.

41. Davies, MJ: Pathology of the conducting tissue of the heart. London, Butterworths, 1971.

42. Glasser, SP, Clark, PI, Applebaum, HJ: Occurrence of frequent complex arrhythmias detected by ambulatory monitoring. Findings in an apparently healthy asymptomatic elderly population. Chest 75:565–568, 1979.

43. Fleg, JL: Ventricular arrhythmias in the elderly: Prevalence, mechanisms, and therapeutic implications. Geriatrics 43:23–29, 1988.

44. Martin, A, Benbow, LJ, Butrous, G, et al: Five-year follow-up of 106 elderly subjects by means of long-term ambulatory cardiac monitoring. Eur Heart J 55:592, 1984.

45. Madsen, JK: Ischaemic heart disease and prodromes of sudden cardiac death. Is it possible to identify high risk groups for sudden cardiac death? Br Heart J 54:27–32, 1985.

46. Aronow, WS and Epstein, S: Usefulness of silent ischemia, ventricular tachycardia and complex ventricular arrhythmias in predicting new coronary events in elderly patients with coronary artery disease or systemic hypertension. Am J Cardiol 65:511–512, 1990.

47. Glazer, MD, Hill, RD, Wenger, NK: Dx and Tx of the elderly patient with atherosclerotic coronary heart disease. Geriatrics 10:45–54, 1985.

48. Rich, MW and Freedland, KE: Effect of DRGs on three-month readmission rate of geriatric patients with congestive heart failure. Am J Public Health 78:680–682, 1988.

49. Furberg, CD, Yusuf, F, Thom, TJ: Potential for altering the natural history of congestive heart failure: Need for large clinical trials. Am J Cardiol 55:45A–55A, 1985.

50. Limacher, MC, Johnstone, DI, Rousseau, MF, et al: Differences between men and women with left ventricular dysfunction. Circulation 83:733, 1991.

51. Plotnick, GD, Kelemen, MH, Garrett, RB, et al: Acute cardiogenic pulmonary edema in the elderly: Factors predicting in-hospital and one-year mortality. South Med J 75:565–569, 1982.

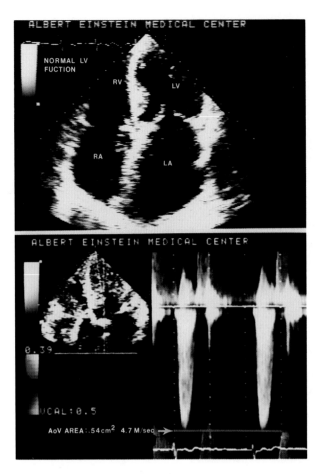

**Figure 7–2.** *Upper panel:* Apical 4-chamber view in a patient with senile aortic stenosis and normal LV function. Left atrium (LA) is enlarged. *Lower panel:* Apical 5-chamber view with CW Doppler beam directed through the calcified aortic valve leaflet. The maximal gradient recorded across the aortic valve measures 88 mm Hg. Aortic valve area calculated by the continuity equation is 0.54 cm². Abbreviations: LV = left ventricle. RV = right ventricle. RA = right atrium.

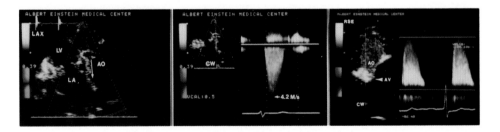

**Figure 7–3.** Eccentric directed jet in a patient with senile aortic stenosis and markedly post stenotic dilated proximal aorta. *Left hand panel:* demonstrates an eccentric color flow jet directed towards the posterior aortic wall obtained in the parasternal long-axis view. *Middle panel:* color CW directed Doppler measurement of aortic stenosis gradient. The maximal gradient across the aortic valve measures 71 mm Hg. *Right hand panel:* right parasternal view (RSE) of eccentrically directed color jets with CW directed Doppler measurement. The maximal gradient measures 64 mm Hg. Abbreviations: LAX = long axis view. AO = aorta. LA = left atrium. AV = aortic valve. CW = continuous wave Doppler.

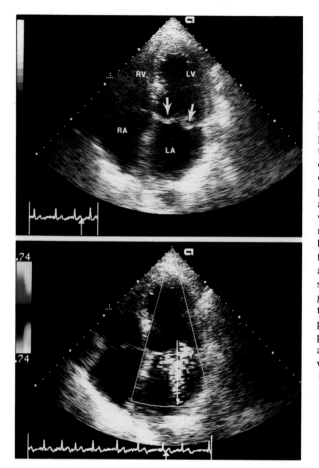

**Figure 7–7.** *Upper panel:* Apical 4-chambered view in an elderly patient with marked mitral valve prolapse of both anterior and posterior leaflets *(arrows)*. This view demonstrated the most apparent displacement of both anterior and posterior leaflets into the left atrium (LA) but the displacement was also apparent in the parasternal long axis and apical 2-chambered views. *Lower panel:* Color flow Doppler obtained from the apical 4-chambered view in the same patient. Significant mitral regurgitation is demonstrated with the mosaic jet extending to the posterior left atrial wall and occupying at least 50% of the left atrial area. Abbreviations: LV = left ventricle. RA = right atrium. RV = right ventricle.

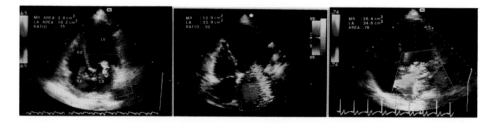

**Figure 7–8.** Color flow Doppler echocardiogram obtained in the apical 4-chambered views in patients with mild *(left hand panel)*, moderate *(middle panel)* and severe mitral regurgitation *(right hand panel)*. See text for explanation.

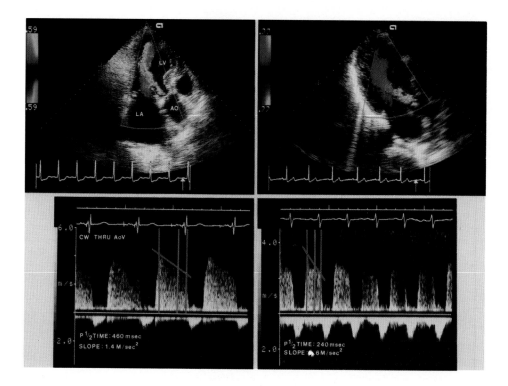

**Figure 7–10.** *Upper panel:* Color flow Doppler studies obtained from the apical 2-chambered views in a patient with mild aortic regurgitation *(left-hand panel)* and a patient with severe aortic regurgitation *(right-hand panel). Lower panel:* Corresponding continuous wave Doppler profiles of same patients demonstrating corresponding pressure half-time (p ½) measurements and deceleration slope velocities. Abbreviations: LV = left ventricle. AO = aorta. LA = left atrium.

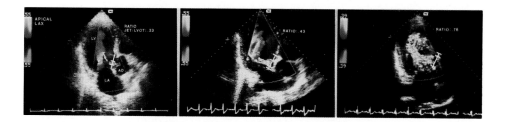

**Figure 7–11.** Color flow Doppler echocardiogram obtained from the apical 2-chambered views in patients with minimal *(left-hand panel)*, mild to moderate *(middle panel)* and severe aortic regurgitation *(right-hand panel)*. See text for explanation. Abbreviations: LV = left ventricle. AO = aorta. LA = left atrium.

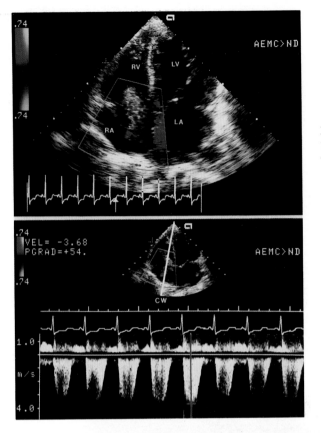

**Figure 7–12.** *Upper panel:* Color flow Doppler echocardiogram obtained in a older patient with pulmonary hypertension and moderately severe tricuspid regurgitation. *Lower panel:* Continuous wave Doppler (CW) in same patient demonstrating a maximal gradient of 54 mm Hg. The pulmonary systolic pressure is calculated to be 68 mm Hg. Abbreviations: LV = left ventricle. LA = left atrium. RV = right ventricle. RA = right atrium.

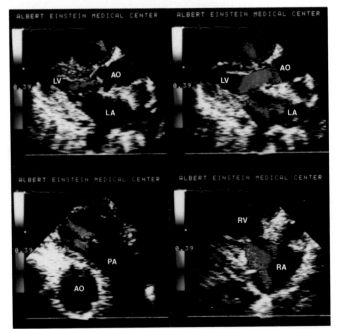

**Figure 7–13.** Color Doppler echocardiogram obtained in an 80-year-old patient demonstrating aortic regurgitation *(left-hand upper panel)*, mitral regurgitation *(right-hand upper panel)* obtained in the parasternal long axis views, pulmonic regurgitation *(left-hand lower panel)* obtained in the parasternal short axis view, and tricuspid regurgitation *(right-hand lower panel)* obtained in the right ventricular inflow view. Abbreviations: AO = aorta. LV = left atrium. PA = pulmonary artery. RV = right ventricle. RA = right atrium.

# CHAPTER 7

# Evaluation of Valvular Heart Disease in Patients Older Than Age 65*

*Morris N. Kotler, M.D.*
*Larry E. Jacobs, M.D.*
*With Technical Assistance of Alfred Ioli*

The major cause of death in the elderly is attributed to cardiovascular disease, accounting for 40% of deaths in individuals older than 75 years of age and rising to 48% in those older than the age of 85. Ischemic heart disease and hypertensive heart disease are the most common causes of death in the elderly, especially when related to congestive heart failure. Degenerative calcific changes of the atrioventricular valves commonly occur; in one series reported by Pomerance,[1] these changes were the second most common cause of congestive heart failure in the elderly. In patients without congestive heart failure, significant degenerative calcific changes in heart valves occurred in 29% of patients, with approximately 9% of patients having critical aortic stenosis.[2] However, it is not always possible to separate the etiologies of congestive heart failure in the elderly because multiple pathologic entities frequently coexist and contribute to the overall clinical syndrome.

## PATHOLOGIC CHANGES THAT OCCUR IN HEART VALVES IN THE ELDERLY

With advancing age, the cardiac valves thicken and become more opaque.[3,4] The degree of change is, in part, genetically determined and, in part, age-related. As more and more individuals live longer in the United States and throughout the world and as new treatment modalities such as valvuloplasty evolve, the prevalence and significance of valvular abnormalities in the elderly become more important. In an autopsy study of 805 patients ranging in age from 10 to 96 years, Pomerance[5] reviewed the aging changes that occur in heart valves. The anterior leaflet of the

*This study was supported in part by: The Women's League for Medical Research, Albert Einstein Medical Center, Philadelphia, PA 19141.

mitral valve generally develops two types of changes that occur with increasing age, that is, nodular thickening at the free edges and lipid deposition. In addition, the posterior leaflet develops changes that occur with age, which include annular calcification, small puckered scars, diffuse opacification of the leaflet, and ballooning deformity. The noduli arantii in the aortic valve develop fenestrations and calcification. According to Pomerance,[5] the development of noduli arantii in the aortic valve and nodularity of the anterior leaflet of the mitral valve represent reactions to local injuries. In contrast to changes involving left-sided valves, minimal changes occur in the tricuspid and pulmonary valves.

## CALCIFIC AORTIC STENOSIS OF THE ELDERLY

### AGING CHANGES

During the process of aging, the aortic valve progressively thickens, especially at the base, with opaque ridges and central nodular corpora arantii appearing along the line of closure. Histologic examination of these plaques reveals fine sudanophilic droplets that have a foamy appearance. The lipids appear to be similar to those found in fatty streaks, but thrombosis, calcification, and hemorrhage are not encountered. In addition, the collagen in elderly valves is denser staining; it is variable and the parallel orientation is lost. Microscopic calcification can occur in patients older than 40 years of age. With regard to degenerative changes, there are two main forms, calcification and mucoid degeneration. Both these processes affect the left-sided valves and are not very commonly found in the right-sided valves. In many patients older than the age of 75, calcification first appears in the fibrosa at the base of the aortic cusp. The development appears to be related to repeated mechanical stresses that occur with normal valve action. With increasing severity of calcification, the deposits extend toward the free margin of the cusp, but rarely do they involve the free edges.[6] On histologic examination, these solid zones of calcification expand and occasionally break through the fibrosa. Thin-wall vascular channels and scanty chronic inflammatory cell infiltrate may be present adjacent to the calcified regions. Although degenerative calcification is responsible for the majority of patients presenting with clinical aortic stenosis in the elderly, some patients with congenital bicuspid valves develop extensive calcification and present with symptoms later on in life. In general, aortic stenosis in patients younger than 60 years of age may occur as a result of a bicuspid aortic valve or of previous rheumatic heart disease. In the age group 60 to 75 years, calcification involving congenital bicuspid valves and degenerative aortic stenosis occurs most frequently, whereas in patients older than the age of 75, degenerative calcification is responsible for the majority of cases. Senile aortic stenosis is characterized morphologically by a trileaflet aortic valve free of commissural fusion, with calcified nodular excrescences within the valve pockets that restrict motion (Fig. 7–1). At the Mayo Clinic, senile aortic stenosis comprised half the cases operated upon.[7]

### CLINICAL FEATURES

In the vast majority of patients older than age 65, an ejection systolic murmur is heard in the aortic area, frequently radiating to the base of the neck (Table 7–1). Many elderly patients have aortic ejection murmurs due to "aortic sclerosis" without evidence of significant stenosis. However, isolated significant aortic valve ste-

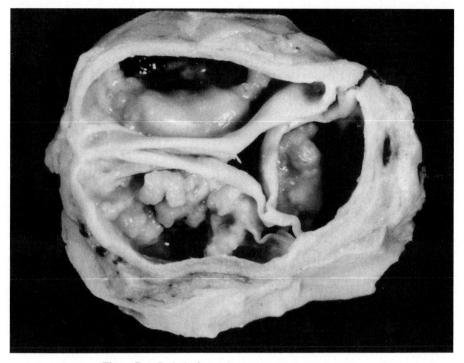

**Figure 7–1.** Pathologic specimen of senile aortic stenosis.

nosis is not uncommon in patients older than the age of 80 years and accounted for 13% in one series.[8] In that particular group, women predominated. In addition, in 40% of the patients with significant aortic stenosis the severity was not suspected by the referring physician.[8] A harsh or rasping ejection systolic murmur is frequently heard in the second right intercostal space and generally occurs as a result of the disturbance of flow caused by the high velocity jet. The murmur frequently radiates to the base of the neck. In many instances, a loud high frequency musical systolic murmur can be heard at the cardiac apex. This high pitched murmur frequently may be mistaken for the murmur of mitral regurgitation. The high frequency components selectively radiate to the apex (the so-called Gallavardin phenomenon).[9] In many instances in the elderly patient, as a result of a rigid aorta or hypertension, the pulse pressure is increased. As a result, the aortic component of the second sound may not be markedly decreased in intensity, the murmur may peak earlier in systole, and the carotid pulses may not demonstrate the typical pulses parvus et tardus (a slow rising pulse that is small and sustained). Therefore, physical examination may underestimate the severity of aortic stenosis in the elderly.[10] In addition, a fourth heart sound, which is frequently audible in severe aortic stenosis in younger patients, is commonly auscultated in the elderly patient without aortic stenosis, as a result of the aging phenomenon or noncompliance of the left ventricle. If the patient has all the typical physical findings consistent with severe aortic stenosis, generally the echocardiography Doppler findings support the diagnosis. In patients with critical aortic stenosis and a low cardiac output, the physical findings may be unimpressive and the severity of the stenosis may not be appreciated clinically.

**Table 7–1.** Clinical Differentiation of Aortic Sclerosis, Senile Calcific Aortic Stenosis, and Hypertrophic Obstructive Cardiomyopathy

| Clinical Parameter | Aortic Sclerosis | Senile Calcific Aortic Stenosis | Hypertrophic Obstructive Cardiomyopathy |
|---|---|---|---|
| Carotid Pulse | Normal to hyperkinetic | *Parvus et tardus* to slightly diminished | Brisk upstroke—sometimes bisferious |
| Apical Impulse | Normal to mildly forceful or sustained if hypertension is present | Forceful sustained | Forceful, double or triple |
| Sounds | Second sound normal to increased in hypertension; S$_4$ frequently present | Second sound single; S$_4$ present; S$_3$ present if left ventricular dysfunction present | Second sound normal or paradoxically split; S$_4$ |
| Systolic Murmur | Second right sternal border radiating to neck and to apex, peaks early in systole | Second right sternal border; radiating to neck and to apex where it is frequently high pitched; peaks in midsystole in presence of hypertension but usually long and peaks late in systole in nonhypertensive patients | Third or fourth left sternal border and apex may mimic mitral regurgitation |
| Amyl Nitrite | ← → | → ← | ← → |
| Valsalva | ← → | → ← | → ← |
| Squatting | | | |
| Isometric Handgrip | | | |
| Regurgitant Diastolic Murmur | ± | ± | Occasionally audible if associated calcific, aortic sclerosis present |
| ECG | Normal to LVH if hypertension present | LVH "strain pattern" | LVH, strain pattern, deep septal Q waves; rarely WPW pattern |
| Chest Roentgenogram | | | |
| Cardiothoracic Ratio | NL | NL – ↑ | NL – ↑ |
| Poststenotic Dilation | — | ↑↑ | — |
| Calcified Valve | Minimal | Generally extensive | Unless associated aortic valve sclerosis present |

ECG = electrocardiogram; LVH = left ventricular hypertrophy; NL = normal ; WPW = Wolff-Parkinson-White Syndrome

## ECHOCARDIOGRAPHIC DOPPLER FEATURES

Two-dimensional echocardiography is useful in determining the degree of aortic valve thickness, calcification, and the degree of restriction of motion.[11] In addition, left ventricular function, the degree of left ventricular hypertrophy, and the extent of poststenotic dilation of the aorta can be accurately assessed. Evaluation of morphology may be important for patients being considered for balloon valvuloplasty. When the aortic valve is heavily calcified and restricted in motion, two-dimensional echocardiography and even aortic root angiography is unable to differentiate a calcified congenitally bicuspid aortic valve from a heavily calcified tricuspid aortic valve. However, a catheter-based intravascular ultrasound system can differentiate a bicuspid from a tricuspid valve in adults with calcific aortic stenosis.[12] Valvuloplasty is best performed in patients with senile degenerative disease or in patients with rheumatic heart disease without dense calcification.[13] If the aortic valve leaflets are moderately thickened and/or calcified and restricted in motion by echocardiography, further evaluation with Doppler ultrasound is mandatory.

### Doppler Echocardiography

Doppler ultrasound provides a noninvasive technique that allows clinicians to gather information regarding pressure differences and blood flow in the heart and great vessels. Therefore in aortic stenosis the transvalvular gradient and aortic valvular orifice area can be determined. With continuous-wave Doppler, the ultrasound beam is directed parallel to the flow jet so that the velocity of blood flow distal to the stenotic jet is obtained[14] (Fig. 7–2). To obtain the maximal velocity of flow, the transducer is placed at the apex and the right parasternal or suprasternal position. More recently, color Doppler has been found to be useful, especially in older patients with eccentrically directed flow jets (Fig. 7–3).[15] Color-flow–guided CW Doppler allows more accurate determination of transvalvular gradients.[15] Using the modified Bernoulli equation,[16,17] the maximal instantaneous (and mean transvalvular pressure gradients) can be obtained by the formula $\triangle P = 4V^2$, with P representing the pressure gradient and V the velocity of transvalvular blood flow measured by continuous-wave Doppler echocardiography. In comparison with cardiac catheterization, the Doppler-determined maximal instantaneous gradient always exceeds the peak-to-peak gradient obtained at cardiac catheterization.[11,14] The correlation of Doppler-derived gradient measurements with cardiac catheterization measurements has been validated by simultaneous Doppler echocardiographic and dual catheterization studies.[14] The correlations between maximal instantaneous and mean gradients measured by Doppler echocardiography and those measured by dual catheters in the left ventricle and aorta have been excellent.[14] Thus it appears that the most reliable expression of severity of aortic stenosis by Doppler echocardiography is the mean gradient. However, because gradients are dependent on flow and the status of the left ventricle, the severity of aortic stenosis by Doppler echocardiography determination of gradients alone may be unreliable (Fig. 7–4).[18] Therefore, determination of aortic valve area by Doppler echocardiography using the continuity equation is recommended as the most useful noninvasive test for assessing the severity of aortic stenosis.[18] The continuity equation is derived as follows:

$$A_1 \times V_1 = A_2 \times V_2$$

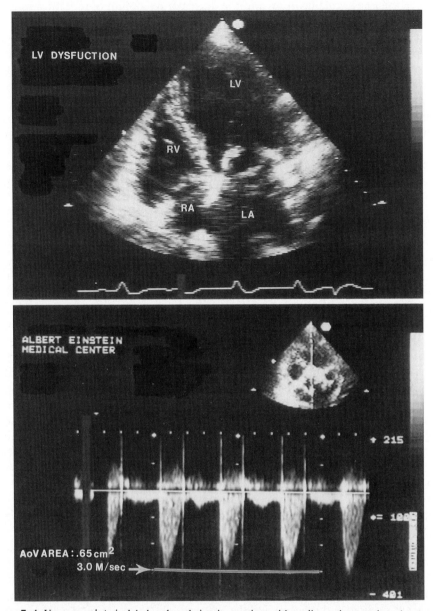

**Figure 7–4.** *Upper panel:* Apical 4-chambered view in a patient with senile aortic stenosis and severe left ventricular (LV) dysfunction. The left ventricle is significantly dilated and the mitral leaflets and posterior submitral annulus is calcified. *Lower panel:* CW Doppler in same patient obtained from the apical 5-chambered view. The maximal gradient measures 36 mmHg but the aortic valve (AOV) area as determined by the continuity equation measures 0.65 cm$^2$. Abbreviations: LV = left ventricle; LA = left atrium; RV = right ventricle; RA = right atrium.

where $A_1$ = cross-sectional area of the left ventricular outflow tract; $A_2$ = the cross-sectional area of the stenotic valve; $V_2$ = the mean velocity of blood flow distal to the obstruction; and $V_1$ = mean velocity of blood flow proximal to the obstruction. Thus, the continuity equation can be re-arranged:

$$A_2 = A_1 \times \frac{V_1}{V_2}$$

The two Doppler velocity measurements can be readily made with CW Doppler measuring the distal stenotic jet and pulsed-wave Doppler measuring the mean velocity proximal to the obstruction. $A_1$ is derived from the midsystolic diameter[10] of the left ventricular outflow tract directly underneath the aortic valve leaflets in the parasternal view. Thus, the final form of the continuity equations is:

$$A_2 = 0.875D^2 \frac{V_1}{V_2}$$

A simplified formula for predicting the severity of aortic stenosis can be accomplished by measuring the ratio of $V_1$ to $V_2$. Severe aortic stenosis can be reliably predicted if the ratio $V_1/V_2$ is less than 0.25.[18] This ratio is independent of cardiac output. A new fractional shortening/velocity ratio has recently been proposed as a simplified method of determining aortic valve area in patients with clinically significant aortic stenosis.[19] Maximal flow is determined in the usual manner by the continuous-wave Doppler spectral tracing and using the modified Bernoulli equation, $P = 4V^2$. Percent fractional shortening (%FS) is calculated as $EDD - \frac{ESD}{EDD}$ × 100, where EDD is the end-diastolic and ESD is the end-systolic dimension measured by M-mode echocardiography at the midpapillary muscle level.

FRACTIONAL SHORTENING VELOCITY EQUATION. (Aortic Area = $\frac{\%FS}{4V^2}$) minimally underestimates the severity of aortic stenosis. However, using an appropriate regression formula, the correlations with the Gorlin formula at cardiac catheterization were excellent.[19] The ratio was highly sensitive (90% to 96%) and has a positive accuracy of 90% to 92% in predicting significant aortic valvular stenosis.[19]

VALUE OF DOPPLER ECHOCARDIOGRAPHY IN PATIENTS UNDERGOING AORTIC BALLOON VALVULOPLASTY. Because percutaneous transluminal balloon valvuloplasty is being undertaken in many elderly patients, it is essential that precise hemodynamic parameters be monitored before and after valvuloplasty.[20-25] Although valve orifice dimensions and leaflet mobility increase in the majority of patients acutely, the long-term results have been disappointing.[22,23] A high secondary mortality rate of 29% to 38% occurs, which may be related to the severity of left ventricular impairment and to either insufficient valve dilation or subsequent restenosis (as well as coexistent morbid medical conditions).[22,23] Therefore in some centers the technique is offered as a palliative procedure so as to allow either general anesthesia for noncardiac surgery[26] or as a means of improving the patient's condition as a prelude for aortic valve replacement. The mechanisms of successful dilation include fracture of calcified nodules, separation of fused commissures, and grossly inapparent microfractures with increase in leaflet mobility.[21] Immediate hemodynamic assessment by Doppler-derived aortic valve area may be inaccurate because of transient left ventricular dysfunction and reduced cardiac output related to the procedure.[27] When Doppler-derived aortic valve area is performed more than 24 to 48 hours after balloon valvuloplasty, the correlation between Doppler-derived aortic valve area and cardiac catheterization-derived aortic area was excellent.[27] Doppler-derived aortic valve area appears to be an ideal technique for longer-term follow-up for detecting restenosis.

In severe aortic stenosis of the elderly, mild aortic regurgitation is not uncommon because the valves are heavily calcified and are associated with some deformity in leaflet closure. For the most part, aortic regurgitation is mild and does not affect the determination of the aortic valve area by the continuity equation.

### DIFFERENTIATION OF HYPERTROPHIC OBSTRUCTIVE CARDIOMYOPATHY IN THE ELDERLY FROM AORTIC STENOSIS

A substantial proportion of patients with hypertrophic cardiomyopathy (HCM) may be diagnosed only late in life. Although elderly patients with HCM may have similar signs and symptoms compared with younger patients, some differences are apparent. Elderly patients have predominately an ovoid cavity contour with normal septal curvature.[28] In contrast, in younger patients, a markedly abnormal cardiac shape with a crescent V-shaped left ventricular cavity and a reversed curvature of the interventricular system is present.

In addition, a major difference between HCM in the elderly compared with younger patients is that in the former, there is a much lower proportion with a family history of the disease and a higher incidence of mild hypertension.[28] From the clinical point of view, most of these patients have a harsh ejection-type systolic murmur, maximum at the left sternal border in the third intercostal space, radiating poorly up into the neck, but if there is associated aortic valve thickening, the murmur often will radiate up into the neck (see Table 7–1). The second sound is well preserved and the carotid pulses are bounding. A bisferious pulse is frequently palpated. Generally, using the Valsalva maneuver or the squatting position may allow differentiation from aortic stenosis. However, in the elderly, it is not always possible to obtain cooperation with regard to the performance of these maneuvers,[10] but two-dimensional echocardiography and Doppler usually will permit differentiation of HCM from aortic stenosis.

Patients with HCM have a significant degree of myocardial hypertrophy, with hyperkinetic hyperdynamic contraction frequently leading to cavity obliteration.[29] In those patients with HCM and outflow tract obstruction, the two-dimensional echocardiography Doppler features consist of asymmetric septal hypertrophy and systolic anterior motion of the anterior mitral leaflet, which frequently abuts against the septum (Fig. 7–5).[30] In addition, the Doppler flow velocity profile demonstrates a relatively high blood velocity early in systole, with further late systolic acceleration ("ski-slope appearance") reflecting the late systolic gradient (see Figure 7–5).[31] Variants of HCM include apical hypertrophy[32] and midventricular obstruction,[33] which may be found in the elderly. In older patients, there is a tendency toward less hypertrophy than in younger patients.[28]

Patients with genetically determined HCM should be differentiated from hypertensive HCM of the elderly.[34] In the latter syndrome, patients present with

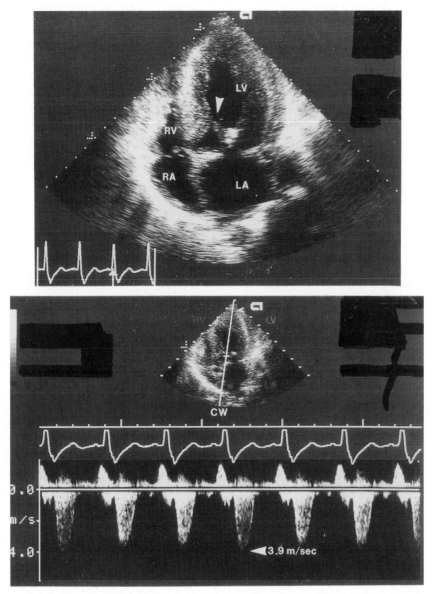

**Figure 7–5.** *Upper panel:* Apical 4-chambered view in an elderly patient with hypertrophic cardiomyopathy. Note the ovoid left ventricular (LV) cavity and the markedly thickened proximal interventricular septum. In addition, systolic anterior motion of the mitral valve is present *(arrow)* with focal thickening and/or calcification of the anterior mitral valve leaflet. *Lower panel:* Continuous wave (CW) Doppler of same patient with maximal gradient of 61 mmHg measured across the left ventricular outflow tract. In contrast to patients with calcific aortic stenosis the gradient peaks later in systole. Abbreviations: LA = left atrium; RA = right atrium; RV = right ventricle.

hypertension and/or symptoms of heart failure. Cardiac function is characterized by excessive left ventricular contraction, concentric hypertrophy (increased ejection fraction), and abnormal diastolic function but does not include features of outflow obstruction.[34]

## MITRAL REGURGITATION

The mitral apparatus consists of the left atrial wall, mitral annulus, mitral leaflets, chordae tendineae, papillary muscles, and left ventricular wall; and each of these components and the intimate interrelationship between these structures, may contribute to the development of mitral regurgitation.[35]

In the elderly, mitral regurgitation may result from organic valvular disease, cardiomyopathy, or ischemic heart disease. With the decline in the incidence of rheumatic heart disease, the most frequent cause of isolated mitral regurgitation in adults is leaflet prolapse. However, in the elderly, mitral annular calcification, a common degenerative condition, also is frequently associated with mitral regurgitation.[36]

Patients with severe chronic mitral regurgitation may present with atrial fibrillation and congestive heart failure. In patients with acute mitral regurgitation secondary to ruptured chordae tendineae or torn leaflet secondary to bacterial endocarditis, the presenting clinical feature is commonly acute pulmonary edema, especially in the presence of sinus rhythm.[39] In chronic severe mitral regurgitation, the left ventricular impulse is hyperdynamic and displaced at the apex. In addition, a holosystolic murmur is present at the apex and frequently radiates to the axilla. A third heart sound is frequently audible, often accompanied by a short mid-diastolic rumble. Left ventricular hypertrophy is commonly found by electrocardiogram (ECG), and x-ray shows an enlarged heart with an enlarged left atrium.

Structural abnormalities of the valve apparatus are easily recognized by two-dimensional echocardiography. Hence, two-dimensional echocardiography allows differentiation of organic valvular disease from a myopathic cause.[37]

### MITRAL ANNULAR CALCIFICATION OF THE ELDERLY

Calcific aortic stenosis and mitral annular calcification are chronic degenerative processes that often coexist.[38-41] In a recent echocardiographic study of 553 octogenarian patients, mitral annular calcification was found in 59% of the group.[42] Generally, women are more affected than men, with the relative incidence being about 4:1.[43]

Mitral annular calcification is regarded as a degenerative change and may be related to the pull of the left ventricular myocardium and aortic and mitral valves on their attachments to the cardiac skeleton. Pathologically, the gross appearance varies from small nodules to consummation of the entire mitral annulus into a rigid C-shape or J-shape structure measuring up to 2 cm in thickness. Calcification frequently can extend into the subvalvular region forming a prominent ridge of the posterior cusp that causes it to be stretched. Generally, mitral annular calcification is unrelated to rheumatic heart disease, rheumatoid disease, or any other form of cardiac inflammation but has been found to be associated with hypertension, aortic stenosis, HCM, coronary artery disease, mitral valve prolapse, Marfan's syndrome, Hurler's syndrome, mitral valve replacement, and chronic renal failure.[44] Metastatic calcification also can involve the annulus, and severe annular calcification occurs in patients with hypercalcemia, especially in renal failure patients.[45,46] Rarely, the mass may erode through the atrial surface and cause erosion of the leaflets producing thrombotic or infective endocarditis. On rare occasions, the annulus may show a central softening resembling a mycotic abscess. Pathologically, the annular calcification may be extensive enough to erode through the central portion of the conduction bundle producing conduction abnormalities and/or heart block.[47] Clinically patients with severe mitral annular calcification may present with heart block, embolic phenomenon including thromboembolic cerebral vascular events and mitral regurgitation, and on rare occasions with clinical and pathologic findings of mitral stenosis.[48] Several studies have reported an increased incidence of mitral regurgitation in patients with mitral annular calcification.[43,49] There are two possible reasons as to why mitral regurgitation may occur in these patients. First, the ability of the mitral annulus to reduce its circumference during systole is impaired. Second, the calcific mass frequently extends into the area between the posterior leaflet causing distortion and elevation of the posterior leaflet, thus making less mitral valvular tissue available for coaptation.[36] Although mitral regurgitation murmurs have been reported to occur in 33% to 100% of patients with annular calcification, clinically significant regurgitation is much less common.[47] It should be remembered that many patients have associated aortic valve sclerosis or stenosis with a high pitched musical murmur at the apex that is often mistaken for mitral regurgitation.[9] The importance of quantitating the severity of mitral annular calcification has been borne out recently in a study of 553 octogenarian patients who underwent Doppler echocardiography.[42] Mild mitral annular calcification was defined as an echodensity involving less than one-third of the posterior mitral annular circumference on the parasternal short axis view and usually associated with < 3 mm width of echodensity. Moderate MAC involved one-third to two-thirds of the posterior annular circumference (3 to 5 mm in width) and severe MAC with echodensity greater than two-thirds of the posterior annular circumference > 5 mm in width (Fig. 7–6).[49] Only patients with moderate and severe mitral annular calcification had significant mitral regurgitation.[42] A markedly increased incidence of atrial fibrillation in patients with mitral annular calcification has been reported;[49,56] many have enlarged left atria presumably on the basis of an increase in left atrial pressure. However, when comparing a group of patients older than the age of 80 with and without mitral annular calcification, the incidence of atrial fibrillation was found to be identical or higher in the group without the condition.[42] Other associated abnormalities, such as left ventricular hypertrophy, conduction abnormalities, and mitral regurgitation are more common only in the severe form of mitral annular calcification.[42] Therefore, in the majority of elderly patients with mild and moderate mitral annular calcification, its presence represents merely an aging process. Thus, only patients with severe mitral annular calcification have an increased incidence of associated cardiac abnormalities.

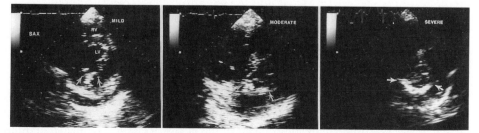

**Figure 7–6.** Parasternal short axis view of patients with mild, moderate, and severe mitral annular calcification. The arrows delineate the extent of mitral annular calcification. See text for explanation.

## MITRAL VALVE PROLAPSE

Elderly patients with mitral valve prolapse are more likely to present with a holosystolic murmur as opposed to an isolated click or late systolic murmur found in younger patients.[51] Elderly male patients usually predominate as compared with the younger population in whom females have the greatest incidence of mitral valve prolapse.

M-mode and two-dimensional echocardiography has revealed a variety of abnormalities in mitral valve prolapse. The quantitative echocardiographic assessment of the degree of prolapse, leaflet thickness, and leaflet and annular size has correlated with subsequent morbid events such as endocarditis, thromboembolism, sudden death, and the need for surgical valve repair or replacement.[52,53] Generally, the need for valve replacement occurs in elderly male patients. Sudden hemodynamic deterioration in patients with mitral valve prolapse frequently results from chordal rupture, a not uncommon presentation in the elderly. Ruptured chordae tendineae can be readily recognized by echocardiography.[54] Because two-dimensional echocardiography may overestimate mitral valve prolapse or mitral valve buckling into the left atrium, especially in the apical four-chambered view, some investigators insist that the clinical syndrome depends on the classic findings of a mid-to-late systolic click, late systolic murmur, holosystolic murmur, and/or a combination of findings.[55,56] In a recent study, a nonplanar saddle-shaped mitral annulus may produce an apparent bowing of the leaflets toward the atrial side of the annulus in the apical four-chamber view, thus leading to the apparent over-diagnosis of the disorder.[57] In these patients, the apical two-chamber or apical long-axis view and the parasternal long axis view reveal no evidence of bowing of the leaflets toward the atrial side of the annulus. Thus, most investigators insist that the diagnosis of mitral valve prolapse be limited to those patients with late systolic prolapse by M-mode or two-dimensional echocardiographic evidence of systolic arching or bowing of one or both of the valve leaflets superior to the mitral annulus into the left atrium seen in the parasternal long-axis view.[11,58] Shown in Figure 7–7 is a significant mitral valve prolapse obtained in the apical four-chambered view. In addition, exaggerated motion of the posterior mitral annulus has been reported.[58]

## ASSESSMENT OF MITRAL REGURGITATION BY DOPPLER ECHOCARDIOGRAPHY

The earlier time-consuming and laborious technique of pulsed-wave Doppler mapping of the regurgitant signal into the left atrium has largely been replaced by color flow mapping. With color flow Doppler, turbulence and aliasing associated with high-velocity flow produces a mosaic appearance.

Several studies have correlated the jet area[59] by color flow or the maximal jet area to left atrial area[60] in different tomographic views (Fig. 7–8).

In a correlative study of 47 patients undergoing cardiac catheterization and left ventriculography, Doppler color flow imaging jet areas were compared. Jet area was measured as the largest clearly definable flow disturbance in the parasternal and apical areas. Maximal jet area and mean of the largest jet area (average jet area) in two views and the ratio of both maximal jet area and mean jet area to left atrial area was determined. All patients with an average jet area $> 8$ cm$^2$ demonstrated severe mitral regurgitation. A maximal jet area $> 8$ cm$^2$ predicted severe mitral regurgitation with a sensitivity of 82% and a specificity of 94%. A maximal jet area $< 4$ cm$^2$ predicted mild mitral regurgitation with a sensitivity of 85% and a specificity of 75%. Of all the Doppler color flow measurements, maximal jet area ($r = 0.76$) correlated best with angiographic grades of mitral regurgitation. However, there was a limited correlation of jet area with regurgitant volume and fraction and no correlation with hemodynamic variables.[59]

When compared with angiography, using the ratio of maximal jet area to left atrial area, Helmcke and associates[60] demonstrated that a ratio of 0.2 corresponded to angiographic grade I (mild), a ratio between 0.2 and 0.4 corresponded to grade II (moderate), and a ratio of greater than 0.4 corresponded to grade III (severe regurgitation). However, jet area by color is affected by a variety of variables including hemodynamic factors such as loading conditions and technical factors. The latter include gain setting, transducer position and angulation, and direction of jets and hence the need to obtain multiple off-axis views. In addition to color flow mapping, some investigators have graded the severity of mitral regurgitation by the strength of the regurgitant signal relative to the anterograde signal on a continuous-wave Doppler spectral display as well as the relation between the mitral and aortic anterograde velocity time integrals.[61] Mitral regurgitation is frequently detected in up to 5% to 50% of normal subjects.[61] In a recently reported study in octogenarian patients, mitral regurgitation was detected by Doppler echocardiography in 60% of patients studied.[8]

## MITRAL STENOSIS

With the declining incidence of acute rheumatic fever, mitral stenosis is being encountered less frequently in the United States. However, occasional patients with rheumatic mitral stenosis present with clinical symptoms late in life. The majority of patients with rheumatic heart disease present with clinical manifestations usually in middle-aged life. In the elderly, calcification of the leaflets and commissures frequently occurs. In contrast, in younger patients commissural fusion occurs and the leaflets are thin and mobile. About one-third of elderly patients with rheumatic disease have mitral stenosis and two-thirds have predominant mitral regurgitation, with many patients having a mixed picture.[62] In the elderly, extensive mitral annular calcification in the presence of a small hypertrophied left ventricle has been shown to be a cause of nonrheumatic mitral valve stenosis.[48] These patients have demonstrated end-diastolic gradients across the mitral valve by cardiac catheterization. In the elderly, patients with rheumatic mitral stenosis may present with atrial fibrillation, congestive heart failure and/or pulmonary hypertension, or with thromboembolic complications. In many instances, so-called silent mitral stenosis may be present. Clues that suggest mitral stenosis include the presence of a loud first heart sound, signs of pulmonary hypertension, right-axis deviation in the presence of atrial fibrillation on ECG, and an enlarged left atrium on x-ray with straightening of the left heart border and enlarged pulmonary arteries. A mid-diastolic rumble may sometimes be audible especially in the left lateral decubitus position. The combination of ischemic heart disease and mitral stenosis in the elderly is particularly ominous.[63] These patients may present with severe, intractable pulmonary edema when they become ischemic.

The echocardiographic features of rheumatic mitral stenosis include reduced excursion of the anterior mitral valve leaflet at its tip, with doming of the body portion of the leaflet best visualized in the parasternal long-axis view.[64] The posterior leaflet is frequently restricted in its motion. Additional findings include thickening and/or calcification of the valvular and subvalvular apparatus.[11,65] The left atrium is usually enlarged, and the right ventricle and right atrium are frequently enlarged. Although left atrial thrombus may be detected in the left atrium by transthoracic echocardiography,[66] usually transesophageal echocardiography is required to demonstrate thrombus in the left atrial appendage.[67]

The mitral orifice area can be planimetered by direct measurement of the orifice as obtained in the parasternal short-axis views. Careful attention to obtaining optimal views of the smallest orifice by scanning superiorly or inferiorly is required. Suboptimal images, dense calcification, or predominant subvalvular obstruction may limit two-dimensional echocardiography as a reliable means of estimating the severity of mitral stenosis.[68] Recently, a scoring system that is based on valve mobility, valve thickness, valve calcification, and subvalvular thickness (grades I through IV) has been introduced to assess suitability of the valve for valvuloplasty.[69,70] Generally, a score of 8 or less has a favorable chance of a satisfactory result. In most instances, valvuloplasty is generally not as satisfactory in the elderly as in the young because most elderly patients with mitral stenosis have severe calcification of the valve, decreased mobility, and subvalvular fibrosis. Percutaneous transluminal mitral commissurotomy is most successful in patients with pliable leaflets and least successful in patients with thickened and calcified valves.[71] Doppler echocardiography provides hemodynamic assessment of the severity of obstruction to mitral inflow. Continuous-wave Doppler exhibits an increased diastolic flow velocity with a reduced diastolic velocity decay slope (Fig. 7–9).[72,73] Using color flow Doppler, correct alignment of the continuous-wave cursor to obtain the maximal velocity of the jet is helpful especially in abnormally directed jets.[74] The transvalvular mitral pressure gradient (both maximal and mean) measured by Doppler echocardiography has been correlated with pressure gradients obtained by cardiac catheterization.[72,75]

The pressure half-time method is useful in calculating the mitral valve area.[76] The pressure half-time is the time required for the initial diastolic gradient to decline by 50%. The pressure half-time is obtained from the Doppler velocity profile by dividing peak velocity by the $\frac{\sqrt{2}}{2}$ (0.72) and then measuring the time from peak velocity to the time velocity has decreased to 72% of peak. The more prolonged the half-time the more severe the reduction in orifice area (see Fig. 7–9).[76] Generally, mitral valve area equals 220 divided by pressure half-time.

In most instances, the mitral valve area determined by the pressure half-time correlates well with the mitral valve area obtained by the Gorlin formula at catheterization.[76,77] The pressure half-time is independent of heart rate and the presence of mitral regurgitation.[78]

The mitral valve area by the pressure half-time method may be unreliable in patients with combined aortic regurgitation and mitral stenosis. The aortic regurgitant blood may interfere with the calculation of the valve area from the pressure gradient half-time.[79] In addition, in patients undergoing balloon mitral valvuloplasty the immediate calculation of mitral valve area by the pressure half-time method may be inaccurate because of the acute changes in left atrial compliance associated with the procedure.[80]

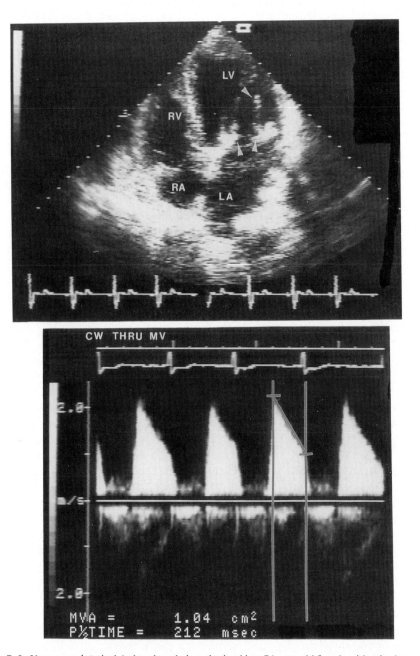

**Figure 7–9.** *Upper panel:* Apical 4-chambered view obtained in a 74-year-old female with mitral stenosis. Both anterior and posterior mitral leaflets are heavily calcified and restricted *(two small arrows)*. In addition, there is subvalvular thickening and/or calcification *(solitary arrow)*. *Lower panel:* Continuous wave (CW) Doppler mitral valve inflow velocity profile. There is increased early diastolic flow velocity as well as a reduced diastolic velocity decay slope. The pressure half-time (p ½) measures 212 msec and the mitral valve area (MVA) is calculated to be 1.04 cm². Abbreviations: LV = left ventricle; LA = left atrium; RV = right ventricle; RA = right atrium.

## AORTIC REGURGITATION

Severe aortic regurgitation is a relatively uncommon finding in the elderly. Although valvular etiologies such as myxomatous degeneration, rheumatic heart disease, and rheumatoid arthritis[81] may cause clinically significant aortic regurgitation, aortic root dilation is a more frequent cause of aortic regurgitation in the elderly. Multiple etiologies of aortic root dilation include syphilitic aortitis, connective disorders (ankylosing spondylitis, rheumatoid arthritis, or giant cell arteritis),[81] idiopathic dilation of the ascending aorta, age-related progressive dilation of the thoracic aorta, and systemic hypertension. In the elderly, approximately 10% of patients with systemic hypertension may have evidence of mild aortic regurgitation,[83] but seldom do these patients require aortic valve replacement for severe aortic regurgitation.[84] In patients with significant aortic regurgitation, idiopathic dilation was the predominant indication for surgical replacement of the aortic valve at the Mayo Clinic.[82] In many instances, cystic medial necrosis is present without any of the other typical features of Marfan's syndrome. Hemodynamic stresses in the elderly including hypertension may contribute to the progressive aortic root dilation. In patients with aortic dissection, either acute or chronic,[48] aortic regurgitation may develop and in some instances is significant.[85]

Although degenerative calcific aortic stenosis is usually associated with mild aortic regurgitation, significant aortic regurgitation is distinctly unusual.[86]

Most elderly patients present with chronic aortic regurgitation, but occasionally acute aortic regurgitation may be encountered in patients with aortic dissection or a ruptured aortic cusp secondary to bacterial endocarditis. Most patients with chronic aortic regurgitation remain asymptomatic for many years. Awareness of pulsation in the neck or in the precordium, palpitation, pounding head, and fatigue may precede symptoms of left ventricular dysfunction or myocardial ischemia. Nocturnal angina associated with hot flashes, sweating, and palpitation may occur in some patients. Physical examination reveals a wide pulse pressure and a collapsing or Corrigan pulse. The cardiac impulse is often displaced laterally and may be sustained. A pulsation in the right parasternal area is often palpated in patients with aortic root dilation.

A high-pitched diastolic decrescendo murmur is usually present in the second right intercostal space with radiation down the right sternum (aortic root disorders) or down the left sternal border (valvular causes of aortic regurgitation). The duration rather than the intensity of the murmur reflects the severity of the aortic regurgitation.[87] Usually a crescendo-decrescendo systolic murmur is audible in the second right or left intercostal space reflecting an increased stroke volume as a result of the aortic regurgitant increase in left ventricular end-diastolic volume. In severe aortic regurgitation, a third heart sound and an apical mid-diastolic or presystolic murmur (Austin Flint murmur) are audible. The ECG frequently shows signs of left ventricular hypertrophy, and significant cardiomegaly and dilation of the ascending aorta are present on x-ray.

Patients presenting with acute regurgitation may not display the typical findings encountered in chronic regurgitation. These patients frequently present with rapidly progressive signs and symptoms of left ventricular dysfunction in the absence of severe cardiomegaly and wide pulse pressure. Frequently, the diastolic murmur is shorter as a result of rapid equilibration of aortic and left ventricular end-diastolic pressure.[88]

## ECHOCARDIOGRAPHY-DOPPLER FINDINGS IN AORTIC REGURGITATION

The characteristic M-mode and two-dimensional echocardiographic findings are diastolic fluttering of the anterior leaflet of the mitral valve and/or interventricular system and left ventricular volume overload.[89,90] In acute severe aortic regurgitation, premature closure of the mitral valve can be detected by M-mode echocardiography.[88] In these patients, left ventricular cavity size is normal and function is often hyperdynamic. Two-dimensional echocardiography is useful in assessing the etiology of aortic regurgitation, especially in differentiating root causes from valvular causes.[91] However, M-mode and two-dimensional echocardiography are not useful for assessing the severity of aortic regurgitation.

Doppler echocardiography is especially useful in detecting the presence of aortic regurgitation and in the semiquantitative assessment of its severity. Diastolic reversal of flow occurs in the left ventricular outflow tract, and both pulsed and continuous-wave Doppler as well as color flow Doppler are extremely sensitive in detecting the presence of aortic regurgitation.

Originally, pulsed-wave mapping of the extent of the regurgitant jet in multiple planes including its height, width, and length were employed to estimate the severity of aortic regurgitation.[11] Some investigators have used the depth of the signal in the left ventricle as an index of severity of aortic regurgitation.[92]

Other investigators have examined the reversal of thoracic aortic flow by pulsed-wave Doppler.[93] If the area of reversal of thoracic aortic flow profile was > 30% of the forward flow profile, moderate to severe aortic regurgitation could be differentiated from mild regurgitation.[93] Continuous-wave Doppler allows measurements of the regurgitant velocity profile. The rate of pressure decline as measured by the deceleration slope correlates with the severity of aortic regurgitation.[94,95] Generally, a diastolic velocity decay slope of greater than 3 m/sec$^2$ suggests severe aortic regurgitation (Fig. 7–10). Other investigators have used pressure half-time measurements of the regurgitant velocity profile.[96] A pressure half-time of < 350 msec generally is associated with severe regurgitation.[96] In severe and especially in acute aortic regurgitation, there is a rapid fall in aortic regurgitant velocity by CW Doppler. This occurs as a result of a rapid decrease in the pressure gradient between the aorta and the left ventricle. As the aortic diastolic pressure decreases rapidly, there is a rapid rise in left ventricular end-diastolic pressure. In addition, the velocity profile allows determination of left ventricular end-diastolic pressure.

Color flow Doppler is probably the most useful and practical Doppler technique to assess the severity of aortic regurgitation. The width of the aortic regurgitant jet divided by the left ventricular outflow tract width in the parasternal long-axis view allows semiquantitation of the severity of aortic regurgitation.[97] A ratio of less than 0.25 (grade I) is considered minimal, 0.25 to 0.46 (grade II) is mild, 0.47 to 0.64 (grade III) is moderate, and 0.65 or greater (grade IV) is considered significant (Fig. 7–11).[97]

The limitations of color flow Doppler semiquantitation of severity of aortic regurgitation are similar to those of mitral regurgitation. Doppler echocardiography is extremely sensitive in detecting aortic regurgitation. In one study in an elderly population, aortic regurgitation was detected in 50% of patients.[8] In another study of elderly patients older than the age of 80, an 89% incidence of aortic regurgitation was detected.[98]

## TRICUSPID REGURGITATION

Tricuspid disease is extremely unusual in elderly patients but occasionally two-dimensional echocardiography may be useful in the diagnosis of tricuspid endocarditis. Tricuspid regurgitation may be encountered in elderly patients[8] especially in patients with heart failure due to a variety of causes. In many instances, the holosystolic murmur at the left sternal border increasing with inspiration may be absent although, if carefully looked for, peripheral signs of tricuspid regurgitation, such as a pulsatile liver or large jugular V waves, are invariably present. Severe tricuspid regurgitation can be recognized by a systolic signal in the right atrium by pulsed-wave or continuous-wave Doppler or by color flow Doppler (Fig. 7–12).[11] In addition, reversal of blood flow into the hepatic veins during systole can be detected by Doppler sampling of the hepatic venous flow.[99] Noninvasive measurement of the pressure in the right side of the heart can be determined by the tricuspid regurgitant signal. The velocity of the tricuspid regurgitant signal accurately reflects the pressure between the right ventricle and right atrium during systole as calculated by the Bernoulli equation $\triangle P = 4V^2$.[100,101] The right atrial pressure can be clinically estimated (by evaluating the jugular venous pulse) or by using an arbitrary value of 14 mmHg. Therefore, the sum of the right atrial pressure and the right ventricular right atrial pressure gradient equals the right ventricular systolic pressure (see Fig. 7–12). In the absence of pulmonic stenosis, the right ventricular systolic pressure is equal to the systolic pulmonary artery pressure.

In one reported series tricuspid regurgitation was detected by echo Doppler in 24% of octogenarian patients studied.[8]

## PULMONARY REGURGITATION

Pulmonary regurgitation is not infrequently detected in normal subjects as well as in those patients with pulmonary hypertension. Pulmonary regurgitation is detected by pulsed-wave Doppler in the region immediately below the valve. Usually color flow Doppler allows detection of a regurgitant jet below the pulmonic valve, best appreciated in the parasternal short-axis view.[11] The extent and width of the jet is directly proportional to the severity of pulmonary regurgitation.[11] A wide regurgitant jet extending deep into the right ventricle in association with right ventricular enlargement suggests severe pulmonary hypertension. In many instances, a diastolic blowing murmur is often inconspicuous or may not be detected. Multivalvular regurgitation of all four valves in elderly patients is not an uncommon finding (Fig. 7–13).[8]

## CONCLUSIONS

In the elderly, valvular heart disease is the next most common cause of congestive heart failure after ischemic and/or hypertensive heart disease. Frequently, signs and symptoms are masked by the inability of elderly patients to cooperate because of their bed ridden status or because of the presence of associated medical conditions (e.g., hypertension). In some instances, critical aortic valve stenosis may be present without the patients being aware of any symptoms. Although clinical evaluation is extremely important in assessing the valvular lesions, Doppler echocardiography has become a powerful tool in assessing the nature, severity, and hemodynamic consequences of valvular disorders.

Valvular disease in the elderly may represent a physical adaptation to aging, whereas in others significant valvular disease represents true pathology. Nevertheless, the implications of valvular heart disease in the elderly are significant with regard to bacterial endocarditis prophylaxis, potential valvuloplasty, or consideration for valvular surgery.

## REFERENCES

1. Pomerance, A: Pathology of the heart without cardiac failure in the aged. Br Heart J 27:697, 1965.
2. Pomerance, A: Cardiac pathology in the elderly. In Brest, AN (ed): Geriatric Cardiology. Philadelphia, FA Davis, 1981, pp 9–54.
3. Davies, MJ, Moore, BP, Brainbridge, MV: The floppy mitral valve: Study of incidence, pathology and complications in surgical, necropsy and forensic material. Br Heart J 40:468, 1978.
4. Both, DC and DeMaria, AM: Valvular heart disease in the elderly. In Messerli, FH (ed): Cardiac Disease in the Elderly. Martinus Nijhoff, Boston, 1981, p 127.
5. Pomerance, A: Aging changes in human heart valves. Br Heart J 29:222, 1967.
6. Bloor, CM: Valvular heart disease in the elderly. In Coodley, EL (ed): Geriatric Heart Disease. Littleton, MA, PSG Publishing 1985, pp 295–303.
7. Passik, CS, Ackermann, DM, Pluth, JR, et al: Temporal changes in the cause of aortic stenosis: A surgical pathologic study of 646 cases. Mayo Clin Proc 62:119, 1987.
8. Zavitsanos, JP, Goldman, AP, Kotler, MN, et al: The Echo Doppler spectrum of valvular abnormalities in the hospitalized octogenarian. Clin Cardiol 11:683, 1988.
9. Henke, RP, March HW, Hultgren, HN: An aid to identification of the murmur of aortic stenosis with atypical localization. Am Heart J 60:354, 1960.
10. Kotler, MN, Mintz, GS, Parry, WR, et al: Bedside diagnosis of organic murmurs in the elderly. Geriatrics 36:107, 1981.
11. Olson, LJ and Tajik, AJ: Echocardiographic evolution of valvular heart disease. In Marcus, ML, Schelbert, HR, Skorton, DJ, et al (eds): Cardiac Imaging. Philadelphia, WB Saunders, 1991, pp 419–448.
12. Isner, JM, Losordo, DW, Rosenfield, K, et al: Catheter-based intravascular ultrasound discriminates bicuspid from tricuspid valves in adults with calcific aortic stenosis. J Am Coll Cardiol 15:1310, 1990.
13. Kennedy, KD, Hauck, AJ, Edwards, WD, et al: Mechanism of reduction of aortic valvular stenosis by percutaneous transluminal balloon valvuloplasty; report of 5 cases and review of literature. Mayo Clin Proc 63:769, 1988.
14. Currie, PJ, Seward, JB, Reeder, GS, et al: Continuous-wave Doppler echocardiographic assessment of severity of calcific aortic stenosis; a simultaneous Doppler-catheter correlative study in 100 adult patients. Circulation 71:1162, 1985.
15. Fan, PH, Kapur, KK, Nanda, NC: Color-guided Doppler echocardiographic assessment of aortic valve stenosis. J Am Coll Cardiol 12:441, 1988.
16. Hegrames, L and Hatle, L: Aortic stenosis in adults; non-invasive estimation of pressure differences by continuous-wave Doppler echocardiography. Br Heart J 54:396, 1985.
17. Hatle, L, Angelsen, BA, Tromsdal, A: Non-invasive assessment of aortic stenosis by Doppler ultrasound. Br Heart J 43:284, 1980.
18. Oh, JK, Taliercio, CP, Holmes, DR Jr, et al: Prediction of the severity of aortic stenosis by Doppler aortic valve area determination: prospective Doppler-catheterization correlation in 100 patients. J Am Coll Cardiol 11:1227, 1988.
19. Mann, DL, Usher, BW, Hammerman, S, et al: The fractional shortening-velocity ratio: Validation of a new echocardiographic Doppler method for identifying patients with significant aortic stenosis. J Am Coll Cardiol 15:1578, 1990.
20. Cribier, A, Savin, T, Berland, J, et al: Percutaneous transluminal balloon valvuloplasty of adult aortic stenosis: Report of 92 cases. J Am Coll Cardiol 9:381, 1987.
21. Safian, RD, Mandell, VS, Thurer, RE, et al: Postmortem and intraoperative balloon valvuloplasty of calcific aortic stenosis in elderly patients: Mechanisms of successful dilation. J Am Coll Cardiol 9:655, 1987.
22. Letac, B, Cribier, A, Konig, R, et al: Aortic stenosis in elderly patients 80 or older: Treatment by percutaneous balloon valvuloplasty in a series of 92 cases. Circulation 80:1514, 1989.

23. Lewin, RF, Dorros, G, King, JF, et al: Percutaneous transluminal aortic valvuloplasty: Acute outcome and follow-up of 125 patients. J Am Coll Cardiol 14:1210, 1989.

24. Stoddard, MF, Vandormael, MG, and Pearson, AC: Immediate and short-term effects of aortic balloon valvuloplasty on left ventricular diastolic function and filling in humans. J Am Coll Cardiol 14:1218, 1989.

25. Berland, J, Cribier, A, Savin, T, et al: Percutaneous balloon valvuloplasty in patients with severe aortic stenosis and low ejection fraction: Immediate results and 1-year follow-up. Circulation 79:1189, 1989.

26. Hayes, SM, Holmes, DR Jr, Nishimura, RA: Palliative percutaneous aortic balloon valvuloplasty before non-cardiac operations and invasive diagnostic procedures. Mayo Clin Proc 64:753, 1989.

27. Nishimura, RA, Holmes, DR Jr, Reeder, GS, et al: Doppler evaluation of results of percutaneous aortic balloon valvuloplasty in calcific aortic stenosis. Circulation 78:791, 1988.

28. Lever, HM, Karam, RF, Currie, PJ, et al: Hypertrophic cardiomyopathy in the elderly; distinctions from the young based on cardiac shape. Circulation 79:580, 1989.

29. Shapiro, LM and McKenna, WJ: Distribution of left ventricular hypertrophy in hypertrophic cardiomyopathy: A two-dimensional echocardiographic study. J Am Coll Cardiol 2:437, 1983.

30. Pollick, C, Rakowski, H, Wigle, ED: Muscular subaortic stenosis: The quantitative relationship between systolic anterior motion and the pressure gradient. Circulation 69:43, 1984.

31. Sasson, Z, Yock, PG, Hatle, LK, et al: Doppler echocardiographic determination of the pressure gradient in hypertrophic cardiomyopathy. J Am Coll Cardiol 11:752, 1988.

32. Louie, EK and Mason, BJ: Apical hypertrophic cardiomyopathy; clinical and two-dimensional echocardiographic assessment. Ann Intern Med 106:663, 1987.

33. Maze, S, Kotler, MN, Parry, WR: Dynamic intracavitary left ventricular obstruction. American Journal of Noninvasive Cardiology 4:76, 1990.

34. Topol, EJ, Traill, TA, Fortuin, NJ: Hypertensive hypertrophic cardiomyopathy of the elderly. N Engl J Med 312:277, 1985.

35. Roberts, WC and Perloff, JK: Mitral valvular disease; a clinicopathologic survey of the conditions causing the mitral valve to function abnormally. Ann Intern Med 77:939, 1972.

36. Nestico, PF, Depace, NL, Morganroth, J, et al: Mitral annular calcification: Clinical, pathophysiology, and echocardiographic review. Am Heart J 107:989, 1984.

37. Mintz, GS, Kotler, MN, Segal, BL, et al: Two-dimensional echocardiographic evaluation of patients with mitral insufficiency. Am J Cardiol 44:670, 1979.

38. Roberts, WC, Braunwald, E, Morrow, AG: Acute severe mitral regurgitation secondary to ruptured chordae tendineae; clinical, hemodynamic, and pathological considerations. Circulation 33:58, 1966.

39. Nair, CK, Sketch, MH, Ahmed, J, et al: Calcific valvular aortic stenosis with and without mitral annular calcium. Am J Cardiol 60:865, 1987.

40. Roberts, WC, Perloff, JK, Constantino, T: Severe valvular aortic stenosis in patients over 65 years of age. Am J Cardiol 27:497, 1971.

41. Nair, CK, Aronow, WS, Stokke, K, et al: Cardiac conduction defects in patients older than 60 years with aortic stenosis with and without mitral anular calcium. Am J Cardiol 53:169, 1986.

42. Kochar, G, Jacobs, LE, Blondheim, DS, et al: Quantifications of mitral annular calcification in octogenarian patients: Innocent bystander or marker of pathology. Echocardiography 8:329, 1991.

43. Korn, D, DeSanctis, RW, Sell, S: Massive calcification of the mitral annulus; a clinicopathological study of 14 cases. N Engl J Med 267:900, 1962.

44. Kotler, MN, Goldman, AP, Parry, WR: Managing the most common nonischemic disorders. Geriatrics 41:45, 1986.

45. Schott, GR, Kotler, MN, Parry, WR, et al: Mitral annular calcification. Arch Intern Med 137:1143, 1977.

46. Nestico, PF, Depace, NL, Kotler, MN, et al: Calcium-phosphorous metabolism in dialysis patients with and without mitral annular calcification. Am J Cardiol 51:497, 1983.

47. Fulkerson, PK, Beaver, BM, Aveson, JC, et al: Calcification of the mitral anulus; etiology, clinical associations, complications and therapy. Am J Med 66:967, 1979.

48. Hammer, WJ, Roberts, WC, deLeon, AC Jr: Mitral stenosis secondary to combined massive mitral annular calcific deposits and small hypertrophic ventricles. Am J Med 64:371, 1978.

49. Nair, CK, Thomson, W, Ryschon, K, et al: Long-term follow-up of patients with echocardiograph-

ically detected mitral anular calcium and comparison with age- and sex-matched control subjects. Am J Cardiol 63:465, 1989.

50. Savage, DD, Garrison, RJ, Castelli, WP, et al: Prevalence of submitral (annular) calcium and its correlates in general population-based sample: The Framingham Study. Am J Cardiol 51:1385, 1983.

51. Tresch, DD, Siegel, R, Meelom, MH, et al: Mitral valve prolapse in the elderly. J Am Geriatr Soc 27:421, 1979.

52. Nishimura, RA, McGoon, MD, Shub, C, et al: Echocardiographically documented mitral-valve prolapse: Long-term follow-up of 237 patients. N Engl J Med 313:1305, 1985.

53. Marks, AR, Choong, CY, Sanfilippo, AJ, et al: Identification of high-risk and low-risk subgroups of patients with mitral-valve prolapse. N Engl J Med 320:1031, 1989.

54. Mintz, GS, Kotler, MN, Segal, BL, et al: Two-dimensional echocardiographic recognition of ruptured chordae tendineae. Circulation 57:244, 1978.

55. Perloff, JK and Child, JS: Clinical and epidemiologic issues in mitral valve prolapse: Overview and perspective. Am Heart J 113:1324, 1987.

56. Devereux, RB: Diagnosis and prognosis of mitral-valve prolapse. N Engl J Med 320:1077, 1989.

57. Levine, RA, Triulzo, MO, Harrigan, P, et al: The relationship of mitral annular shape to the diagnosis of mitral-valve prolapse. Circulation 75:756, 1987.

58. Gilbert, BW, Schotz, RA, Von Ramm, OT, et al: Mitral valve prolapse: Two-dimensional echocardiographic and angiographic correlation. Circulation 54:716, 1976.

59. Spain, MG, Smith, MD, Graybarn, PA, et al: Quantitative assessment of mitral regurgitation by Doppler color-flow imaging; angiographic and hemodynamic correlations. J Am Coll Cardiol 13:585, 1989.

60. Helmcke, F, Nanda, NC, Hsuing, MC, et al: Color Doppler assessment of mitral regurgitation with orthogonal planes. Circulation 75:175, 1987.

61. Popp, RL: Echocardiography. N Engl J Med 323:101, 1990.

62. Hargreaves, T: Rheumatic mitral valve disease in the elderly: incidence found at necropsy. Br Med J 2:342, 1961.

63. Herling, IM, Kotler, MN, Segal, BL, et al: Combined mitral stenosis and coronary artery disease: A clinical syndrome characterized by paroxysmal pulmonary edema with rapid resolution. Am J Cardiol 54:680, 1984.

64. Kotler, MN, Mintz, GS, Segal, BL, et al: Clinical uses of two-dimensional echocardiography. Am J Cardiol 45:1061, 1980.

65. Zanolla, L, Marino, P, Nicolosi, GL, et al: Two-dimensional echocardiographic evaluation of mitral valve calcification; sensitivity and specificity. Chest 82:154, 1982.

66. Depace, N, Kotler, MN, Soulen, R, et al: Two-dimensional echocardiographic detection of intraatrial masses. Am J Cardiol 48:954, 1981.

67. Seward, JB, Khandheira, BK, Oh, JK, et al: Transesophageal echocardiography: Technique, anatomic correlations, implementation, and clinical applications. Mayo Clin Proc 63:649, 1988.

68. Smith, MD, Handshoe, R, Handshoe, S, et al: Comparative accuracy of two-dimensional echocardiography and Doppler pressure half-time methods in assessing severity of mitral stenosis in patients with and without prior commissurotomy. Circulation 73:100, 1986.

69. Wilkins, GT, Weyman, AE, Abascal, VM, et al: Percutaneous balloon dilation of the mitral valve; an analysis of echocardiographic variables related to outcome and mechanism of dilation. Br Heart J 60:299, 1988.

70. Chen, C, Wang, X, Wang, Y, et al: Value of two-dimensional echocardiography in selecting patients and balloon sizes for percutaneous balloon mitral valvuloplasty. J Am Coll Cardiol 14:1651, 1989.

71. Nobuyoshi, M, Hamasaki, N, Kimura, T, et al: Indications, complications and short-term clinical outcome of percutaneous transvenous mitral commissurotomy. Circulation 80:782, 1989.

72. Hatle, L, Brubakk, A, Tromsdal, A, et al: Non-invasive assessment of pressure drop in mitral stenosis by Doppler ultrasound. Br Heart J 40:131, 1978.

73. Holen, J and Simonsen, S: Determination of pressure gradient in mitral stenosis with Doppler echocardiography. Br Heart J 41:529, 1979.

74. Khandheira, BK, Tajik, AJ, Reeder, GS, et al: Doppler color flow imaging: A new technique for visualization and characterization of the blood flow jet in mitral stenosis. Mayo Clin Proc 61:623, 1986.

75. Stamm, RB and Martin RP: Quantification of pressure gradients across stenotic valves by Doppler ultrasound. J Am Coll Cardiol 2:707, 1983.

76. Hatle, L, Angelsen, B, Tromsdal, A: Non-invasive assessment of atrio ventricular pressure half-time by Doppler ultrasound. Circulation 60:1096, 1979.
77. Holen, J, Aaslid, R, Landmark, K, et al: Determination of effective orifice area in mitral stenosis from non-invasive ultrasound Doppler data and mitral flow rate. Acta Med Scand 201:83, 1977.
78. Bryg, RJ, Williams, GA, Labovitz, J, et al: Effect of atrial fibrillation and mitral regurgitation on calculated mitral valve area in mitral stenosis. Am J Cardiol 57:634, 1986.
79. Nakatani, S, Masuyama, T, Kodama, K, et al: Value and limitations of stenotic mitral valve area: Comparison of the pressure half-time and the continuity equation methods. Circulation 77:78, 1988.
80. Thomas, JD, Wilkins, GT, Choong, CY, et al: Inaccuracy of mitral pressure half-time immediately after percutaneous mitral valvotomy: Dependence on transmitral gradient and left atrial and ventricular compliance. Circulation 78:980, 1988.
81. Brandenburg, RO, Fuster, V, Giuliani, ER: Valvular heart disease: When should the patient be referred? Pract Cardiol 5:50, 1979.
82. Olson, LJ, Subramanian, R, Edwards, WD: Surgical pathology of pure aortic insufficiency. A study of 225 cases. Mayo Clin Proc 59:835, 1984.
83. Barlow, J and Kincaid-Smith, P: The auscultatory findings in hypertension. Br Heart J 22:505, 1960.
84. Waller, BF, Zoltick, JM, Rosen, JH, et al: Severe aortic regurgitation from systemic hypertension (without aortic dissection) requiring aortic valve replacement. Analysis of four patients. Am J Cardiol 49:473, 1982.
85. Hirst, AE Jr, Johns VJ Jr, Kime, SW Jr: Dissecting aneurysm of the aorta: A review of 505 cases. Medicine 37:217, 1958.
86. Nylander, E, Ekman, I, Marklund, T, et al: Severe aortic stenosis in elderly patients. Br Heart J 55:480, 1986.
87. Reichek, N, Shelburne, JC, Perloff, JK: Clinical aspects of rheumatic valvular disease. Prog Cardiovasc Dis 15:491, 1973.
88. Morganroth, J, Perloff, JK, Zeldis, SM: Acute severe aortic regurgitation: Pathophysiology, clinical recognition, and management. Ann Intern Med 87:223, 1977.
89. Johnson, AD and Gosink, BB: Oscillation of left ventricular structures in aortic regurgitation. Journal of Clinical Ultrasound 5:21, 1977.
90. McDonald, IG: Echocardiographic assessment of left ventricular function in aortic valve disease. Circulation 53:860, 1976.
91. DePace, NL, Nestico, PF, Kotler, MN, et al: Comparison of echocardiography and angiography in determining the cause of severe aortic regurgitation. Br Heart J 51:36, 1987.
92. Ciobanu, M, Abbasi, AS, Allen, M, et al: Pulsed Doppler echocardiography in the diagnosis and estimation of severity of aortic insufficiency. Am J Cardiol 49:339, 1982.
93. Quinnones, MA, Young, JB, Waggoner, AD, et al: Assessment of pulsed Doppler echocardiography in detection and quantification of aortic and mitral regurgitation. Br Heart J 44:612, 1980.
94. Grayburn, PA, Handshoe, R, Smith, MD, et al: Quantitative assessment of the hemodynamic consequences of aortic regurgitation by means of continuous wave Doppler recordings. J Am Coll Cardiol 10:135, 1987.
95. Labovitz, AJ, Ferrara, RP, Kern, MJ, et al: Quantitative evaluation of aortic insufficiency by continuous wave Doppler echocardiography. J Am Coll Cardiol 8:1341, 1986.
96. Teague, SM, Heinsimer, JA, Anderson, JL, et al: Quantification of aortic regurgitation utilizing continuous wave Doppler ultrasound. J Am Coll Cardiol 8:592, 1986.
97. Perry, GJ, Helmcke, F, Nanda, NC, et al: Evaluation of aortic insufficiency by Doppler color flow mapping. J Am Coll Cardiol 9:952, 1987.
98. Akasaka, T, Yoshikawa, J, Joshida, K, et al: Age-related valvular regurgitation. A study by pulsed Doppler echocardiography. Circulation 76:262, 1967.
99. Pennestri, F, Loperfido, F, Salvatori, MP, et al: Assessment of tricuspid regurgitation by pulsed Doppler ultrasonography of the hepatic veins. Am J Cardiol 54:363, 1986.
100. Currie, PJ, Seward, JB, Chan, KL, et al: Continuous wave Doppler determination of right ventricular pressure. A simultaneous Doppler-catheterization study in 127 patients. J Am Coll Cardiol 6:750, 1985.
101. Yock, PG and Popp, RL: Noninvasive estimation of right ventricular systolic pressure by Doppler ultrasound in patients with tricuspid regurgitation. Circulation 70:657, 1984.

# CHAPTER 8

# Pericardial Disease in the Elderly

*Nanette K. Wenger, M.D.*

Pericardial disease in elderly patients differs little from that encountered in their younger counterparts, save that the etiologic forms reflect the prevalence of systemic diseases in an elderly population. Pericardial disease may present as pericarditis; this may be accompanied by pericardial effusion, which may progress to cardiac tamponade; and constrictive pericarditis may result.

## ACUTE PERICARDITIS

### CLINICAL PRESENTATION

Acute pericarditis is typically manifest as a chest pain syndrome, and one that must be differentiated from acute myocardial infarction, which is a very frequent clinical problem in the elderly. The pain of acute pericarditis is described as sharp, often substernal but may radiate to the back and to the scapulae, frequently accentuated by respiration and swallowing, and can be ameliorated by sitting up and leaning forward.

A pericardial friction rub is often audible, with a three-component rub (atrial systole, ventricular systole, and ventricular diastole) being classic, although at times only a ventricular systolic component can be heard. The pericardial friction rub is best detected between the lower left sternal border and the cardiac apex.

It is important to differentiate the electrocardiographic abnormalities of acute pericarditis from those of acute myocardial infarction (Table 8–1).[1]

### ETIOLOGY

Pericarditis may be infective, with a frequent etiologic agent being the coxsackievirus; often a history of prior respiratory infection is obtained. Although a virus is rarely isolated, the diagnosis can be made retrospectively by demonstration of elevated serum viral titers. However, viral pericarditis is less common than in a younger population. Tuberculous pericarditis must be considered in elderly residents in nursing homes, where the transmission of tuberculosis is frequent. Purulent pericarditis may occur in association with systemic staphylococcal or pneu-

**Table 8-1.** Comparison of ECG Abnormalities Encountered
in Acute Pericarditis and Acute MI

| ECG Abnormalities | Acute Pericarditis | Acute MI |
|---|---|---|
| ST abnormalities | Diffuse | Localized |
| Elevated ST-segment configuration | Concave upward | Concave downward (convex) |
| Reciprocal ST-segment changes | Absent, except in leads aVR and V1 | Present |
| PR-segment displacement | PR depression, except in leads aVR and V1 (where the PR segment is elevated) | PR generally isoelectric in the absence of atrial infarction |
| ST-T serial changes | Initial abnormal ST phase and subsequent abnormal T phase | Concomitant ST-T abnormalities |
| Q waves | Absent | Present (with Q-wave MI) |
| QT prolongation | Absent | Present |
| Electrical alternans | Present with cardiac tamponade | Absent |

ECG = electrocardiogram; MI = myocardial infarction

mococcal infection, particularly pneumonia; and pericarditis may be caused by virtually any organism causing systemic sepsis or transmitted from a contiguous organ system, for example, the lung.

Pericarditis often occurs in association with acute myocardial infarction and can be detected by the appearance of a friction rub. It more commonly complicates large anterior Q-wave infarctions[2] with concomitant congestive heart failure and is associated with an adverse prognosis.[3] The appearance of a pericardial friction rub in the course of acute myocardial infarction is a relative contraindication to anticoagulation, in that pericardial bleeding may result in cardiac tamponade. Pericarditis also has been described following coronary angioplasty,[4] presumably due to coronary dissection at the percutaneous transluminal coronary angioplasty (PTCA) site with epicardial/pericardial hematoma formation.

As more elderly patients undergo dialysis for chronic renal failure, uremic pericarditis is increasingly encountered; dialysis pericarditis also can occur in the absence of azotemia. Pericarditis also may result from chest trauma and is common after cardiac surgery, both as acute postoperative pericarditis and as the delayed and probably immune-mediated postpericardiotomy syndrome. Both Dressler's (late postinfarction) syndrome[5] and the postpericardiotomy syndrome tend to be relapsing, with the cyclic recurrences characterized by chest pain, fever, pericardial rub, and the variable presence of pericardial and pleural effusions.

The frequent use of pharmacotherapy in an elderly population is associated with complications of drug therapy; iatrogenic pericarditis may be secondary to hydralazine, procainamide, minoxidil,[6] as well as a variety of other drugs and may result from therapeutic radiation as well.[7] Less commonly, pericarditis complicates collagen vascular disease. A pericardial rub has been described in up to one-fourth of patients with rheumatoid arthritis, both with and without pericardial effusion; however, constrictive pericarditis is rare, < 1%. Echocardiographic studies suggest that asymptomatic pericarditis may occur frequently,[8] and clinically manifest pericarditis is described to indicate an adverse prognosis.[9]

Acute pericarditis also may occur with acute aortic dissection, as blood dissects backward into the pericardial space; the size of the hemorrhagic effusion may vary.

Pericarditis also has occurred as a complication of penetrating peptic ulcer,[10] esophageal sclerotherapy,[11] and subdiaphragmatic abscess.[12]

## THERAPY

The therapy for viral pericarditis is symptomatic, with reasonably rapid response frequently described to salicylates, ibuprofen, and short-term corticosteroid hormones. Purulent pericarditis requires surgical drainage of the effusion and appropriate antibiotic therapy.[13] Recent reports suggest that some patients with tuberculous pericarditis can be managed with combined antituberculous therapy (rifampin, isoniazid, and ethambutol) rather than with surgical drainage, without an increase in subsequent cardiac tamponade or in late pericardial constriction.[14]

Uremic pericarditis responds to an increased schedule of dialysis; drug-related pericarditis to discontinuation of the offending agent; and postoperative or immune-related postpericardiotomy syndrome to salicylates or corticosteroid hormones. Although resolution of uremic effusions may be aided and hastened by the use of corticosteroid hormones, they increase the risk of bleeding. Neoplastic pericarditis may respond to chemotherapy, hormonal therapy, immunosuppressive drugs, and/or therapeutic radiation. Institution of or increase in the dosage of corticosteroid hormones or other immunosuppressive drugs is indicated for the pericarditis of collagen vascular disease.

## PERICARDIAL EFFUSION AND CARDIAC TAMPONADE

### ETIOLOGY

Pericardial effusion occurs when fluid production by the pericardium is more rapid than fluid resorption. Pericardial fluid may be serous, hemorrhagic or purulent, or combinations of these may be present.

Pericardial effusion can result from most etiologies of pericardial disease— infection, tumor, postinfarction or postpericardiotomy syndromes, drug reactions, therapeutic radiation, trauma, collagen vascular disease, renal insufficiency and chronic dialysis, aortic dissection, and so on. In an elderly patient receiving regular hemodialysis, pericardial tamponade was due to a tuberculous pericardial effusion, suggesting the need to especially consider this diagnosis in immunocompromised hosts.[15]

Neoplastic effusions are most commonly due to bronchogenic carcinoma, carcinoma of the breast, or lymphoma. The effusion occurring after therapeutic radiation is due mainly to blockage of the lymphatic drainage from the pericardium.

Rheumatoid arthritis is the predominant collagen vascular disease producing pericardial effusion in the elderly, in contrast to the more frequent occurrence of lupus pericardial effusion in a younger population; cardiac tamponade also has been described.[16]

Pericardial effusion due to myxedema should be suspected in elderly women, in whom the occurrence of hypothyroidism is frequent; this condition is manifest as effusion without symptomatic pericarditis, although low voltage on the electrocardiogram (ECG) is characteristic. The effusion is often large and may have a high cholesterol content, the so-called gold paint appearance.

## CLINICAL PRESENTATION

Noncompressing pericardial effusion is typically asymptomatic, is often suspected because pericarditis is diagnosed, and may be heralded by enlargement of the cardiac silhouette or evidence of elevation of the jugular venous pressure. Echocardiography is diagnostic.

A pericardial rub may persist despite fluid accumulation, as may the pain of pericarditis. With neoplastic pericardial effusion, although a friction rub is often audible, ECG evidence of pericarditis is uncommon.

Whereas low voltage on the ECG is common with pericardial effusion, the presence of effusion does not predictably alter the QRS voltage of the ECG. With sizable pericardial effusion, electrical alternans may be evident on the ECG, generally manifest as alternating voltage of the QRS complex; occasionally total alternans (alternation of the P, QRS, and T complexes) occurs. Electrical alternans disappears promptly when the pericardial fluid is removed, as it correlates at least in part with the swinging of the heart within the large pericardial effusion (as demonstrated echocardiographically).

The clinical presentation consists of elevation of the jugular venous pressure without evidence of tricuspid regurgitation; no murmur or $S_3$ is audible; and there is radiographic evidence of enlargement of the cardiac silhouette in the presence of clear lung fields, although a pleural effusion may be present.

Two-dimensional echocardiography can define the presence of pericardial effusion by demonstration of an echo-free space between the heart and pericardium. It can quantify the amount and location of the effusion and identify impending cardiac tamponade; the latter is suggested by a large effusion, with resultant diastolic collapse of the right atrium and/or right ventricle. Echo-Doppler evidence of markedly decreased mitral and aortic valve flow velocities on inspiration further suggests impending tamponade. Abnormalities of the pericardium also can be detected. Serial echocardiography is of value in following the course of pericardial effusion and in deciding when intervention is warranted.

Cardiac tamponade is a medical emergency, as the increased intrapericardial pressure limits ventricular filling and stroke volume, and thereby curtails an adequate cardiac output, despite the compensatory tachycardia.[17] There is resultant hypotension and elevation of the jugular venous pressure. A characteristic feature is pulsus paradoxus, wherein the pulse is not truly paradoxic but rather demonstrates an exaggeration of the normal inspiratory decline in systemic blood pressure and pulse pressure.

The speed of development of cardiac tamponade is variable; however, it occurs precipitously in the setting of cardiac rupture resulting from acute myocardial infarction, a complication encountered predominantly in the elderly. Cardiac rupture may be heralded by chest pain; electromechanical dissociation is characteristic, and shock rapidly supervenes. Prompt aspiration of blood from the pericardium may be lifesaving if surgical correction can be immediately accomplished. Chronic effusive-constrictive pericarditis due to silent myocardial infarction and intrapericardial hemorrhage due to a leaking left ventricular pseudoaneurysm was described in an elderly woman. Radionuclide imaging suggested the diagnosis, which was confirmed by angiography and surgery.[18]

THERAPY

The medical treatment of pericardial effusion is that of the underlying pericarditis. Pericardiocentesis should not be routine;[19] it is indicated for diagnosis when purulent pericardial effusion is suspected or therapeutically for impending cardiac tamponade. At times, in patients with systemic neoplasm, pericardiocentesis with examination of the fluid can help differentiate among malignant pericardial effusion, effusion secondary to therapeutic radiation, or that due to drug therapy.

In general, purulent pericardial effusion is treated with surgical drainage.[13] This is also recommended when the pericardial effusion is malignant,[20,21] in that the rapid reaccumulation following pericardiocentesis limits the ability of sclerosing or chemotherapeutic agents injected into the pericardium to be effective in obliterating the pericardial space and limiting the rapid reaccumulation of fluid with resulting cardiac tamponade. The need for repeated pericardiocentesis for large recurrent effusion carries the risks of pneumothorax and of infection; further, sclerosing agents cause pain. Alternatively, an indwelling pericardial catheter may enable longer-term drainage[23,24] if the frequently hemorrhagic or viscous fluid does not become loculated. The surgical approach allows pericardial tissue to be examined and pericardial cultures to be performed for diagnostic purposes.

Thyroid hormone replacement causes resolution of myxedematous effusion, and the euthyroid state is associated with an increase in ECG voltage.

The management of impending cardiac tamponade involves the urgent removal of pericardial fluid, either by pericardiocentesis or by surgical drainage. Subxiphoid insertion of a needle into the pericardium, typically guided by electrocardiographic or echocardiographic control, enables removal of fluid and relief of the hemodynamic abnormalities of tamponade. Removal of even small amounts of pericardial fluid can produce striking hemodynamic improvement. Often a soft catheter is inserted via the needle into the pericardium for continued drainage. Surgical drainage can be accomplished by open thoracotomy, which has the advantage of permitting removal of a sizable amount of pericardium to prevent late constriction and enables the lysing of pericardial adhesions when present. More limited subxiphoid extrapleural surgical drainage also has been effective and entails less morbidity.

## CONSTRICTIVE PERICARDITIS

### ETIOLOGY

Constrictive pericarditis is a late result of a variety of etiologies of pericarditis, but is less common in the elderly than is acute pericarditis or pericardial effusion. Constriction may occur after viral pericarditis or postoperative pericarditis; deposition of calcium is prominent with constriction due to tuberculous pericarditis. As patients with chronic renal disease live to older age, pericardial constriction due to this cause will increase in incidence. Constrictive pericarditis as a result of coronary bypass procedures and other cardiac surgery is likely to increase among the elderly as cardiac surgical procedures are increasingly undertaken in this age group; currently, at least one-third of all coronary bypass operations in the United States are performed in patients aged 65 years and older. Similarly, as chemotherapy and therapeutic radiation improve the prognosis of many forms of neoplasm in the elderly population, the effects of these therapies in producing constrictive pericarditis are more likely to be encountered. Long-duration severe rheumatoid arthritis and prior episodes of pleuropericardial disease are risk factors for the development of constrictive pericarditis,[16] which occurs more commonly in men.

## CLINICAL PRESENTATION

Ventricular filling is markedly limited by pericardial constriction, with resultant equalization of filling pressures of the right and left sides of the heart, and elevation of the jugular venous pressure; pulse volume and cardiac output are decreased.[17]

Often the presenting symptoms of dyspnea, fatigue, and exhaustion are attributed to the underlying clinical problem rather than to the development of constrictive pericarditis. Chest pain is characteristically absent. The jugular venous pressure may further increase during inspiration (known as the Kussmaul sign); and the jugular venous pulse shows prominent x and y descents. The precordium is quiet, and there are no murmurs, although an $S_3$ or occasionally a pericardial knock is audible. Peripheral edema is common, and hepatomegaly and ascites may be present. The heart size is typically normal on chest x-ray; but pericardial calcium deposition may be detected.

The occurrence of atrial fibrillation may be catastrophic, as a consequence both of the loss of the atrial contribution to ventricular filling and of the rapid ventricular rate.

The echocardiographic findings are not specific for pericardial constriction, but pericardial thickening is common, a marked increase in left ventricular isovolumic relaxation time occurs, and an abrupt termination to left ventricular filling often is evident. Differentiation of constrictive pericarditis from restrictive cardiomyopathy may be difficult, even with the newer noninvasive imaging techniques and at cardiac catheterization; cardiac amyloid can cause restrictive cardiomyopathy in elderly persons. Constrictive pericarditis also may be confused with right ventricular infarction and hepatic cirrhosis, with and without ascites.

## REFERENCES

1. Spodick, DH: The normal and diseased pericardium: Current concepts of pericardial physiology, diagnosis, and treatment. J Am Coll Cardiol 1:240, 1983.
2. Dubois, C, Smeets, JP, Demoulin, JC, et al: Frequency and clinical significance of pericardial friction rubs in the acute phase of myocardial infarction. Eur Heart J 6:766, 1985.
3. Tofler, GH, Muller, JE, Stone, PH, et al: Pericarditis following acute myocardial infarction (abstract). Circulation 78(Suppl II):II-437, 1988.
4. Slack, JD, Pinkerton, CA, Nasser, WK: Acute pericarditis after percutaneous transluminal coronary angioplasty. Am J Cardiol 55:843, 1985.
5. Lichstein, E, Arsura, E, Hollander, G, et al: Current incidence of post myocardial infarction (Dressler's) syndrome. Am J Cardiol 50:1269, 1982.
6. Krehlik, JM, Hindson, DA, Crowley, JJ Jr., et al: Minoxidil-associated pericarditis and fatal cardiac tamponade. West J Med 143:527, 1985.
7. Schneider, JS and Edwards, JE: Irradiation induced pericarditis. Chest 75:560, 1979.
8. Hara KS, Ballard, DJ, Ilstrup DM, et al: Rheumatoid pericarditis: Clinical features and survival. Medicine 69:81, 1990.
9. Jurik, AG and Graudal, H: Pericarditis in rheumatoid arthritis. A clinical and radiological study. Rheumatology International 6:37, 1986.
10. West, AB, Nolan, N, O'Briain, DS: Benign peptic ulcers penetrating pericardium and heart: Clinicopathological features and factors favoring survival. Gastroenterology 94:1478, 1988.
11. Lewis, P, Johnstone, D, Celestin, LR: Pericarditis complicating esophageal sclerotherapy. Gastroenterology 96:1625, 1989.

12. Horton, JM and Tucker, WS Jr: Pericarditis with effusion and tamponade complicating left subdiaphragmatic abscesses. West J Med 149:213, 1988.

13. Symbas, PN, Ware, RE, DiOrio, DA, et al: Purulent pericarditis: A review of diagnostic and surgical principles. South Med J 67:46, 1974.

14. Long, R, Younes, M, Patton, N, et al: Tuberculous pericarditis: Long-term outcome in patients who received medical therapy alone. Am Heart J 117:1133, 1989.

15. Kudoh, Y, Kijima, T, Sugita, J, et al: Tuberculosis on regular hemodialysis: A case of pericardial tamponade. Jpn Circ J 53:416, 1989.

16. Kelly, CA, Bourke, JP, Malcolm, A, et al: Chronic pericardial disease in patients with rheumatoid arthritis: A longitudinal study. Q J Med 75:461, 1990.

17. Shabetai, R, Fowler, NO, Guntheroth, WG: The hemodynamics of cardiac tamponade and constrictive pericarditis. Am J Cardiol 26:480, 1970.

18. Sehgal, E, Sherman, W, Isom, OW, et al: Left ventricular pseudoaneurysm causing superior vena caval obstruction and effusive-constrictive pericarditis. J Nucl Med 28:918, 1987.

19. Permanyer-Miralda, G, Sagrista-Sauleda, J, Soler-Soler, J: Primary acute pericardial disease: A prospective series of 231 consecutive patients. Am J Cardiol 56:623, 1985.

20. Hawkins, JW and Vacek, JL: What constitutes definitive therapy of malignant pericardial effusion? "Medical" versus surgical treatment. Am Heart J 118:428, 1989.

21. Little, AG, Kremser, PC, Wade, JL, et al: Operation for diagnosis and treatment of pericardial effusions. Surgery 96:738, 1984.

22. Shepherd, FA, Morgan, C, Evans, WK, et al: Medical management of malignant pericardial effusion by tetracycline sclerosis. Am J Cardiol 60:1161, 1987.

23. Kopecky, SL, Callahan, JA, Tajik, AJ, et al: Percutaneous pericardial catheter drainage: Report of 42 consecutive cases. Am J Cardiol 58:633, 1986.

24. Nawa, S, Irie, H, Takata, K, et al: A new method for continuous pericardiocentesis-percutaneous pericardial drainage via a sheath-introducer. Jpn J Surg 18:224, 1988.

# CHAPTER 9

# Cardiomyopathies in the Elderly

*Richard J. Backes, M.D.*
*Bernard J. Gersh, M.B., Ch.B., D.Phil.*

Cardiomyopathies are defined as a group of diseases of heart muscle of unknown cause or causes. From a practical standpoint, however, a pathophysiologic or behavioral classification is useful: 1) In *dilated cardiomyopathy,* there is predominant impairment of left ventricular systolic function usually, but not invariably, associated with dilation of the ventricle. 2) *Hypertrophic cardiomyopathy* is characterized by normal or small chamber size, increased wall thickness, hyperdynamic systolic function, and impaired diastolic filling characteristics. Hypertrophic cardiomyopathy may be further subdivided into obstructive and nonobstructive forms on the basis of obstruction to flow in the left ventricular outflow tract. 3) In *restrictive cardiomyopathy,* there is an increase in left ventricular stiffness and early diastolic dysfunction, with various degrees of systolic dysfunction, particularly in the later stages.

Traditionally, the cardiomyopathies (particularly hypertrophic cardiomyopathy and idiopathic dilated cardiomyopathy) have been viewed as diseases primarily of younger patients. Nonetheless, heart failure is common in the elderly, and its prevalence increases markedly with increasing age from the sixth decade onward. It also has become increasingly apparent that the cardiomyopathies are an important contributor to the development of heart failure in the elderly, and it is likely that these conditions have been underdiagnosed in the past. Furthermore, increasing evidence emphasizes the heterogeneity of the cardiomyopathies, including differences in clinical presentation, pathophysiologic mechanisms, and natural history among younger and older patients. Accordingly, this chapter reviews similarities and differences in these entities between young and old patients.

## DILATED CARDIOMYOPATHY

### EPIDEMIOLOGY

Dilated cardiomyopathy (DCM) was previously believed to be a rare condition in the elderly. Several large series suggested that approximately 10% of patients with DCM were 60 years of age or older.[1-3] Recently, however, population-based data

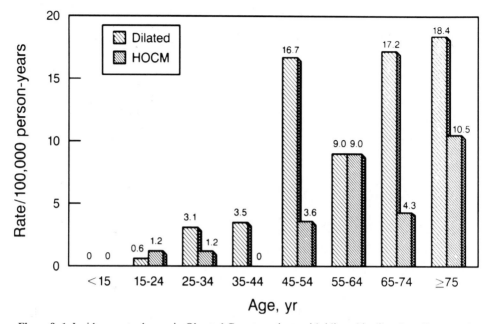

**Figure 9–1.** Incidence rates by age in Olmsted County patients with idiopathic dilated cardiomyopathy and hypertrophic obstructive cardiomyopathy *(HOCM)*. (Data from Codd et al.[5])

suggest that there may have been referral bias in the earlier studies. A retrospective study from Denmark showed an overall incidence of 7.3 per 1 million population per year, with patients older than 60 forming 29.3% of the total.[4] Codd and coworkers,[5] in a population-based study in Olmsted County, Minnesota, documented overall adjusted incidence rates that were highest in the patients older than 75 years (Fig. 9–1). Adjusted prevalence rates were also highest in the elderly group; whereas overall rates were 58.0 per 100,000 in men and 19.4 per 100,000 in women; rates in those older than 75 were 237.5 per 100,000 for men and 35.0 per 100,000 for women.

Reasons for the apparent increase in incidence and prevalence rates of DCM in the elderly are twofold: the demographics of our aging population and previous erroneous diagnoses of coronary artery disease, hypertension, valvular heart disease, and others as the cause of heart failure.

## EFFECT OF AGE ON PROGNOSIS

Natural history studies of DCM, initially published from large referral centers, documented a very poor prognosis (Table 9–1).[6,7] Fuster and coworkers[8] noted that 77% of 104 patients with DCM were dead at a mean follow-up of 11 years, with two-thirds of the deaths occurring in the first 2 years. Kopecky and Gersh[9] summarized the cumulative mortality in 10 large series (1105 patients) and noted a mean survival of 57% at 5 years.

More recent population-based data, however, suggest that the overall prognosis of DCM may not be as dismal as previously thought. Sugrue and colleagues[10] recently compared survival in 41 Olmsted County patients who had DCM with that in referral center patients with DCM. Baseline patient characteristics were similar

**Table 9–1.** Cumulative Mortality in
Dilated Cardiomyopathy

| First Author | No. of Patients | Mortality (%) by Follow-up Years | | | | | | |
|---|---|---|---|---|---|---|---|---|
| | | 1 | 2 | 3 | 4 | 5 | 8 | 10 |
| MacArthur[46] | 146 | | | | 56 | | | |
| Schwarz[53] | 68 | | | 34 | | | | |
| Gauazzi[52] | 137 | | | | | 55 | | |
| Unverferth[44] | 69 | 35 | | | | | | |
| Fuster[43] | 104 | 31 | | | | 62 | | 72 |
| Ogasawara[51] | 65 | | | | | 60 | | |
| Franciosa[49] | 87 | 23 | 48 | | | | | |
| Kuhn[45] | 258 | | | | 29 | 49 | 79 | |
| Figulla[47] | 56 | 17 | | 28 | | | | |
| Segal[59] | 115 | 12 | 18 | | | | | |
| Total: | 1,105 | Mean: 24 | 33 | 30 | | 57 | | |

*Source:* From Kopecky and Gersh.[9] By permission of Year Book Medical Publishers. Reference numbers in table are from this source.

in the two groups, but survival was much better in the population-based cohort: 95% compared with 69 (*P* < 0.001) at 1 year and 80% compared with 36% (*P* < 0.001) at 5 years.

Even though left ventricular systolic function, in addition to unidentified factors, is the major determinant of survival in DCM, older age per se is a powerful independent marker of an adverse prognosis. Fuster and coworkers[8] noted that 97% of patients older than 55 but only 66% of those younger than 55 were dead at a mean follow-up of 11 years. Sugrue and associates[10] estimated that 5-year survival rates were 71% for patients older than 54 and 89% for patients younger than 54. Data on the natural history of dilated cardiomyopathy in the "old, old," that is, patients older than 75 to 80 years, are not currently available.

## AGE AND THERAPY

The treatment of symptomatic DCM can be divided into several categories: treatment of myocarditis (if present), medical management of pulmonary congestion and low cardiac output, use of antiarrhythmic drugs and treatment of conduction disease, anticoagulation, and transplantation.

The link between acute myocarditis and DCM has confused physicians for years. Early reports on the incidence of inflammatory myocarditis by endomyocardial biopsy varied between 0% and 67%,[11] a reflection of different patient populations and the lack of a standardized morphologic definition of myocarditis.

The adoption of the Dallas criteria has helped ensure greater uniformity in diagnosing myocarditis.[12] Nonetheless, the role of routine endomyocardial biopsy in patients with suspected idiopathic DCM requires further clarification, and the diagnostic criteria themselves are still on trial. A critical determinant of the future place of endomyocardial biopsy requires documentation of the efficacy or noneffi-cacy of immunosuppressive therapy in patients with DCM in whom there is biopsy evidence of inflammatory myocarditis.[13,14] More definitive answers may be forthcoming from the Myocarditis Treatment Trial, but even if such therapy is proven to be effective in younger patients, the risk-benefit ratio still must be determined in the elderly, inasmuch as there is some evidence from experience with cardiac transplantation that older patients do not tolerate immunosuppressive therapy as well as their younger counterparts.[15,16]

The same drugs, including diuretics, digitalis, and vasodilators, used to treat heart failure in younger patients are used in older patients. The elderly, however, require meticulous attention to detail because of the increased potential for drug-induced side effects.

### Digitalis

Advanced age has long been known to be a risk factor for digitalis intoxication. Although an earlier study suggested that age per se enhanced sensitivity to digitalis compounds,[17] the causes are multifactorial and most likely the result of an association with the multiple physiologic changes that occur with aging. With age, a decrease in total body water and lean body mass and a concomitant increase in body fat lead to a reduction in the volume of distribution of water-soluble drugs (e.g., digoxin), with a resultant increase in plasma concentrations for any given dose.[18] The half-life of digoxin is prolonged in the elderly because of a reduction in glomerular filtration rate, tubular secretion, and renal blood flow.[19] Moreover, drug-drug interactions with quinidine, amiodarone, verapamil, and others can increase the risk of digitalis intoxication.[20–22]

### Vasodilators and Diuretics

The elderly may be extremely sensitive to drugs that reduce preload and afterload (for example, vasodilators and diuretics), because their potential to cause orthostatic hypotension and falls is enhanced. Falls are a serious complication of drug therapy, currently being the sixth leading cause of death in the elderly;[23] and one study documented that in patients older than age 80, 56% of falls were associated with severe injury.[24] Falls also may have a substantial impact on the functional independence of the elderly, because another study found that a history of recent falls was a frequent precipitant of nursing home admissions.[25] The elderly are extremely sensitive to preload reduction; contributory factors include diminished orthostatic responses (including changes in baroreflex sensitivity), reduction in ventricular compliance, chronotropic incompetence, and concomitant diseases (such as cerebrovascular disease).

### Beta-blocking Agents

The precise role of $\beta$-adrenergic receptor blocking agents in the treatment of DCM is unclear. In the elderly, however, the number of pacemaker cells in the sinus node is reduced by approximately 90%, and this reduction enhances the potential for marked depression of sinoatrial function.[26]

### Anticoagulants

Anticoagulants are clearly beneficial in preventing embolic events in patients with DCM, especially those in atrial fibrillation. Fuster and associates[8] noted embolic events in 18% of patients not receiving anticoagulants, whereas there were no embolic events in patients receiving anticoagulant therapy.[9,27] However, the risk of anticoagulation in the elderly is increased, particularly in those with associated diseases, for example, malignant lesions, hypertension, and cerebrovascular disease, and in those who are frail, are unsteady, or have disturbances in gait.[28] Therefore, risk-benefit ratios must be taken into account before anticoagulants are used in the elderly. In the recent Stroke Prevention in Atrial Fibrillation Trial[27] of anticoagulants in patients with nonrheumatic atrial fibrillation, the benefit of warfarin and aspirin over placebo was noted only in patients younger than 75 years. Further data on patients older than age 75 years are forthcoming.

### Antiarrhythmic Agents

Ventricular ectopy is ubiquitous in patients with DCM. More importantly, at least 50% of patients with DCM have documented ventricular tachycardia on Holter monitoring, and sudden death is the most common form of death. However, no randomized, controlled trials in any age group document a survival benefit with antiarrhythmic agents in patients with congestive heart failure, and the role of electrophysiologic testing to guide therapy remains uncertain.[29-36] The increasing use of implantable defibrillators is an encouraging option for all age groups.

### Cardiac Transplantation

The ultimate treatment for DCM—cardiac transplantation—is occasionally an option for the elderly. Although absolute age limits do not currently exist and the age of patients considered for transplantation is increasing, the scarcity of donors (at least in the United States) and priorities attached to the allocation of limited resources dictate patterns of practice. In reality, relatively few patients older than the age of 65 undergo cardiac transplantation in this country.

## HYPERTROPHIC CARDIOMYOPATHY

### EPIDEMIOLOGY

Traditionally, hypertrophic obstructive cardiomyopathy (HOCM) has been recognized as a disease of younger patients. This awareness may, in part, reflect referral trends, because mostly younger, sicker patients were seen at the few major centers that had expertise in this disease during the 1960s and 1970s. For example, in a large series from Hammersmith General Hospital, only 3% of 234 patients were older than age 60.[37] Nonetheless, even the earlier literature contains numerous reports of hypertrophic cardiomyopathy in the elderly.[38,39] Whiting and colleagues[40] noted that 32% of patients with HOCM at the Massachusetts General Hospital were older than age 60, and in a community hospital-based series, Petrin and Tavel[41] documented that 83% of patients were older than age 40. Lever and associates[42] from the Cleveland Clinic Foundation emphasized that there were more patients with hypertrophic cardiomyopathy older than age 65 than younger than age 40. This finding is reinforced by a recent population-based epidemiologic study from Olmsted County, Minnesota, which documented that the highest incidence and prevalence of hypertrophic cardiomyopathy were in patients older than 75 years and that the next closest age group in frequency was 55 to 64 years[5] (see Fig. 9–1).

### MORPHOLOGY

The first published description of the morphologic features of hypertrophic cardiomyopathy was in 1958 by Teare,[43] who observed an association between asymmetric hypertrophy of the interventricular septum and sudden unexpected death in young adults. During the 1970s, it became apparent that the entity of "asymmetric septal hypertrophy" was but one aspect of a diverse morphologic spectrum. Echocardiographic surveys documented that hypertrophy could involve any region of the left ventricular wall, and in some patients, occurrence was symmetric.[44–46] Consequently, the definition of hypertrophic cardiomyopathy was expanded to include a hypertrophied, nondilated left ventricle in the absence of a cardiac or systemic disease that in itself could produce left ventricular hypertrophy.[47]

With the increasing recognition of the frequency of HOCM in the elderly and the use of more sophisticated imaging techniques, attention has been drawn to the clinical and structural differences in hypertrophic cardiomyopathy in older and younger patients. In many patients, the differences are substantial enough to have raised the question whether HOCM in the elderly is a separate disease entity or a modified form or expression of the disease encountered in younger patients. To address this issue, Lever and associates,[42] using two-dimensional echocardiography, compared the structural characteristics of HOCM in older and younger patients (using age 65 as a cutoff). Septal hypertrophy, systolic anterior motion of the mitral valve, and outflow tract gradients were similar in the two groups. However, the extent of hypertrophy, as determined by septal and free-wall measurements, was greater in younger patients. Of particular importance was the significant difference in cardiac shape between the two groups. Of the elderly patients, 86% had normal septal curvature and an ovoid left ventricle, and 54% had a proximal septal bulge (in addition to an ovoid left ventricle). In contrast, none of the younger patients had a proximal septal bulge, and 75% of them had reversed septal curvature with a distinctive crescent-shaped left ventricular cavity (Fig. 9–2).

The explanation for these age-related structural differences remains unclear. Wigle and colleagues[48] suggested that the pattern of septal curvature and ventricular shape in the elderly represented a milder form of the disease, which could explain why these patients lived to an advanced age. An alternative explanation is that the septal bulge and the pattern of hypertrophy may be exaggerations of the normal aging process. In an autopsy series from the Mayo Clinic, Kitzman and coworkers[49]

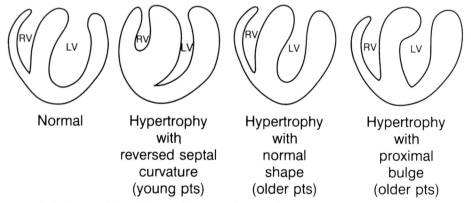

| Normal | Hypertrophy with reversed septal curvature (young pts) | Hypertrophy with normal shape (older pts) | Hypertrophy with proximal bulge (older pts) |

**Figure 9–2.** Characteristics of the septal curvature in normal persons and young and old patients with hypertrophic obstructive cardiomyopathy. LV = left ventricle; RV = right ventricle. (From Lever et al,[42] with permission of the American Heart Association.)

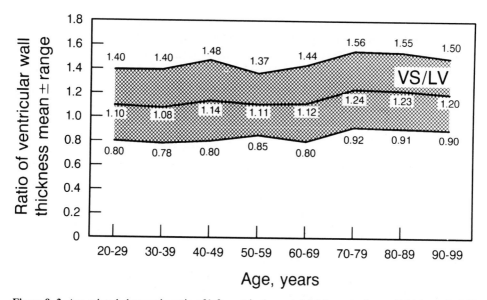

**Figure 9–3.** Age-related changes in ratio of left ventricular septal thickness to free-wall thickness in 765 normal subjects. VS/LV = ratio of ventricular septal to left ventricular wall thickness. (From Kitzman et al,[49] with permission of Mayo Foundation.)

observed that even in "normal" hearts, there was a significant increase with age in the ratio of septal thickness to free-wall thickness (Fig. 9–3). Goor and associates[50] described the development of a "sigmoid septum" in normal elderly patients. These investigators noted that with advancing age, there was a tendency toward a rightward shift of the aorta in relationship to the ventricular septum, which led to the development of a subaortic bulge in the septum that could create left ventricular outflow tract narrowing.

In summary, the morphologic features of HOCM in the young generally consist of a markedly abnormal and hypertrophied ventricular septum, with reversal of normal septal curvature and a distinctive crescent-shaped left ventricular cavity. In contrast, in most elderly patients with hypertrophic cardiomyopathy, a normal ovoid-shaped left ventricle is maintained but there is an exaggerated proximal septal ridge or bulge.

## RELATIONSHIP BETWEEN HYPERTENSION AND HOCM IN THE ELDERLY

The relationship between systemic hypertension and HOCM in the elderly is controversial. It is likely that hypertension in some patients modifies the pathophysiologic anatomy of hypertrophic cardiomyopathy in addition to the extent of left ventricular hypertrophy. What is more debatable but remains a subject of great interest is whether mild hypertension is the inciting stimulus to "inappropriate hypertrophy." If it were, the implication would be that hypertension could be the cause of overt hypertrophic cardiomyopathy in genetically "predisposed" individuals. The controversy dates back to 1957 when Brock[51] described an elderly patient with severe left ventricular hypertrophy causing a left ventricular outflow tract gradient simulating severe aortic stenosis. Brock concluded that the subvalvular obstruction was secondary to severe hypertension. In a subsequent report of six patients with probable hypertrophic cardiomyopathy, he observed that only two had a history of systemic hypertension.[52] However, in 1979, Petrin and Tavel[41] again postulated that hypertension was the etiologic factor in HOCM in the elderly.

In 1985, Topol and coworkers[53] defined the entity of "hypertensive hypertrophic cardiomyopathy of the elderly" in their description of a group of 21 elderly patients (mostly black and female) who had what appeared to be a distinct clinical syndrome. All these patients had severe concentric left ventricular hypertrophy on echocardiography, with reduced cavity size, excessive systolic ejection, and impaired diastolic function. All had a history of hypertension; most were receiving antihypertensive therapy, and at presentation, all had clinical evidence of pulmonary congestion. Subsequent symptomatic improvement during treatment with $\beta$-blocking or calcium channel blocking agents was noted, whereas afterload-reducing agents and diuretics caused significant hypotension. The systolic and diastolic flow abnormalities in this syndrome were further delineated by Pearson and associates[54] using Doppler echocardiography. Seventeen patients with a history of systemic hypertension and evidence of HOCM were compared with age-matched control subjects. Left ventricular filling was characterized by an increased peak atrial velocity and a reduced ratio of initial peak velocity to velocity at the time of atrial contraction in the study group. Left ventricular outflow tract velocities were increased in 14 of the 17 study patients, with peak velocities ranging from 1.2 to 5.0 m/sec, corresponding to a peak intraventricular gradient between 16 and 100 mmHg. It was concluded that these hemodynamic characteristics would support the use of agents with negative inotropic properties for the treatment of congestive heart failure in patients with this syndrome.

An important study by Karam and associates[55] compared 39 patients who had hypertension and HOCM with 39 age- and gender-matched patients with HOCM but without hypertension in an attempt to categorize more precisely the role of hypertension in hypertrophic cardiomyopathy. There were no clinical or electrocardiographic differences between the two groups. Two-dimensional echocardiographic studies showed that there was no difference in the incidence or severity of systolic anterior motion of the mitral valve, mitral annular calcification, septal thickness, or left ventricular outflow tract gradients. The only difference was related to the extent of hypertrophy involving the posterior wall: 54% of the hypertensive group had a posterior wall thickness greater than 13 mm as opposed to 31% in the nonhypertensive group ($P = 0.02$). The authors concluded that hypertension could increase the severity of left ventricular hypertrophy but was *not* the primary cause of hypertrophic cardiomyopathy, and they suggested that the syndrome be named "hypertrophic cardiomyopathy with hypertension."

Lewis and Maron[56] implied that the mechanism of dynamic left ventricular outflow tract obstruction may differ between younger and older patients. That is, obstruction in the elderly is caused primarily by anterior displacement of the mitral valve as a result of mitral annular calcification and systolic posterior excursion of the ventricular septum, whereas in younger patients, obstruction is due primarily to systolic anterior motion of the mitral valve.

In summary, it is likely that some of the differences in hypertrophic cardiomyopathy between younger and older patients are simply a reflection of the wide spectrum and heterogeneity of this disease. In some patients, survival to old age probably represents the natural history of a more benign form of the same disease that affects younger patients. In other older patients, the morphologic characteristics could be the result of different pathophysiologic processes or a separate disease entity. The cause remains speculative, but HOCM in some elderly patients may be the end result of an "inappropriate" or "excessive" response to multiple stimuli associated with aging, which usually would result in milder degrees of left ventricular hypertrophy, for example, hypertension, loss of aortic compliance, and age-related changes in mean septal to left ventricular free-wall thickness. It is unlikely that hypertension is the primary cause of hypertrophic cardiomyopathy in the elderly, but the entity of "hypertensive hypertrophic cardiomyopathy" in patients with mild-to-moderate hypertension can certainly be included within the spectrum of hypertrophic cardiomyopathy.

## EFFECT OF AGE ON PROGNOSIS

Most natural history studies, which involve mainly younger patients with severe symptoms referred to tertiary care institutions, have emphasized the generally poor prognosis of HOCM.[57,58] In contrast, a recent study on an outpatient population (mean age, 44 years) implied a more benign prognosis than originally suggested.[59] In a recent Mayo Clinic study confined to patients aged 65 years and older with HOCM, a comparison of their outcome with that of an age- and sex-matched control population suggested that the course is relatively benign in most of the elderly.[60] Although 75% of the patients were symptomatic at presentation, with chest pain, dyspnea, or syncope, the respective 97% and 50% 1-year and 5-year survival rates were not significantly different from those in the age- and sex-matched control population. Nonetheless, not all patients had a benign clinical course, and numerous clinical and echocardiographic variables were examined for their relationship to prognosis. The only clinical variable associated with decreased survival was the severity of dyspnea. Among patients with New York Heart Association (NYHA) functional class I or II dyspnea at presentation, only 18 had progression to class III or IV during the follow-up period, but among patients presenting with class III symptoms, the 1-year mortality was 36%. The only echocardiographic variables associated with an adverse outcome were a left atrial size of 42 mm or larger and a septal thickness of 20 mm or more (Fig. 9–4). These results are consistent with those of McKenna and colleagues,[37] who noted that severe dyspnea was an adverse prognostic feature in younger patients with HOCM. Lewis and Maron[56] followed the clinical course of 52 elderly patients with HOCM who had severe symptoms and documented a high incidence of progressive symptoms, failure of medical therapy, and progression to surgical correction.

In summary, the prognosis for elderly patients with hypertrophic cardiomyopathy is generally favorable, but among the elderly are those with severe disease characterized by advanced symptoms and certain echocardiographic features documenting increased left atrial size and ventricular septal thickness. This subgroup of patients has an adverse prognosis.

## MEDICAL AND SURGICAL TREATMENT OF HOCM IN THE ELDERLY

In many patients, HOCM can be effectively treated medically; however, as discussed previously, the elderly are, in general, less tolerant of medications, especially some of those used to treat this disease such as beta-blocking agents, calcium channel blockers, disopyramide (Norpace), and amiodarone. Conduction disturbances,

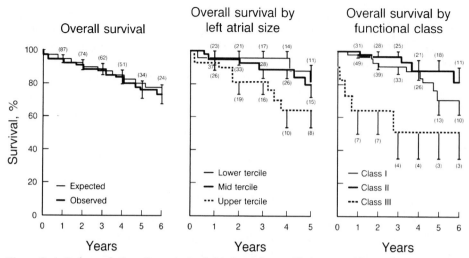

**Figure 9–4.** *Left panel:* Overall survival of elderly patients with hypertrophic cardiomyopathy and expected survival of an age- and sex-matched control group. No significant difference (*P* = 0.28) in survival was noted. *Middle panel:* Relationship of left atrial size to cardiac mortality. Patients were divided into terciles on the basis of indexed left atrial size. Lower tercile: indexed left atrial size <22 mm/m$^2$ (*n* = 31). Mid tercile: indexed left atrial size between 22 and 26 mm/m$^2$ (*n* = 31). Upper tercile: indexed left atrial size >26 mm/m$^2$ (*n* = 32). Survival free from cardiac death is shown for each tercile. On multivariate analysis, indexed left atrial size was independently associated with cardiac death (*P* < 0.05). *Right panel:* Survival of elderly patients with hypertrophic cardiomyopathy by New York Heart Association functional class dyspnea at presentation. (From Fay et al,[60] with permission of the American College of Cardiology.)

orthostatic hypotension with subsequent falls, and pulmonary edema if left ventricular function is depressed are all potential side effects. Supraventricular rhythm disturbances, in general, and atrial fibrillation, in particular, are very common in elderly patients with HOCM and can very rapidly lead to clinical deterioration. Therefore, prompt treatment with direct-current cardioversion, if necessary, is an integral part of the medical management of these patients.[61,62] Ventricular arrhythmias are also relatively common in HOCM, although more so in younger patients.[63–65] In view of the relatively favorable prognosis of HOCM in the elderly and the side effects of amiodarone, we would not routinely advocate therapy for asymptomatic nonsustained ventricular tachycardia, despite evidence that this may be beneficial in younger patients.[66] However, amiodarone may be helpful in patients with symptomatic sustained ventricular arrhythmias, as is the use of implantable cardioverter-defibrillators in all age groups.

The increasing longevity of the U.S. population has resulted in a marked increase in the use of cardiac surgery in the elderly, including the operative treatment of HOCM. Surgery for HOCM is generally reserved for patients who cannot tolerate drug treatment, those who continue to have severe symptoms despite maximal medical therapy, and those with associated cardiac diseases requiring operation, for example, coronary artery disease and aortic stenosis.

The first operation for the relief of subvalvular obstruction due to HOCM was performed in 1959,[67] and by 1968 the procedure of choice for this disease became transaortic left ventricular septal myectomy and myotomy.[68] Surgical experience with HOCM at the National Institutes of Health (NIH) in patients older than 65 years was reported by Maron and colleagues[69] in 1978. This series comprised 20 patients with severe symptoms (NYHA functional class III or IV dyspnea), all of whom had intraventricular gradients, either at rest or on provocation, greater than 50 mmHg. Two postoperative deaths occurred, one on the second day and one after 4 years, both from myocardial infarction. Of the remaining 18 patients, 16 had significant functional improvement for up to 6 years, and 7 patients were asymptomatic at follow-up. The overall results were similar to the experience from NIH with younger patients, and the conclusion was that age per se should not be a contraindication to operative intervention.[70] Although 12 patients in this series had hypertension, only 2 had coronary artery disease, and no patient had significant valvular heart disease or underwent coronary bypass surgery. The absence of associated diseases in this initial series is presumably a reflection of the selection criteria prevalent at that time.

Cooper and associates[71] updated the NIH surgical experience on HOCM in the elderly in 1987. Of 52 patients older than 65 years undergoing surgery, 42 had significant obstructive coronary artery disease (narrowing in at least one major artery). Hospital mortality was 8% in the patients without coronary artery disease (similar to the 8.6% hospital mortality in younger patients undergoing operative intervention) and 27% in patients with coronary artery disease, all related to an acquired ventricular septal defect. Three patients underwent valve replacement (two aortic and one tricuspid), and all three died in the early postoperative period. Of hospital survivors, 85% had significant symptomatic improvement (at least one NYHA functional class), and 78% continued to show improvement at an average follow-up of 4.5 years. The authors concluded that operative treatment in elderly patients with HOCM provided good palliation with acceptable operative mortality and recognized that associated cardiac conditions considerably increased the operative risk.

The importance of acquired ventricular septal defects as a cause of early mortality was further expounded by Siegman and coworkers,[72] who noted that 5 of 24 patients who underwent combined myectomy-myotomy and coronary artery bypass grafting had postoperative ventricular septal defects. Of these five patients, two died and two required a second operation to repair the defect. The authors subsequently recommended considering mitral valve repair as a preferable operation to myotomy-myectomy in patients with a preoperative septum less than 20 mm in thickness.

The Mayo Clinic experience with operative treatment of HOCM was reported in 1989.[73] From May 1972 through April 1987, 83 patients younger than 65 years and 32 who were 65 or older underwent surgery. Operative mortality was 1.2% in patients younger than 65 and 15.6% in those 65 or older. The cumulative 5-year survival was 95% ± 3% in patients younger than 65 and 63% ± 13% in those 65 or older (Fig. 9–5). Although not stratified by age, the need for associated procedures substantially increased the late mortality—to 50% in patients having concomitant aortic valve replacement and 30% in patients undergoing coronary bypass surgery. Symptomatic improvement was substantial, although this was not stratified according to age; 90% of patients had improvement in their symptoms, and 73% were free of symptoms at last follow-up (mean, 5.1 years). Because of the higher hospital and overall mortality, it was recommended that surgical relief of outflow tract obstruction in the elderly be reserved for highly symptomatic patients who do not have a response to maximal medical management.

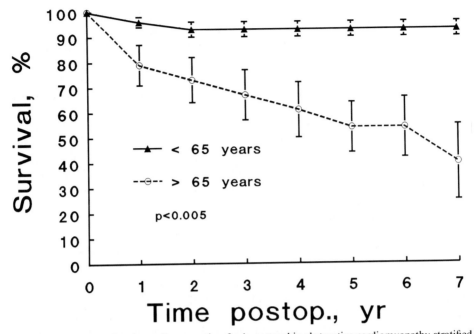

**Figure 9–5.** Survival of patients after operation for hypertrophic obstructive cardiomyopathy stratified by age above and below 65 years. Younger patients had significantly ($P < 0.005$) better late survival. This analysis includes operative deaths, but findings were similar when only hospital survivors were analyzed. (From Mohr et al,[73] with permission of C.V. Mosby Company.)

In summary, surgical treatment of HOCM in the elderly is feasible, and hospital survivors have an excellent symptomatic outcome. Determinants of operative mortality appear to be related to associated medical diseases requiring additional cardiovascular procedures, for example, coronary artery bypass and valve replacement.

## RESTRICTIVE CARDIOMYOPATHY

### GENERAL PRINCIPLES AND ASSOCIATION WITH HEART FAILURE

The restrictive cardiomyopathies, in general, can be characterized by abnormalities in diastolic function with well-preserved systolic function, at least during the earlier phases of the disease. Characterization of the restrictive cardiomyopathies has been hampered by multiple definitions that include pathologic,[74,75] clinical,[76] and hemodynamic[77] criteria. More recently, the term "restrictive cardiac disease" was proposed as a unifying definition that would encompass the multiple disorders with similar pathophysiologic and hemodynamic features (Table 9–2). Subcategories would include primary restrictive cardiomyopathy (either with or without eosinophilia) and secondary restrictive disease due to specific causes, for example, infiltration.

Restrictive cardiac disease is characterized by an abnormality of diastolic filling that culminates in a high filling pressure for any change in ventricular volume, resulting in low forward output and signs of pulmonary congestion and right-sided

**Table 9-2.** Differential Diagnosis
of Restrictive Cardiac Disease

Primary restrictive cardiomyopathy
  With eosinophilia
  Hypereosinophilic syndrome
  Eosinophilic myocarditis
  Endomyocardial fibrosis
  Noneosinophilic form
Secondary restrictive cardiac disease with a specific cause
  Infiltrative
    Amyloidosis
    Hemochromatosis
    Pseudoxanthoma
    Sarcoidosis
    Post-transplantation
Constrictive pericarditis

*Source:* From Nishimura and Warnes,[78] with permission of Current Science.

failure.[78] The most typical hemodynamic abnormality is rapid early left ventricular filling, with the bulk of filling completed in early diastole.[79] Doppler echocardiography, by providing noninvasive measurements of flow across the mitral and tricuspid valves, has greatly increased our understanding of the hemodynamic profiles encountered in restrictive heart disease.

The pattern of mitral valve inflow continually depends on the left atrial-left ventricular pressure gradient and begins with an early initial diastolic velocity (E wave) as the left ventricular pressure decreases below left atrial pressure. Then, as left ventricular pressure begins to rise, mitral flow velocity decelerates and the rate of decrease is measured by the deceleration time. At the time of atrial contraction, there is a further increase in velocity (A wave) as left atrial pressure again exceeds left ventricular pressure (Fig. 9-6).[80]

In general, patterns of mitral flow can be placed in three clinically distinguishable categories: 1) normal, in which the E-wave velocity exceeds the A-wave velocity; 2) abnormal relaxation, in which a decreased E wave, prolonged deceleration time, and higher A wave represent the increased role of left atrial contraction in ventricular filling; and 3) restriction, in which the E velocity increases and the deceleration time decreases because of a high initial left atrial-left ventricular pressure gradient (see Fig. 9-6).[81-83]

These abnormalities in diastolic function have been useful prognostic indicators in patients with cardiac amyloidosis.[84] Nonetheless, it must be appreciated that the physiologic changes associated with "normal" aging may result in progressive alteration of diastolic properties of the myocardium over time. With increasing age, the isovolumic relaxation period is prolonged, the E velocity is decreased, and the A velocity is increased.[82,83] Inasmuch as "normal" valves for the general population (including the elderly) are not completely standardized, a "gray zone" remains between filling patterns deemed physiologic and those considered pathologic.

Aging changes in diastolic filling patterns have also been noted by use of radionuclide angiography. Iskandrian and Hakki[85] noted age-related declines in resting and exercise peak filling rates. Clements and coworkers[86] showed that peak filling

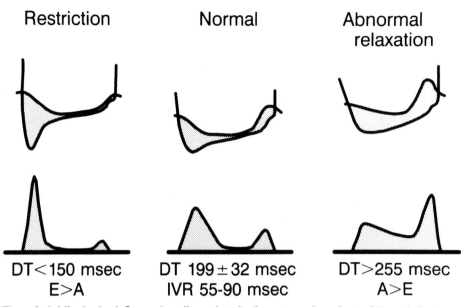

**Figure 9–6.** Mitral valve inflow and cardiac catheterization patterns in patients with restrictive hemodynamics, normal subjects, and patients with abnormal relaxation. $A$ = velocity at time of atrial contraction; $DT$ = deceleration time; $E$ = initial peak velocity; $IVR$ = isovolumic relaxation period. (Modified from Nishimura et al.[83])

rates and time-to-peak filling rates were negatively correlated with age and that atrial filling fraction and filling duration were increased with age. These data further emphasize the difficulty of distinguishing between age-related and disease-related changes in diastolic function.

The entity of "diastolic dysfunction," particularly in the elderly, is of more than academic interest. Radionuclide studies have documented normal systolic function in 30% to 40% of patients referred with a history of congestive heart failure.[87,88] Recognition of "diastolic heart failure" or restrictive heart disease is essential, because the treatment of this entity differs markedly from the conventional approach to patients with heart failure due to primary systolic dysfunction.[89] For example, arterial vasodilators and digitalis may be harmful in patients with diastolic disease, but calcium channel and $\beta$-blocking agents have been shown to improve left ventricular relaxation. Through this mechanism and by a slowing of the heart rate, improvement in clinical symptoms and prolongation of exercise time have been noted.[90–92]

### DIFFERENTIAL DIAGNOSIS OF RESTRICTIVE HEART DISEASE

Documentation of diastolic dysfunction or restrictive cardiac physiology should prompt a search for secondary causes, for example, infiltrative diseases. If none is found, a diagnosis of primary restrictive cardiomyopathy can be made.

Primary restrictive cardiomyopathy with eosinophilia previously included the entities of Löffler's syndrome, endomyocardial fibroelastosis, hypereosinophilia syndrome, and others. It has been postulated that these conditions are all manifestations of the same syndrome occurring at different stages in the clinical course.[93]

Despite medical therapy, patients with eosinophilic heart disease generally have progressive deterioration and die at a relatively young age.[94]

Primary restrictive cardiomyopathy without eosinophilia has been described mainly in middle-aged patients from the United States.[95] Endomyocardial biopsy reveals scattered fibrosis as the lone morphologic substrate for the classic restrictive hemodynamics. No specific data are available on the frequency of this entity in the elderly, but it is likely that it is more common than originally thought, because Doppler echocardiography heightens our awareness of abnormal diastolic filling patterns.

Difficulties arise, however, because a large number of patients occupy a "gray zone." The borders between diastolic changes that occur normally with aging, those that occur secondary to hypertension, and those associated with a restrictive cardiomyopathy are ill-defined. It may be that many patients with "diastolic dysfunction" secondary to hypertension may actually have mild restrictive cardiomyopathy. Only further study will help in these distinctions.

Restrictive cardiac disease secondary to a specific cause is much more common than the primary types, and the prototype of this disorder is amyloid heart disease. Amyloidosis is characterized by the extracellular deposition of insoluble fibrillar proteins.[96] The fibrils are composed of immunoglobulin light chains, non-immunoglobulin proteins,[97] or, as recently described, a prealbumin-like protein.[98]

## Amyloidosis

Amyloidosis can present as several clinicopathologic entities, including acquired systemic, organ-limited, and localized deposition. Acquired systemic amyloidosis includes heredofamilial amyloidosis and that associated with multiple myeloma, chronic infections, or other inflammatory conditions. Organ-limited amyloidosis can be limited to the renal, neural, or cardiac system, with cardiac involvement increasing with advancing age, hence the term "senile cardiac amyloid."[99] Unlike systemic amyloidosis, senile cardiac amyloid is a frequent postmortem finding in patients older than 80 years old and is generally thought to be a nonspecific and clinically insignificant finding.[100] Autopsy studies, however, have suggested that there may be an association between senile cardiac amyloid and congestive heart failure or arrhythmias.[101–103]

Three distinct forms of senile cardiac amyloidosis cannot be differentiated by light or electron microscopy but can be by immunohistochemical techniques. Isolated atrial amyloid is characterized by local deposits in the atria.[104] Aortic amyloid commonly affects the aorta of elderly patients.[105] Third, senile systemic amyloid involves the lungs, liver, and kidneys in addition to the heart.[106]

The primary structure of the amyloid fibril in senile systemic amyloidosis is similar to human prealbumin.[107] More significantly, antiserum to human prealbumin cross-reacts with the protein and has been used in autopsy studies to differentiate it from other forms of amyloidosis.[108,109]

Olson and colleagues[98] were the first to describe a clinical series of patients with prealbumin senile cardiac amyloidosis. Five patients with NYHA class III dyspnea and clinical evidence of congestive heart failure were described. Four patients underwent echocardiographic evaluation, and all had increased wall thickness and an ejection fraction of less than 40%. All five patients had cardiac catheterization; increased left ventricular diastolic pressures and global left ventricular hypokinesis were universally present. None of the patients had immunoglobulin light chains in serum or urine, and all had negative findings on bone marrow biopsy. The diagnosis was made only by use of immunohistochemical techniques on tissue from endomyocardial biopsy.

At follow-up, four or five patients were alive 12 to 38 months after diagnosis. In comparison, mean survival was 5 months for patients with primary systemic amyloidosis,[110] so that prealbumin senile cardiac amyloidosis appears to be a more benign disease.

## Other Entities

Several other entities may cause restrictive cardiac disease: hemochromatosis with excessive tissue iron deposition, which can result in restrictive or dilated cardiomyopathy and is important to recognize because its effects are potentially reversible;[111] sarcoidosis with multiple granulomas and subsequent scarring of the ventricle;[112] and storage abnormalities, including Gaucher's and Fabry's diseases.[113,114] Fortunately, the process appears to be reversible.[115] Specific data about these entities in elderly patients are unavailable.

# SUMMARY

Cardiomyopathies are an important cause of congestive heart failure in the elderly, and the magnitude of the problem is compounded by changing population demographics and the frequency of congestive heart failure in the elderly. Although the data are far from complete, differences in the clinical presentations and natural history of the cardiomyopathies in older and younger patients are becoming more clearly appreciated.

Dilated cardiomyopathy (DCM) is clearly more common than previously appreciated, and elderly patients have a worse prognosis than their younger counterparts with this disease. The medical management of DCM is often more difficult in the elderly, and the problem is compounded by the relatively infrequent use of cardiac transplantation as a therapeutic option.

Hypertrophic cardiomyopathy is also more common than previously appreciated, and changes in left ventricular structure often create difficulties in differentiating pathologic states from physiologic. Fortunately, the prognosis for HOCM is more favorable in the elderly than in younger patients and may be partly accounted for by the different structure of the left ventricle. If needed, surgery is an option for elderly patients with medically refractory HOCM, but particular attention must be paid to the presence and severity of associated cardiovascular disease.

Restrictive cardiomyopathy with diastolic dysfunction is increasingly recognized as a cause of congestive heart failure. The differentiation from systolic dysfunction is crucial, because the treatments are so markedly different. Age-related changes in diastolic function are becoming more apparent and better characterized, but standardization of age-related "normal" values is still not available. The diagnosis of restrictive heart disease should stimulate a search for an underlying cause, inasmuch as restrictive cardiomyopathy remains a diagnosis of exclusion.

Advances in noninvasive imaging have led to a resurgence of interest and have enhanced our knowledge of the cardiomyopathies. Further investigation should proceed in conjunction with studies aimed at defining the characteristics and variables of "normal" aging. For the present, the enigmatic, poorly identified "cardiomyopathies" remain a problem for both young and old.

# REFERENCES

1. Torp, A: Incidence of congestive cardiomyopathy. Postgrad Med J 54:435, 1978.
2. Dock, W: Cardiomyopathies of the senescent and senile. Cardiovasc Clin 4(1):361, 1972.
3. Segal, JP, Stapleton, JF, McClellan, JR, et al: Idiopathic cardiomyopathy: Clinical features, prognosis and therapy. Curr Probl Cardiol 3(6):1, 1978.
4. Bagger, JP, Baandrup, U, Rasmussen, K, et al: Cardiomyopathy in western Denmark. Br Heart J 52:327, 1984.
5. Codd, MB, Sugrue, DD, Gersh, BJ, et al: Epidemiology of idiopathic dilated and hypertrophic cardiomyopathy: A population-based study in Olmsted County, Minnesota, 1975–1984. Circulation 80:564, 1989.
6. Franciosa, JA, Wilen, M, Ziesche, S, et al: Survival in men with severe chronic left ventricular failure due to either coronary heart disease or idiopathic dilated cardiomyopathy. Am J Cardiol 51:831, 1983.
7. Unverferth, DV, Magorien, RD, Moeschberger, ML, et al: Factors influencing the one-year mortality of dilated cardiomyopathy. Am J Cardiol 54:147, 1984.
8. Fuster, V, Gersh, BJ, Giuliani, ER, et al: The natural history of idiopathic dilated cardiomyopathy. Am J Cardiol 47:525, 1981.
9. Kopecky, SL and Gersh, BJ: Dilated cardiomyopathy and myocarditis: Natural history, etiology, clinical manifestations, and management. Curr Probl Cardiol 12:569, 1987.
10. Sugrue, DD, Codd, MB, Melton, LJ, et al: The natural history of idiopathic dilated cardiomyopathy: A comparison of population-based and referred cohorts (abstract). Circulation 78(Suppl 2):II-585, 1988.
11. Dec, GW Jr, Palacios, IF, Fallon, JT, et al: Active myocarditis in the spectrum of acute dilated cardiomyopathies: Clinical features, histologic correlates, and clinical outcome. N Engl J Med 312:885, 1985.
12. Aretz, HT, Billingham, ME, Edwards, WD, et al: Myocarditis: A histopathologic definition and classification. Am J Cardiovasc Pathol 1:3, 1986.
13. Latham, RD, Mulrow, JP, Virmani, R, et al: Efficacy of prednisone therapy for new onset idiopathic dilated cardiomyopathy (abstract). J Am Coll Cardiol 9(Suppl):143A, 1987.
14. Parrillo, JE, Cunnion, RE, Epstein, SE, et al: A prospective, randomized, controlled trial of prednisone for dilated cardiomyopathy. N Engl J Med 321:1061, 1989.
15. Griepp, RB: A decade of human heart transplantation. Transplant Proc 11:285, 1980.
16. Kahan, BD: Immunosuppressive therapy with cyclosporine for cardiac transplantation. Circulation 75:40, 1987.
17. Dall, JLC: Digitalis intoxication in elderly patients. Lancet 1:194, 1965.
18. Vestal, RE: Drug use in the elderly: A review of problems and special considerations. Drugs 16:358, 1978.
19. Crooks, J, O'Malley, K, Stevenson, IH: Pharmacokinetics in the elderly. Clin Pharmacokinet 1:280, 1976.
20. Marcus, FI: Pharmacokinetic interactions between digoxin and other drugs. J Am Coll Cardiol 5:82A, 1985.
21. Kuhlmann, J and Marcin, S: Effects of verapamil on pharmacokinetics and pharmacodynamics of digitoxin in patients. Am Heart J 110:1245, 1985.
22. Moysey, JO, Jaggarao, NSV, Grundy, EN, et al: Amiodarone increases plasma digoxin concentrations. Br Med J 282:272, 1981.
23. Campbell, AJ, Reinken, J, Allan, BC, et al: Falls in old age: A study of frequency and related clinical factors. Age Ageing 10:264, 1981.
24. Gryfe, CI, Amies, A, Ashley, MJ: A longitudinal study of falls in an elderly population: I. Incidence and morbidity. Age Ageing 6:201, 1977.
25. Lipsitz, LA: Orthostatic hypotension in the elderly. N Engl J Med 321:952, 1989.
26. Feldman, RD, Limbirde, LE, Nadeau, J, et al: Alterations in leukocyte $\beta$-receptor affinity with aging: A potential explanation for altered $\beta$-adrenergic sensitivity in the elderly. N Engl J Med 310:815, 1984.
27. Stroke Prevention in Atrial Fibrillation Study Group Investigators: Preliminary report of the stroke prevention in atrial fibrillation study. N Engl J Med 322:863, 1989.
28. Levine, MN, Raskob, G, Hirsch, J: Hemorrhagic complications of long-term anticoagulant therapy. Chest 95(Suppl):26S, 1989.
29. Anderson, KP, Freedman, RA, Mason, JW: Sudden death in idiopathic dilated cardiomyopathy (editorial). Ann Intern Med 107:104, 1987.

30. Bigger, JT Jr: Why patients with congestive heart failure die: Arrhythmias and sudden cardiac death. Circulation 75(Suppl IV):IV-28, 1987.

31. Neri, R, Mestroni, L, Salvi, A, et al: Ventricular arrhythmias in dilated cardiomyopathy: Efficacy of amiodarone. Am Heart J 113:707, 1987.

32. Rae, AP, Spielman, SR, Kutalek, SP, et al: Electrophysiologic assessment of antiarrhythmic drug efficacy for ventricular tachyarrhythmias associated with dilated cardiomyopathy. Am J Cardiol 59:291, 1987.

33. Gonska, B-D, Bethge, K-P, Kreuzer, H: Programmed ventricular stimulation in coronary artery disease and dilated cardiomyopathy: Influence of the underlying heart disease on the results of electrophysiologic testing. Clin Cardiol 10:294, 1987.

34. Kron, J, Hart, M, Schual-Berke, S, et al: Idiopathic dilated cardiomyopathy: Role of programmed electrical stimulation and Holter monitoring in predicting those at risk of sudden death. Chest 93:85, 1988.

35. Milner, PG, Dimarco, JP, Lerman, BB: Electrophysiological evaluation of sustained ventricular tachyarrhythmias in idiopathic dilated cardiomyopathy. PACE 11:562, 1988.

36. Poll, DS, Marchlinski, FE, Buxton, AE, Josephson, ME: Usefulness of programmed stimulation in idiopathic dilated cardiomyopathy. Am J Cardiol 58:992, 1986.

37. McKenna, W, Deanfield, J, Faruqui, A, et al: Prognosis in hypertrophic cardiomyopathy: Role of age and clinical, electrocardiographic and hemodynamic features. Am J Cardiol 47:532, 1981.

38. Sanders, CA, Austen, WG, Jordan, JC, et al: Idiopathic hypertrophic subaortic stenosis in two elderly siblings. N Engl J Med 274:1254, 1966.

39. Shenoy, MM, Khanna, A, Nejat, M, et al: Hypertrophic cardiomyopathy in the elderly: A frequently misdiagnosed disease. Arch Intern Med 146:658, 1986.

40. Whiting, RB, Powell, WJ Jr, Dinsmore, RE, et al: Idiopathic hypertrophic subaortic stenosis in the elderly. N Engl J Med 285:196, 1971.

41. Petrin, TJ and Tavel, ME: Idiopathic hypertrophic subaortic stenosis as observed in a large community hospital: Relation to age and history of hypertension. J Am Geriatr Soc 27:43, 1979.

42. Lever, HM, Karam, RF, Currie, PJ, et al: Hypertrophic cardiomyopathy in the elderly: Distinctions from the young based on cardiac shape. Circulation 79:580, 1989.

43. Teare, D: Asymmetrical hypertrophy of the heart in young adults. Br Heart J 20:1, 1958.

44. Shapiro, LM and McKenna, WJ: Distribution of left ventricular hypertrophy in hypertrophic cardiomyopathy: A two-dimensional echocardiographic study. J Am Coll Cardiol 2:437, 1983.

45. Ciró, E, Nichols, PF III, Maron, BJ: Heterogeneous morphologic expression of genetically transmitted hypertrophic cardiomyopathy: Two-dimensional echocardiographic analysis. Circulation 67:1227, 1983.

46. Maron, BJ, Gottdiener, JS, Epstein, SE: Patterns and significance of distribution of left ventricular hypertrophy in hypertrophic cardiomyopathy: A wide angle, two dimensional echocardiographic study of 125 patients. Am J Cardiol 48:418, 1981.

47. Maron, BJ and Epstein, SE: Hypertrophic cardiomyopathy. Recent observations regarding the specificity of three hallmarks of the disease: Asymmetric septal hypertrophy, septal disorganization and systolic anterior motion of the anterior mitral leaflet. Am J Cardiol 45:141, 1980.

48. Wigle, ED, Sasson, Z, Henderson, MA, et al: Hypertrophic cardiomyopathy. The importance of the site and the extent of hypertrophy. A review. Prog Cardiovasc Dis 28:1, 1985.

49. Kitzman, DW, Scholz, DG, Hagen, PT, et al: Age-related changes in normal human hearts during the first 10 decades of life. Part II (Maturity): A quantitative anatomic study of 765 specimens from subjects 20 to 99 years old. Mayo Clin Proc 63:137, 1988.

50. Goor, D, Lillehei, CW, Edwards, JE: The "sigmoid septum": Variation in the contour of the left ventricular outlet. Am J Roentgenol Radiat Ther Nucl Med 107:366, 1969.

51. Brock, R: Functional obstruction of the left ventricle (acquired aortic subvalvar stenosis). Guy Hosp Rep 106:221, 1957.

52. Brock, R: Functional obstruction of the left ventricle (acquired aortic subvalvar stenosis). Guy Hosp Rep 108:126, 1959.

53. Topol, EJ, Traill, TA, Fortuin, NJ: Hypertensive hypertrophic cardiomyopathy of the elderly. N Engl J Med 312:277, 1985.

54. Pearson, AC, Gudipati, CV, Labovitz, AJ: Systolic and diastolic flow abnormalities in elderly patients with hypertensive hypertrophic cardiomyopathy. J Am Coll Cardiol 12:989, 1988.

55. Karam, R, Lever, HM, Healy, BP: Hypertensive hypertrophic cardiomyopathy or hypertrophic cardiomyopathy with hypertension?: A study of 78 patients. J Am Coll Cardiol 13:580, 1989.

56. Lewis, JF and Maron, BJ: Elderly patients with hypertrophic cardiomyopathy: A subset with distinctive left ventricular morphology and progressive clinical course late in life. J Am Coll Cardiol 13:36, 1989.

57. Wigle, ED: Hypertrophic cardiomyopathy: A 1987 viewpoint (editorial). Circulation 75:311, 1987.

58. McKenna, WJ, Goodwin, JF: The natural history of hypertrophic cardiomyopathy. Curr Probl Cardiol 6(4):1, 1981.

59. Spirito, P, Chiarella, F, Carratino, L, et al: Clinical course and prognosis of hypertrophic cardiomyopathy in an outpatient population. N Engl J Med 320:749, 1989.

60. Fay, WP, Taliercio, CP, Ilstrup, DM, et al: Natural history of hypertrophic cardiomyopathy in the elderly. J Am Coll Cardiol 16:821, 1990.

61. Savage, DD, Seides, SF, Maron, BJ, et al: Prevalence of arrhythmias during 24-hour electrocardiographic monitoring and exercise testing in patients with obstructive and nonobstructive hypertrophic cardiomyopathy. Circulation 59:866, 1979.

62. McKenna, WJ, England, D, Doi, YL, et al: Arrhythmia in hypertrophic cardiomyopathy. I: Influence on prognosis. Br Heart J 46:168, 1981.

63. Fananapazir, L, Tracy, CM, Leon, MB, et al: Electrophysiologic abnormalities in patients with hypertrophic cardiomyopathy: A consecutive analysis in 155 patients. Circulation 80:1259, 1989.

64. Maron, BJ, Roberts, WC, Epstein, SE: Sudden death in hypertrophic cardiomyopathy: A profile of 78 patients. Circulation 65:1388, 1982.

65. Kowey, PR, Eisenberg, R, Engel, TR: Sustained arrhythmias in hypertrophic obstructive cardiomyopathy. N Engl J Med 310:1566, 1984.

66. McKenna, WJ, Adams, KM, Poloniecki, JD, et al: Long term survival with amiodarone in patients with hypertrophic cardiomyopathy and ventricular tachycardia. Circulation 80(Suppl 2):II-7, 1989.

67. Kirklin, JW and Ellis, FH Jr: Surgical relief of diffuse subvalvular aortic stenosis. Circulation 24:739, 1961.

68. Morrow, AG: Hypertrophic subaortic stenosis: Operative methods utilized to relieve left ventricular outflow obstruction. J Thorac Cardiovasc Surg 76:423, 1978.

69. Maron, BJ, Merrill, WH, Freier, PA, et al: Long-term clinical course and symptomatic status of patients after operation for hypertrophic subaortic stenosis. Circulation 57:1205, 1978.

70. Maron, BJ, Koch, J-P, Kent, KM, et al: Results of surgery for idiopathic hypertrophic subaortic stenosis. J Cardiovasc Med 5:145, 1980.

71. Cooper, MM, McIntosh, CL, Tucker, E, et al: Operation for hypertrophic subaortic stenosis in the aged. Ann Thorac Surg 44:370, 1987.

72. Siegman, IL, Maron, BJ, Permut, LC, et al: Results of operation for coexistent obstructive hypertrophic cardiomyopathy and coronary artery disease. J Am Coll Cardiol 13:1527, 1989.

73. Mohr, R, Schaff, HV, Danielson, GK, et al: The outcome of surgical treatment of hypertrophic obstructive cardiomyopathy: Experience over 15 years. J Thorac Cardiovasc Surg 97:666, 1989.

74. Roberts, WC and Ferrans, VJ: Pathologic anatomy of the cardiomyopathies: Idiopathic dilated and hypertrophic types, infiltrative types, and endomyocardial disease with and without eosinophilia. Hum Pathol 6:287, 1975.

75. Edwards, WD: Cardiomyopathies. Hum Pathol 18:625, 1987.

76. Goodwin, JF: The frontiers of cardiomyopathy. Br Heart J 48:1, 1982.

77. Benotti, JR, Grossman, W, and Cohn, PF: Clinical profile of restrictive cardiomyopathy. Circulation 61:1206, 1980.

78. Nishimura, RA and Warnes, CA: Restrictive cardiomyopathy: Further understanding by Doppler echocardiography. Curr Opin Cardiol 4:396, 1989.

79. Chew, CYC, Ziady, GM, Raphael, MJ, et al: Primary restrictive cardiomyopathy: Non-tropical endomyocardial fibrosis and hypereosinophilic heart disease. Br Heart J 39:399, 1977.

80. Appleton, CP, Hatle, LK, Popp, RL: Demonstration of restrictive ventricular physiology by Doppler echocardiography. J Am Coll Cardiol 11:757, 1988.

81. Klein, AL, Oh, JK, Miller, FA, et al: Two-dimensional and Doppler echocardiographic assessment of infiltrative cardiomyopathy. J Am Soc Echocardiography 1:48, 1988.

82. Nishimura, RA, Housmans, PR, Hatle, LK, et al: Assessment of diastolic function of the heart: Background and current applications of Doppler echocardiography. Part I. Physiologic and pathophysiologic features. Mayo Clin Proc 64:71, 1989.

83. Nishimura, RA, Abel, MD, Hatle, LK, et al: Assessment of diastolic function of the heart: Back-

ground and current applications of Doppler echocardiography. Part II. Clinical studies. Mayo Clin Proc 64:181, 1989.

84. Klein, AL, Hatle, LK, Taliercio, CP, et al: Doppler diastolic filling variables predict outcome in cardiac amyloidosis (abstract). Circulation 78(Suppl 2):II-115, 1988.

85. Iskandrian, AS and Hakki, A-H: Age-related changes in left ventricular diastolic performance. Am Heart J 112:75, 1986.

86. Clements, IP, Sinak, LJ, Gibbons, RJ, et al: Determination of diastolic function by radionuclide ventriculography. Mayo Clin Proc 65:1007, 1990.

87. Dougherty, AH, Naccarelli, GV, Gray, EL, et al: Congestive heart failure with normal systolic function. Am J Cardiol 54:778, 1984.

88. Soufer, R, Wohlgelernter, D, Vita, NA, et al: Intact systolic left ventricular function in clinical congestive heart failure. Am J Cardiol 55:1032, 1985.

89. Gaasch, WH: Diastolic dysfunction of the left ventricle: Importance to the clinician. Adv Intern Med 35:311, 1990.

90. Setaro, JF, Schulman, DS, Black, HR, et al: Congestive heart failure and intact systolic function: Improvement in clinical status, diastolic filling, and exercise capacity with verapamil (abstract). Clin Res 36:316A, 1988.

91. Hess, OM, Murakami, T, Krayenbuehl, HP: Does verapamil improve left ventricular relaxation in patients with myocardial hypertrophy? Circulation 74:530, 1986.

92. Fouad, FM, Slominski, MJ, Tarazi, RC, et al: Alterations in left ventricular filling with beta-adrenergic blockade. Am J Cardiol 51:161, 1983.

93. Olsen, EG: Endomyocardial fibrosis and Löffler's endocarditis parietalis fibroplastica. Postgrad Med J 53:538, 1977.

94. Shaper, AG, Hutt, MSR, Coles, RM: Necropsy study of endomyocardial fibrosis and rheumatic heart disease in Uganda 1950–1965. Br Heart J 30:391, 1968.

95. Siegel, RJ, Shah, PK, Fishbein, MC: Idiopathic restrictive cardiomyopathy. Circulation 70:165, 1984.

96. Kyle, RA: Amyloidosis. Clin Haematol 11(1):151, 1982.

97. Glenner, GG: Amyloid deposits and amyloidosis: The $\beta$-fibrilloses (first of two parts). N Engl J Med 302:1283, 1980.

98. Olson, LJ, Gertz, MA, Edwards, WD, et al: Senile cardiac amyloidosis with myocardial dysfunction: Diagnosis by endomyocardial biopsy and immunohistochemistry. N Engl J Med 317:738, 1987.

99. Fogo, A and Virmani, R: Cardiac amyloidosis. Primary Cardiology 10:54, 1984.

100. Cornwell, GG III, Murdoch, WL, Kyle, RA, et al: Frequency and distribution of senile cardiovascular amyloid: A clinicopathologic correlation. Am J Med 75:618, 1983.

101. Pomerance, A: Senile cardiac amyloidosis. Br Heart J 27:711, 1965.

102. Hodkinson, HM and Pomerance, A: The clinical significance of senile cardiac amyloidosis: A prospective clinico-pathological study. Q J Med 46:381, 1977.

103. Smith, TJ, Kyle, RA, Lie, JT: Clinical significance of histopathologic patterns of cardiac amyloidosis. Mayo Clin Proc 59:547, 1984.

104. Westermark, P, Johansson, B, Natvig, JB: Senile cardiac amyloidosis: Evidence of two different amyloid substances in the ageing heart. Scand J Immunol 10:303, 1979.

105. Cornwell, GG III, Westermark, P, Murdoch, W, et al: Senile aortic amyloid: A third distinctive type of age-related cardiovascular amyloid. Am J Pathol 108:135, 1982.

106. Pitkänen, P, Westermark, P, Cornwell, GG III: Senile systemic amyloidosis. Am J Pathol 117:391, 1984.

107. Sletten, K, Westermark, P, Natvig, JB: Senile cardiac amyloidosis is related to prealbumin. Scand J Immunol 12:503, 1980.

108. Husby, G, Ranløv, PJ, Sletten, K, et al: The amyloid in familial amyloid cardiomyopathy of Danish origin is related to pre-albumin. Clin Exp Immunol 60:207, 1985.

109. Cornwell, GG III, Sletten, K, Olofsson, BO, et al: Prealbumin: Its association with amyloid. J Clin Pathol 40:226, 1987.

110. Cueto-Garcia, L, Reeder, GS, Kyle, RA, et al: Echocardiographic findings in systemic amyloidosis: Spectrum of cardiac involvement and relation to survival. J Am Coll Cardiol 6:737, 1985.

111. Olson, LJ, Edwards, WD, McCall, JT, et al: Cardiac iron deposition in idiopathic hemochromatosis: Histologic and analytic assessment of 14 hearts from autopsy. J Am Coll Cardiol 10:1239, 1987.

112. Swanton, RH: Sarcoidosis of the heart. Eur Heart J 9(Suppl G):169, 1988.

113. Goldman, ME, Cantor, R, Schwartz, MF, et al: Echocardiographic abnormalities and disease severity in Fabry's disease. J Am Coll Cardiol 7:1157, 1986.
114. Platzker, Y, Fisman, E-Z, Pines, A, et al: Unusual echocardiographic pattern in Gaucher's disease. Cardiology 72:144, 1985.
115. Young, JB, Leon, CA, Short, D III, et al: Evolution of hemodynamics after orthotopic heart and heart-lung transplantation: Early restrictive patterns persisting in occult fashion. Journal of Heart Transplantation 6:34, 1987.

# CHAPTER 10

# Congestive Heart Failure in the Elderly

*Dennis Tighe, MD*
*Albert N. Brest, MD*

The syndrome of congestive heart failure (CHF) is a major health issue in our aging population. The prevalence of heart failure rises exponentially with advancing age.[1-3] As of 1987, 12.2% of the American population (about 30 million persons) was older than 65 years. Those reaching this age could expect to live an average of another 16.9 years and, by the year 2030, it is estimated that one in four persons will be 65 years or older.[4] Because of physiologic effects of normal aging on all organ systems and the coexistence of other chronic systemic diseases, the diagnosis and treatment of CHF in the elderly can be difficult. This chapter will review key aspects of normal cardiovascular aging as well as the epidemiology, etiology, clinical presentation, and therapy of CHF in the elderly population.

## HUMAN AGING AND CARDIOVASCULAR FUNCTION

To understand the effect of disease processes on the cardiovascular system of elderly subjects, it is important to appreciate expected normal age-related changes. It is equally important to recognize that the elderly are a diverse population and the rate of decline of cardiovascular function with aging varies markedly among individuals.[5] In addition, studies evaluating normal aging also must take into account occult disease processes, such as coronary atherosclerosis, which have been noted to afflict a high percentage of elderly individuals in autopsy series. Asymptomatic ischemia may cause marked ventricular dysfunction, especially during stress. Accounting for differences in life style is also of paramount importance in understanding cardiovascular aging. In general, the level of habitual physical exercise declines with aging in unselected populations.[6] However, chronic exercise confers a training effect on the cardiovascular reserve such that peak cardiac output can differ as much as 75% in individuals leading an active, independent life style versus a sedentary condition. Against this background, physiologic and morphologic processes affecting the aging cardiovascular system will be summarized.

With advancing age, both *in vivo* and *in vitro* studies have documented an increase in arterial stiffness.[7] This increased stiffness appears to result from changes in the vascular media including a reduction in the amount of elastic tissue and an increase in collagen content and/or change in molecular structure.[5] As a result, the aortic wall becomes thickened and less distensible, leading in turn to a rise in arterial pulse pressure. To compensate for this loss of elasticity, the aorta undergoes progressive dilation and elongation (increased volume) to accommodate the ejected blood volume with less change in radius. Decreased diastolic recoil does not adequately sustain forward aortic blood flow in diastole and when coupled with a larger end-diastolic aortic blood volume, impedance to ventricular outflow is increased thereby resulting in myocardial hypertrophy as an adoptive mechanism.

Although resting left ventricular end-diastolic volume is not diminished in healthy individuals, diastolic filling patterns are altered with normal aging. Cardiac hypertrophy and an age-related reduction in left ventricular compliance contribute to a decreased rate of early diastolic filling.[7] As an adaptation, atrial systole contributes significantly to late diastolic ventricular filling, thus maintaining a normal end-diastolic volume albeit at the cost of a higher end-diastolic pressure.[5] Atrioventricular synchrony therefore becomes of paramount importance for the maintenance of cardiac output.

At rest, cardiac output and ejection fraction are maintained in healthy elderly individuals. However, cardiac output and stroke volume are variably affected by exercise depending upon the population studied. With progressive exercise, the maximal heart rate that can be achieved by elderly subjects is less than that in younger individuals. To maintain cardiac output, the elderly compensate via the Frank-Starling mechanism by an increase in left ventricular volume. Data on the change in ejection fraction during exercise in the elderly population are conflicting, with some studies indicating a reduction in ejection fraction related to aging itself. In subjects from the Baltimore Longitudinal Study of Aging, who were rigorously screened for occult cardiac disease, ejection fraction at maximal exercise did not decrease, but it also did not increase to the same extent as in a younger population.[8]

In addition to the aforementioned physiologic changes, a number of morphologic changes occur in the normal aging heart, some of which may mimic or even produce cardiac disease.[9,10] Myocardial changes include lipofuscin deposits, basophilic degeneration, and increased subepicardial fat. Focal amyloid deposition increases in incidence after the age of 60 years and generally is considered an incidental autopsy finding (involving the atria to a greater extent than the ventricles) although in some cases it may lead to significant myocardial dysfunction. Age-related changes in the conduction system include a decrease in the number of functioning sinus node cells along with connective tissue depositions in the node and fibrosis of the atrioventricular (A-V) node, His bundle, and bundle branches. Valvular involvement includes a high incidence of mitral annular calcification that may progress in some cases to cause mitral regurgitation, conduction defects, and, in rare instances, mitral stenosis. Calcific deposits frequently involve the bases of the aortic valve cusps and, if severe enough, can cause calcific aortic stenosis.

## EPIDEMIOLOGY OF CONGESTIVE HEART FAILURE

Congestive heart failure in the elderly is a common clinical syndrome associated with a poor prognosis. Numerous epidemiologic studies seem to confirm this impression, but on the whole they are plagued by a lack of consistent diagnostic criteria and a comprehensive follow-up evaluation. In 1971, a 16-year follow-up study was published that evaluated the natural history of CHF in 5192 patients in the Framingham Heart Study who were initially free of disease.[2] This study included specific criteria for a diagnosis of CHF and detailed follow-up at intervals of at least 2 years. One hundred forty two patients were classified as having acquired definite CHF—3.5% of the male population and 2.1% of females. Aging was strikingly associated with increased risk for heart failure—by the seventh decade the incidence of CHF among men was eight times that in the fifth decade. The Framingham investigators also noted that approximately 60% of those with new onset CHF had an underlying chronic disease or serious illness at the time of diagnosis. The 5-year mortality after the onset of CHF in men was 62% and in women 42% despite therapy.

In 1982, more than 1.5 million final hospital discharges with a diagnosis of CHF were made. Currently, it is estimated that approximately 3 million people have CHF in the United States (approximately 1% of the population).[11] Hospital figures from 1982 indicate that the rate of hospitalization in elderly patients for CHF approaches 20 per 1000 population.[1] Congestive heart failure is now the most common hospital discharge diagnosis among elderly patients.[11]

Prognosis in CHF is related clearly to the degree of underlying myocardial dysfunction. For those patients in New York Heart Association (NYHA) classes I to III, 1-year and 5-year mortality rates are approximately 25% and 52%. Patients with class IV NYHA heart failure have a grim prognosis, with a 1-year mortality rate of approximately 50%. In most series, 40% to 50% of deaths are noted to occur suddenly.[1]

## ETIOLOGY OF CONGESTIVE HEART FAILURE

The term *congestive heart failure* refers to a syndrome rather than a specific etiologic diagnosis. Congestive heart failure is the end result of a process in which there is a progressive and generally irreversible decline in intrinsic myocardial contractility. Numerous insults to the cardiovascular system such as pressure and/or volume overload, decreased intrinsic contractility, loss of heart muscle mass, and/or restriction of diastolic filling can all lead to the same clinical endpoint and are obvious causes of the syndrome of CHF.[12] As already noted, with normal aging there appears to be a loss of cardiovascular reserve especially with exercise. Also, in addition to specific cardiovascular pathology, one must remember that critical insults to other organ systems as well as other predisposing factors can place added burdens on the cardiovascular system and they too must be recognized for effective diagnosis and management.

In the elderly population, the most common causes of heart failure are coronary artery disease, hypertension, valvular heart disease, and cardiomyopathy. Until recently, hypertension was considered the dominant risk factor for the development of CHF because data from the Framingham Heart Study indicated that in up to 75% of cases this disorder preceded a diagnosis of cardiac failure.[2] Enhanced awareness and aggressive therapy have contributed to a decline in the relative incidence of this risk factor. Presently, the most important cause of heart failure in the elderly is ischemic heart disease.

Coronary artery disease has effects on both systolic and diastolic heart function. Myocardial infarction and subsequent scar formation leads to a loss of muscle mass and reduction in pumping capability and reserve capacity of the ventricle.[13]

A classic autopsy study of myocardial changes associated with cardiogenic shock has documented that loss of myocardium and subsequent decline in ventricular function is an additive process that is due to recent as well as remote infarctions, with a total loss of left ventricular myocardium > 40% producing the cardiogenic shock syndrome.[14] Ischemia without infarction also has important effects on left ventricular function. Ischemic muscle loses its ability to contract normally, thereby contributing to regional ventricular wall motion abnormalities and decreased cardiac output. In addition, ischemic muscle contributes to enhanced myocardial stiffness, necessitating elevated pressures to maintain left ventricular filling.[12] Fleg and colleagues[15] recently demonstrated in an asymptomatic population (mean age 60 years) that exercise-induced silent myocardial ischemia increases progressively with age and its presence identifies a subgroup of patients with a high risk of coronary events during a 5-year follow-up period.

Aneurysm formation is an additional mechanism by which coronary disease can contribute to the development of congestive failure. Because aneurysms exhibit paradoxic systolic expansion, they tend to trap a given volume of blood that cannot be ejected. Aneurysms also tend to increase ventricular size, thereby increasing ventricular wall stress.

Valvular heart disease is an important cause of CHF in the elderly.[16] The most common valvular lesion requiring valve replacement in the elderly population is severe calcific aortic stenosis. Pathologic studies have documented a distinct shift in the etiology of aortic stenosis. Formerly, postinflammatory (rheumatic) disease was considered the prime cause.[17] Currently, however, the majority of patients younger than 70 years old have calcification of a congenital bicuspid valve as the primary etiology and, among patients older than 70 years, degenerative calcification of a tricuspid aortic valve is the leading cause of aortic stenosis.[18] In a recent review, Lombard and Selzer[19] found in a primarily older population that 38.6% of patients with critical aortic stenosis present initially with symptoms of impending or overt left ventricular failure. Approximately 60% have concomitant coronary disease. Importantly, the physical examination is often atypical in the elderly population because the "classic" features of aortic stenosis often are not present.[19]

Abnormalities of the mitral valve apparatus involving the leaflets, annulus, chordae tendineae, and papillary muscles can cause mitral regurgitation on an acute or chronic basis, leading to left ventricular failure. Important causes of mitral regurgitation in the elderly include ischemic papillary muscle dysfunction and/or rupture, mitral annular calcification, myxomatous degeneration of the valve leaflets, and infective endocarditis.[16] Mitral stenosis is a less important cause of heart failure in the elderly because its primary cause is rheumatic heart disease, and this abnormality is usually manifest at a younger age. Rarely, severe mitral annular calcification may impede left ventricular filling.

Cardiomyopathic processes have been considered uncommon in the elderly population. It has been noted, however, that at least 10% of cases of idiopathic dilated cardiomyopathy in a number of large series occur in elderly patients.[20] If one includes the secondary causes of dilated cardiomyopathy such as alcohol abuse, chemotherapeutic drugs including anthracyclines, radiation toxicity, nutrition deficiencies, diabetes mellitus, and acute myocarditis, then this entity may be a major cause of heart failure in the elderly.[21] Restrictive (infiltrative) cardiomyopathies appear to be uncommon in the elderly but processes such as amyloidosis, hemochromatosis, sarcoidosis, and neoplastic infiltration should be considered, and differentiation from constrictive pericardial disease must be made.

Hypertrophic cardiomyopathy deserves special mention. For many years it was felt that this disorder is rare in the elderly.[22] Recent studies have documented that the diagnosis is frequently not suspected and potentially harmful medications are prescribed because of the mistaken impression that symptoms are due to systolic dysfunction.[23] Hypertensive hypertrophic cardiomyopathy of the elderly has been described by Topol and associates[24] as a syndrome including severe concentric cardiac hypertrophy, small left ventricular cavity, and supernormal indexes of systolic function in a cohort of hypertensive elderly patients presenting with signs and symptoms of pulmonary congestion. Echocardiography allows prompt recognition of this syndrome.

Congenital cardiac lesions such as atrial septal defect and patent ductus arteriosus can have long-lived natural histories and should be considered as causes of congestive failure in the elderly population given the appropriate clinical setting. In addition, some long-term survivors of corrective operations for congenital cardiac lesions are now entering the geriatric age group, and the problems related to these corrections likely will have an impact upon cardiac function.

Conduction disturbances as well as tachyarrhythmias and bradyarrhythmias are common and significant entities precipitating heart failure in the elderly population. Conduction disturbances can result from a number of disorders including myocardial infarction, fibrosis of the conduction system, calcification due to perivalvular deposits, loss of functioning nodal cells, and drug therapy administered for other conditions. Bradyarrhythmias, especially severe sinus bradycardia associated with the sick sinus node syndrome can be intermittent and can lead to repeated bouts of congestive failure. Tachyarrhythmias such as atrial fibrillation and atrial flutter are very common in the elderly, and the resultant loss of atrial contribution to ventricular filling can be a significant detriment.

Primary processes involving other organ systems but having a major secondary effect on a cardiovascular system with marginal reserve must be recognized. Important causes of high output cardiac failure such as anemia, nutrition deficiencies, Paget's disease of bone, A-V fistula, and febrile reactions due to infectious processes are common in the elderly population. Endocrinologic diseases, especially thyroid disease, may present atypically in the elderly. Hyperthyroidism has a high prevalence in the elderly and its presentation usually lacks the more classic findings noted in younger patients such as exophthalmos, heat intolerance, and increased appetite. In fact, atrial fibrillation due to hyperthyroidism occurs almost exclusively in the elderly population.[25] Many of these elderly patients present with an apathetic state. Hypothyroidism has been documented in up to 12% of elderly hospitalized patients.[26] Frequently, these patients present with nonspecific symptoms and the diagnosis is often overlooked.

Renal function declines with normal aging.[27] Disease processes affecting the kidney may speed this decline and contribute to excessive fluid and sodium retention. The inability of the kidney to handle the added sodium and volume load predisposes to pulmonary congestion. Physiologic and structural changes also take place in the lung with normal aging. Ventilatory function and diffusing capacity decline progressively after the age of 35 years. Pulmonary disorders such as chronic obstructive pulmonary disease, thromboembolism, fibrosis, and rarely primary pulmonary hypertension may have significant secondary effects on the myocardium with marginal reserve.[28]

The ability of medications to contribute to congestive failure must not be overlooked. Negative inotropic agents such as beta-blockers, calcium channel blockers,

and antiarrhythmic drugs may precipitate or exacerbate congestive failure. Nonsteroidal anti-inflammatory drugs are commonly prescribed to elderly patients and can contribute to renal dysfunction, sodium retention, and hypertension. In fact, elderly patients tend to come under the care of different specialists who sometimes prescribe a variety of medications that may cause deleterious cardiovascular effects. Medical noncompliance along with dietary excesses and substance abuse also must be explored and recognized in this population.

## CLINICAL PRESENTATION

As in the general population, the history and physical examination are of paramount importance in recognizing CHF in the elderly population and in discovering underlying cardiovascular pathology and precipitating causes. The most prominent manifestation of congestive failure is dyspnea, usually manifest initially with exertion and subsequently progressing to orthopnea, paroxysmal nocturnal dyspnea, and pulmonary edema. However, commonly dyspnea in the elderly also may be a manifestation of underlying pulmonary parenchymal or vascular disease and must be differentiated. Sodium and fluid retention, which present as weight gain, peripheral edema, nocturia, and symptoms referable to the gastrointestinal tract, are common in CHF, but these symptoms must be differentiated from underlying renal, hepatic, and gastrointestinal pathology. Neck vein distention often points to cardiac etiology in these cases, whereas isolated peripheral edema can be a manifestation of numerous noncardiac entities that are common in the elderly.[13]

Nonspecific symptoms such as fatigue, weakness, tachycardia, constipation, and cerebral symptoms may be presenting complaints of congestive failure in the elderly and they frequently draw attention away from the cardiovascular system. A recent study has revealed that among elderly patients admitted to a general medical service with acute confusion, CHF is frequently found as the precipitating event.[29] Thus, a high level of suspicion must be maintained to make the correct diagnosis under these circumstances.

Diagnostic studies to determine the etiology of congestive failure are similar to those used in a younger population and are guided by history, physical examination, and clinical suspicion. In general, one should not hesitate to recommend invasive diagnostic tests in the elderly population when they are the sole means to establish a firm diagnosis or to confirm suspicion based on noninvasive studies. This is especially true when crucial management decisions regarding invasive therapeutic procedures have to be made.

## MEDICAL MANAGEMENT OF CONGESTIVE HEART FAILURE

Appropriate management of the elderly patient with CHF begins with recognition of the underlying cardiac disorder and of any contributing extracardiac conditions, and their reversal to the extent possible. In addition, specific attention must be directed to the primary physiologic determinants of cardiac function, that is, heart rate, myocardial contractility, afterload, and preload. Although these determinants provide the means of compensation for the failing myocardium, it is also well recognized that they may have a significant detrimental effect when overcom-

pensation occurs. Improvement in cardiac performance can be achieved with specific interventions designed to reverse mechanisms of overcompensation.

Adjunctive therapy for CHF consists of nonpharmacologic therapies such as fluid and sodium restriction along with reduction of cardiac workload by restricting physical activity. When these means fail, specific drug therapy to counteract the detrimental effects of overcompensation of the primary determinants of cardiac performance is generally initiated.

Diuretic agents are of fundamental importance in congestive failure. Neurohormonal and hemodynamic effects on the kidney initiated by myocardial failure promote the retention of sodium and water, leading to extracellular fluid volume expansion. Subsequently, cardiac filling pressures rise, leading to cardiac dilatation and peripheral and central congestion. A number of classes of diuretic agents is available, each having specific actions on a particular segment of the nephron.

Thiazides and related agents act at the distal cortical diluting segment to induce natriuresis. They are the diuretic agents of choice in cardiac edema of mild-to-moderate severity, but are generally ineffective when the glomular filtration rate is < 30 ml/min. A major side effect, particularly in the elderly, is significant hypokalemia. It is very important to recognize and treat this disorder promptly as well as diuretic-induced hyponatremia.[30]

Potassium-sparing diuretics block exchange of sodium and potassium in the distal convoluted tubule and cortical collecting duct. In general, these agents are weak diuretics and when used alone are ineffective in the management of congestive failure. When used with thiazides or loop diuretics, however, the potassium-sparing agents enhance the effectiveness of the more potent diuretics and they reduce the likelihood of diuretic-induced hypokalemia. Conversely, in combination with angiotensin converting enzyme (ACE) inhibitors or in the presence of renal insufficiency, the potassium-sparing agents may lead to clinically significant hyperkalemia. Thus, serum potassium monitoring is important in all patients receiving diuretic therapy.

Loop diuretics inhibit sodium chloride reabsorption in the ascending limb of the loop of Henle and are capable of inducing a natriuresis of up to 20% of the filtered load of sodium.[31] These agents tend to be effective even in the presence of impaired renal function. Intravenous furosemide administration to patients with chronic heart failure has been documented to cause both a rise in venous capacitance decreasing preload and an increase in systemic vascular resistance that can lead to transient worsening of symptoms.[32] In general, loop diuretics are the agents of choice in congestive failure resistant to other diuretic agents, in renal insufficiency, and in acute pulmonary edema. Side effects include a blunted response with nonsteroidal anti-inflammatory drugs, ototoxicity, and the rare occurrence of sinus exit block or increased A-V block in the presence of underlying conduction disturbances.[33]

Digitalis glycosides are widely used in the treatment of CHF although their role in this disorder has been called into question. There is little controversy about using digitalis in patients with ventricular dysfunction and coexisting atrial fibrillation with a rapid ventricular response. In patients with mild congestive failure and normal sinus rhythm, digitalis preparations have been withdrawn without significant effect in some studies, but many of these studies have been noted to have serious deficiencies.[34] Lee and associates[35] compared the effects of oral digoxin and placebo in a group of outpatients in sinus rhythm with CHF in a randomized, double-blind,

crossover protocol. Those patients with more severe and chronic heart failure, ventricular dilatation, and a third heart sound derived a clinically significant benefit from digoxin therapy. A recent study from the Captopril Digoxin Multicenter Research Group comparing the effects of captopril and digoxin treatment in patients with mild-to-moderate heart failure on maintenance diuretic therapy has shown that captopril resulted in improved exercise time, improved NYHA classification, and decreased frequency of ventricular premature beats versus digoxin.[36] Digoxin treatment increased ejection fraction more than in the captopril-treated group. These data suggest that digoxin has benefits in patients with sinus rhythm and significant ventricular dysfunction, but it may be more appropriate to begin therapy with ACE inhibitors than with digoxin.

Digoxin has significant side effects and must be used cautiously in the elderly population. The major digoxin reservoir in the body is the skeletal muscle mass. In the elderly population, skeletal muscle mass is decreased and thus the volume of distribution of digoxin is reduced, contributing to a significant rise in serum digoxin levels. Approximately 70% of digoxin elimination occurs through the kidneys. A decline in renal function with aging is well documented and digoxin clearance from plasma may be decreased by as much as 40% in an elderly population in the absence of underlying renal disease. It is important to appreciate that in the elderly, a decline in muscle mass with aging may result in "normal" values for serum creatinine even when renal function is significantly impaired. Digoxin levels are also influenced by various drugs including quinidine, amiodarone, propafenone, and verapamil. It is extremely important therefore to monitor serum digoxin levels closely in the elderly population. Studies have shown that 5% to 7% of geriatric outpatients have evidence of digitalis toxicity; the side effects most frequently encountered are cardiac rhythm or conduction disturbances, visual changes, anorexia, nausea, and vomiting.[37] In the subset of patients with primarily diastolic myocardial dysfunction, digitalis may cause a worsening of clinical symptoms and should not be employed.

Vasodilator drugs can have profound effects in CHF because in this condition both venous and arterial beds are inappropriately constricted via neurohormonal mechanisms to provide compensation for the failing myocardium. Nitrates function primarily as venodilators thereby increasing venous capacitance and reducing central venous blood volume to decrease preload. Nitrates tend to be most effective in those patients with high filling pressures. Anticongestive therapy with nitrates is enhanced when combined with arteriolar vasodilators, as demonstrated in the Veterans Administration Cooperative Study.[38] Development of tolerance to long-acting nitrate preparations leads to an attenuated hemodynamic effect if a nitrate-free interval is not provided.[39]

Arteriolar vasodilators counteract the excessive increase in systemic vascular resistance that occurs as a compensatory mechanism in heart failure. The prototype drugs of this class are hydralazine and minoxidil. The Veterans Administration Cooperative Study evaluated the effects of vasodilator therapy on mortality in a group of men with impaired cardiac function and reduced exercise tolerance already receiving digoxin and diuretics. A beneficial effect on left ventricular function and mortality at 3 years was noted in the group of patients treated with hydralazine and nitrates as opposed to placebo- and prazosin-treated groups.[39] Of importance, side effects were common in the hydralazine-nitrate treatment group, with approximately 20% of patients discontinuing one or both medications; and by 6

months postrandomization only 55% of patients were taking full doses of both drugs. The main side effects of this class of agents include headache, tachycardia, edema, and gastrointestinal upset. As noted by Packer,[40] although arteriolar dilators increased cardiac output in six double-blind, placebo-controlled trials, these agents failed to alleviate symptoms or improve exercise tolerance in patients with chronic CHF.

Angiotensin converting enzyme inhibitors have emerged as the afterload-reducing agents of choice in the therapy of chronic CHF. Numerous studies have shown that ACE inhibitors have beneficial effects on exercise tolerance, NYHA class, and frequency of premature ventricular contractions.[36,41] The CONSENSUS trial studied the effect of enalapril versus placebo on mortality in a population of patients (NYHA class IV) with chronic heart failure receiving conventional medical therapy. This trial was concluded early because of a 31% reduction in mortality in the treated group at 1 year.[41] Drug-related hypotension in the elderly is a potentially serious problem because of the coexistence of cerebrovascular, coronary artery, and renal disease in this population. Hypotension is most frequently noted in patients who are hypovolemic, hyponatremic, or on diuretic therapy.[42] The decline in renal function associated with ACE inhibitors is likely due to significant reduction of the plasma level of angiotensin II with secondary reductions in efferent arteriolar tone.[43] Renal function can be expected to decline most in those patients with pre-existing renal dysfunction, dependence on angiotensin II for the maintenance of glomerular filtration rate, and intravascular volume depletion. Shorter-acting ACE inhibitors may be preferred in this situation. Other potentially serious side effects of ACE inhibitor therapy include bone marrow suppression, hyperkalemia, and angioedema.

Two recent studies have confirmed the role of ACE inhibition on survival in mild to moderate heart failure. Although these studies were not specifically performed in an elderly population, they have important therapeutic implications. The studies of left ventricular dysfunction (SOLVD) treatment trial enrolled patients with overt CHF primarily in NYHA functional classes II and III already taking drugs other than an ACE inhibitor as part of conventional CHF therapy. The investigators found that the addition of enalapril to conventional therapy as opposed to placebo reduced mortality by 16%, the largest reduction occurring in the deaths due to progressive CHF, and reduced recurrent hospitalization for CHF over a following period averaging 41.4 months.[44] The Veterans' Administration Cooperative Vasodilator—Heart Failure Trial II compared the effects of hydralazine and isosorbide dinitrate to enalapril in a cohort of men receiving digoxin and diuretics for mild to moderate CHF. A 28% reduction in mortality in the enalapril cohort as opposed to the hydralazine-isosorbide dinitrate group was noted 2 years postrandomization. The reduction in mortality was attributed to a reduction in sudden death and not to a reduction in progressive pump dysfunction.[45]

In patients with primarily diastolic heart dysfunction, digoxin and vasodilator agents potentially may have serious negative effects and should not be routinely used in this situation.[44] The drugs of choice in diastolic dysfunction appear to be calcium channel blockers and beta-blocking agents. Beta-blocker therapy with metoprolol has been shown to improve functional class, resting ejection fraction, and exercise capacity in a select group of patients with heart failure due to dilated cardiomyopathy.[45] However, in general, beta blockers and calcium antagonists are not routinely recommended but instead should be used cautiously with severe systolic dysfunction. In fact, data from the Multicenter Diltiazem Postinfarction Research Group showed that postinfarction patients with ejection fraction < 40% who received treatment with diltiazem were at increased risk of subsequently developing CHF.[46]

## INTERVENTION MANAGEMENT

Catheter interventions and cardiac surgery in the elderly are discussed elsewhere in this book. In general, age alone should not be considered a specific contraindication to intervention therapy. Cardiac catheterization is commonly performed with few added complications in elderly patients. Although the Coronary Artery Surgery Study registry and a recent study in a group of octogenarians have documented a higher incidence of left main and three-vessel coronary artery disease as compared with younger individuals, many elderly patients have lesions amenable to percutaneous transluminal coronary angioplasty (PTCA).[49,50] With recent technical advances and proper patient selection, the primary success rate of PTCA approaches that achieved in younger patients.[51,52]

In addition to noncardiac illnesses and underlying left ventricular function, age appears to be a significant predictor of both short-term and long-term outcome in cardiac surgical procedures. Edmunds and colleagues[53] reported on a large consecutive series of patients 80 years of age or older undergoing open-heart operations. Within 90 days of surgery, approximately 30% of patients had died, the majority of whom had severe cardiac disease, and almost another 30% experienced postoperative complications that extended their hospital stay. However, in those patients surviving and leaving the hospital, improvement in NYHA or Canadian Cardiovascular Society classification was sustained. Aortocoronary bypass grafting also has been shown to improve survival and symptomatic status in specific higher risk subsets of elderly patients in comparison with medical therapy alone.[54]

## SUMMARY

Congestive heart failure is in large part a disease of patients with advancing age. As our population ages, the incidence and prevalence of this disorder will continue to rise. The etiology of CHF in the elderly is multifactorial and one must take into account normal changes associated with aging, the heterogeneity of the elderly population, and possible noncardiac as well as cardiac disorders.

Therapy must be aimed at the primary pathophysiologic process affecting the heart. Despite a number of therapeutic advances with medical therapy, CHF usually signals a generally irreversible process with a high mortality, especially in those patients with advanced disease. Therefore preventive measures should assume a paramount role in this disorder. Modification of risk factors such as diabetes, smoking, obesity, sedentary life style, and hypercholesterolemia should be aggressively stressed and pursued in patients of all ages. These preventive measures may have a substantial impact on the incidence of CHF in the elderly.

## REFERENCES

1. McFate-Smith, W: Epidemiology of congestive heart failure. Am J Cardiol 55:3A–8A, 1985.
2. McKee, PA, Castelli, WP, McNamara, PM, et al: The natural history of congestive heart failure: The Framingham Study. N Engl J Med 285:1441–1446, 1971.

3. Sutton, GC: Epidemiologic aspects of heart failure. Am Heart J 120:1538–1540, 1990.

4. Butler, RN: The Challenge of Geriatric Medicine. In Wilson, JD, Braunwald, E, Isselbacher, KJ, et al (eds): Harrison's Principles of Internal Medicine, ed 12. McGraw-Hill, New York, 1991, p 16.

5. Lakatta, EG, Mitchell, JE, Pomerance, A, et al: Human Aging: Changes in Structure and Function. J Am Coll Cardiol 10:42A–47A, 1987.

6. McGardy, RB, Barrows, CH, Spanias, A, et al: Nutrient intakes and energy expenditure in men of different ages. J Gerontol 21:581–587, 1966.

7. Lakatta, EG and Gerstenblith, G: Alterations in Circulatory Function. In Hazzard, WR, Andres, R, Bierman, EL, et al (eds): Principles of Geriatric Medicine and Gerontology, ed 2. McGraw-Hill, New York, 1990, pp 445–457.

8. Gerstenblith, G, Frederiksen, J, Yin, FCP, et al: Echocardiographic assessment of a normal aging population. Circulation 56:273–278, 1977.

9. Rodehafles, RJ, Gerstenblith, G, Becker, LC, et al: Exercise Cardiac Output is Maintained with advancing age in healthy human subjects: Cardiac dilatation and increased stroke volume compensate for a diminished heart rate. Circulation 69:203–213, 1984.

10. Waller, BF: The old age heart: Normal aging changes which can produce or mimic cardiac disease. Clin Cardiol 11:513–517, 1988.

11. Parmley, WW: Pathophysiology and current therapy of congestive heart failure. J Am Coll Cardiol 13:721–785, 1989.

12. Parmley, WW: Pathophysiology of congestive heart failure. Am J Cardiol 55:9A–15A, 1985.

13. Wenger, NK, Franciosa, JA, and Wakes, UT: Heart failure. J Am Coll Cardiol 10:73–76A, 1987.

14. Page, DL, Caulfield, JB, Kastor, JA, et al: Myocardial changes associated with cardiogenic shock. N Engl J Med 285:133–137, 1971.

15. Fleg, JL, Gerstenblith, G, Zonderman, AB, et al: Prevalance and prognostic significance of exercise-induced silent myocardial ischemia detected by thallium scintigraphy and electrocardiography in asymptomatic volunteers. Circulation 81:428–436, 1990.

16. Rahimtoola, SH, Cheitlin, MD, Hutter, AM: Valvular and congenital heart disease. J Am Coll Cardiol 10:60A–62A, 1987.

17. Subramanian, R, Olson, LJ, Edwards, WD: Surgical pathology of pure aortic stenosis: A study of 374 cases. Mayo Clin Proc 59:683–690, 1984.

18. Passik, CS, Ackerman, DM, Pluth, JR, et al: Temporal changes in the causes of aortic stenosis: A surgical pathologic study of 646 cases. Mayo Clin Proc 62:119–123, 1987.

19. Lombard, JT and Selzer A: Valvular aortic stenosis: A clinical and hemodynamic profile of patients. Ann Intern Med 106:292–298, 1987.

20. Shah, PM, Abelmann, WM, Gersh, BJ: Cardiomyopathies in the elderly. J Am Coll Cardiol 10:77A–79A, 1987.

21. Johnson, RA and Palacios, I: Dilated cardiomyopathies of the adult. N Engl J Med 307:1051–1058 and 1119–1126, 1982.

22. Brest, AN: Heart failure in the elderly. Mt Sinai J Med (NY) 55:220–225, 1988.

23. Shenoy, MM, Khanna, A, Nejat, M, et al: Hypertrophic cardiomyopathy in the elderly: A frequently misdiagnosed disease. Arch Intern Med 146:658–661, 1986.

24. Topol, EJ, Traill, TA, Fortuin, NJ: Hypertensive hypertrophic cardiomyopathy of the elderly. N Engl J Med 312:277–283, 1985.

25. Gregerman, RI: Thyroid diseases. In Hazzard, WR, Andres, R, Bierman, EL, et al (eds): Principles of Geriatric Medicine and Gerontology, ed 2. McGraw-Hill, New York, 1990, pp 719–738.

26. Livingston, EH, Hershman, JM, Swain, CT, et al: Prevalence of thyroid disease and abnormal thyroid tests in older hospitalized and ambulatory persons. JAGS 35:109–114, 1987.

27. Rowe, JW, Andres, R, Tobin, JD, et al: The effect of age on creatinine clearance in men: A cross-sectional and longitudinal study. J Gerontol 31:155–163, 1976.

28. Burrows, B, Alpert, JS, Ross, JC: Pulmonary heart disease. J Am Coll Cardiol 10:63A–65A, 1987.

29. Rockwood, K: Acute confusion in elderly medical patients. JAGS 37:150–154, 1989.

30. Borland, C, Amadi, A, Murphy, P, et al: Biochemical and clinical correlates of diuretic therapy in the elderly. Age Aging 15:357–363, 1986.

31. Smith, TW, Braunwald, E, Kelly, RA: The management of heart failure. In Braunwald, E (ed): Heart Disease: A Textbook of Cardiovascular Medicine, ed 3. WB Saunders, Philadelphia, 1988, p 512.

32. Francis, GS, Siegel, RM, Goldsmith, SR, et al: Acute vasoconstrictor response to intravenous furo-
    semide in patients with chronic congestive heart failure. Ann Intern Med 103:1–6, 1985.
33. Smith, TW, Braunwald, E, Kelly, RA: The management of heart failure. In Braunwald, E (ed):
    Heart Disease: A Textbook of Cardiovascular Medicine, ed 3. WB Saunders, Philadelphia,
    1988, p 513.
34. Kimmelstiel, C and Benotti, JR: How effective is digitalis in the treatment of congestive heart fail-
    ure? Am Heart J 116:1063–1070, 1988.
35. Lee, DC, Johnson, RA, Bingham, JB, et al: Heart failure in outpatients: A randomized trial of
    digoxin versus placebo. N Engl J Med 306:699–705, 1982.
36. The Captopril-Digoxin Multicenter Research Group: Comparative effects of therapy with captopril
    and digoxin in patients with mild to moderate heart failure. J Am Med Assoc 259:539–544,
    1988.
37. Moosadian, AD, Grieff, VL, Bressler, R, et al: Digitalis in the elderly. JAGS 37:873–882, 1989.
38. Cohn, JW, Archibald, DG, Ziesche, S, et al: Effect of vasodilator therapy on mortality in chronic
    congestive heart failure: Results of a Veterans Administration Cooperative Study. N Engl J Med
    314:1547–1552, 1986.
39. Jordan, RA, Seth, L, Casebott, P, et al: Rapidly developing tolerance to transdermal nitroglycerin
    in congestive heart failure. Ann Intern Med 104:295–298, 1986.
40. Packer, M: Vasodilator and inotropic drugs for the treatment of chronic heart failure: Distinguishing
    hype from hope. J Am Coll Cardiol 12:1299–1317, 1988.
41. The CONSENSUS Trial Study Group: Effects of enalapril on mortality in severe congestive heart
    failure. N Engl J Med 315:1429–1435, 1987.
42. Reid, JL: Angiotensin-converting enzyme inhibitors in the elderly. Br Med J 295:943–944, 1987.
43. Suki, WN: Renal hemodynamic consequences of angiotensin-converting enzyme inhibition in con-
    gestive heart failure. J Am Med Assoc 149:669–673, 1989.
44. The SOLVD Investigators: Effect of enalapril on survival in patients with reduced left ventricular
    ejection fractions and congestive heart failure. N Engl J Med 325:293, 1991.
45. Cohn, J, Johnson, G, Ziesche, S, et al: A comparison of enalapril with hydralazine-isosorbide dini-
    trate in the treatment of congestive heart failure. N Engl J Med 325:303, 1991.
46. Kessler, KM: Heart failure with normal systolic function (editorial). Arch Intern Med 148:2109–
    2111, 1988.
47. Engelmeier, RS, O'Connell, JB, Walsh, R, et al: Improvement in symptoms and exercise tolerance
    by metoprolol in patients with dilated cardiomyopathy: A double-blind, randomized, placebo-
    controlled trial. Circulation 72:536–540, 1985.
48. Goldstein, RE, Boccuzzi, SJ, Creiess, D, et al: Diltiazem increases late-onset congestive heart failure
    in post-infarction patients with early reduction in ejection fraction. Circulation 83:52–60, 1991.
49. Gersh, BJ, Kronmal RA, Frye, RL, et al: Coronary arteriography and coronary artery bypass sur-
    gery: Morbidity and mortality in patients 65 years or older: A report from the Coronary Artery
    Surgery Study. Circulation 67:483–491, 1983.
50. Kowalchuk, GJ, Siu, SC, Lewis, SM: Coronary artery disease in the octogenarian: Angiographic
    spectrum and suitability for revascularization. Am J Cardiol 66:1319–1323, 1990.
51. Kelsey, SF, Miller, DP, Holubkov, R, et al: Results of percutaneous transluminal coronary angio-
    plasty in patients 65 years of age (from the 1985 to 1986 National Heart, Lung, and Blood
    Institute's Coronary Angioplasty Registry). Am J Cardiol 66:1033–1038, 1990.
52. Jeroudi, MO, Kleiman, NS, Minor, ST, et al: Percutaneous transluminal coronary angioplasty in
    octogenarians. Ann Intern Med 113:423–428, 1990.
53. Edmunds, LH, Stephenson, LW, Edie, RN, et al: Open-heart surgery in octogenarians. N Engl J
    Med 319:131–135, 1988.
54. Gersh, BJ, Kronmal, RA, Schaff, HV, et al: Comparison of coronary artery bypass surgery and
    medical therapy in patients 65 years or older. A nonrandomized study from the Coronary
    Artery Surgery Study. N Engl J Med 313:217–224, 1985.

# CHAPTER 11

# Arrhythmias in the Elderly

*Seth J. Rials, MD, PhD*
*Roger A. Marinchak, MD*
*Peter R. Kowey, MD*

The increase in number of elderly persons in the population has made it necessary for the practicing physician to be familiar not only with their cardiovascular abnormalities but also with what constitutes a "normal" variation. The expected norms of the geriatric population are difficult to define, particularly because these patients may have a number of metabolic problems or receive a variety of cardioactive medications that predispose to, or may be mistaken for, a cardiac rhythm abnormality. An example of this problem is the widespread use of antihypertensive agents in the elderly, which may alter the ST segment and T wave by depleting potassium or may slow the heart rate by blocking beta-adrenergic receptors. These changes may prompt the unwary physician to make a diagnosis of ischemic heart disease or sinus node dysfunction when neither exists. The purpose of this chapter is to review pertinent information regarding cardiac arrhythmias in the elderly. We will first review what may be reasonably expected as normal variation in the two tests most frequently used to evaluate the elderly for arrhythmias—the electrocardiogram (ECG) and Holter monitor.

## ELECTROCARDIOGRAM

Electrocardiograms are frequently found to be "abnormal" in elderly patients.[1-4] Common abnormalities include (in decreasing order of frequency): left axis deviation, nonspecific ST-T wave changes, premature atrial depolarizations, PR prolongation, atrial fibrillation, and premature ventricular depolarizations.[1] For practical purposes, these findings, except for atrial fibrillation, have little prognostic importance when observed in the absence of structural heart disease. Conversely, ECGs with abnormalities suggestive of ischemic heart disease or left ventricular hypertrophy are associated with increased mortality in the aged.[2-4] Thus, it is the underlying heart disease and not the specific ECG abnormality that determines prognosis.

## HOLTER MONITOR

Ambulatory monitoring is frequently used to examine the nature and frequency of rhythm disturbances in the elderly. Studies of asymptomatic patients with no known structural heart disease have demonstrated a relatively high incidence (up to 40%) of sinus arrhythmia, supraventricular and ventricular premature beats, or supraventricular tachycardia in the elderly.[5-7] In one study, patients were followed for an average of more than 3 years and no correlation between asymptomatic atrial and ventricular ectopy and subsequent cardiac events was found.[8] In patients with structural heart disease, however, complex ventricular ectopy is associated with increased cardiac mortality.[9,10] All of these studies were limited by small size and by reliance on standard Holter techniques, which have recently been shown to be subject to considerable day-to-day variability.[11] As a result, the clinician must carefully establish the correlation between symptoms and rhythm abnormalities detected by Holter monitoring and then consider the presence or absence of structural heart disease before initiating therapeutic interventions.

## TACHYARRHYTHMIAS

Tacharrhythmias can be classified by mechanism and location.[12] A classification based on mechanism is summarized in Table 11-1. Although three basic etiologies for tachyarrhythmias are listed, some arrhythmias have more than one mechanism (e.g., ventricular tachycardia).

Increased automaticity, or the spontaneous activation of potentially excitable tissue, is best illustrated by sinus tachycardia and by ectopic atrial tachycardia. Arrhythmias due to increased automaticity are characterized by gradual onset and a gradual increase in rate. When termination occurs, it is also gradual. Re-entry arrhythmias require the presence of a relatively slow zone of conduction with critical timing of conduction and refractoriness. Re-entry rhythms are characterized by abrupt onset following premature beats and are usually regular. Common re-entrant rhythms in the elderly are atrial flutter and ventricular tachycardia. Triggered activity is a manifestation of abnormal automaticity and is thought to represent intracellular fluctuations of calcium current. Digitalis compounds, quinidine, and catecholamines have been shown to produce triggered activity *in vitro,* and this mechanism may be responsible for torsade de pointes and certain other

**Table 11-1.** Arrhythmia Classifications

| Automatic | Re-entrant | Chaotic/Triggered |
|---|---|---|
| Sinus tachycardia | Sinoatrial re-entrant tachycardia | Multifocal atrial tachycardia |
| Atrial tachycardia | Intra-atrial re-entrant tachycardia | Atrial fibrillation |
| Junctional tachycardia | A-V nodal re-entrant tachycardia | Ventricular tachycardia* |
| Ventricular tachycardia* | A-V reciprocating tachycardia | Torsade de pointes |
| | Atrial flutter | |
| | Ventricular tachycardia* | |

*Ventricular tachycardia can be due to any of these mechanisms, depending on the cause.
*Source:* From Marinchak, RA, et al: Common Clinical Challenges in Geriatrics, WB Saunders, Philadelphia, 1988, pp 83–110, with permission.

tachycardias. The comprehensive approach to diagnosis of supraventricular[12] and ventricular[13,14] tachyarrhythmias has been reviewed elsewhere and only those comments that are pertinent to the elderly will be mentioned here.

## SINUS TACHYCARDIA

Sinus tachycardia represents a physiologic response to a number of pathologic states, such as pain, fever, anemia, or dehydration, to which the elderly are particularly susceptible. Although very common, sinus tachycardia is frequently misdiagnosed due to a low index of suspicion coupled with difficulty in discerning P waves during ventricular repolarization (P in the T wave). Treatment should be directed at correcting the underlying pathologic state.

## ATRIAL TACHYCARDIA

As previously stated, atrial premature depolarizations are relatively common in clinical practice and almost never require therapy. Paroxysms of atrial tachycardia are less common, and sustained atrial tachycardia outside of the setting of digitalis toxicity is rare, especially in the elderly. Nonetheless, because of their altered renal function, the elderly are very susceptible to digitalis-related automatic atrial tachycardias (also known as paroxysmal atrial tachycardia with block). Treatment consists of drug withdrawal.

## JUNCTIONAL TACHYCARDIA

Tachycardias caused by enhanced automaticity of the atrioventricular (A-V) nodal tissue and proximal His bundle are not an unusual event in the geriatric population, again because digitalis excess is a common problem.[15] Junctional tachycardia can be recognized by a moderate rate (90 to 110 beats/min) and inverted P waves appearing in close proximity to or within the QRS complex. As with other digitalis-related rhythms, treatment usually consists of drug withdrawal only.

## SINOATRIAL AND INTRA-ATRIAL RE-ENTRANT TACHYCARDIA

Re-entry within the perisinus tissue or the specialized atrial tracts that conduct impulses from the atrium to the ventricle is relatively uncommon in clinical practice and is especially uncommon in the elderly. Criteria for diagnosis, such as abrupt initiation and termination of a heart rate (usually 140 to 160 beats/min), and P-wave location (PR < RP interval) should be recognized so that sinoatrial and intra-atrial re-entrant tachycardias are not confused with automatic rhythms. Because the sinus node is largely comprised of cells with slow conduction properties, sinoatrial re-entry can be treated with beta blockers or calcium channel blocking drugs, if treatment is necessary at all. Furthermore, the tendency of these medications to exacerbate sinus node dysfunction should be considered before initiation of therapy. Intra-atrial re-entry may be treated with type 1A antiarrhythmics, which have been shown to be useful in other re-entrant arrhythmias such as atrial flutter. Data to support their use for intra-atrial re-entrant tachycardia, however, are limited.[16,17]

## A-V Nodal Re-entrant Tachycardia

A-V node re-entry tachycardia is the most common form of re-entrant supra-ventricular tachycardia in the general population. A large but imprecisely quanti-fied number of individuals exhibit dual pathways within the A-V node that have physiologically distinct properties of conduction and refractoriness. This configu-ration provides an ideal setting for initiation of a re-entrant arrhythmia. A-V node re-entry is usually initiated by a premature impulse that arrives at the A-V node when one of the pathways is refractory, conducts down the other pathway, then continues in a circus movement between the two pathways with antegrade activa-tion of the ventricles over the His bundle and retrograde activation of the atria. Because the atria and ventricles are activated nearly simultaneously, P waves may not be identifiable or, if seen, will generally be inverted and inscribed on the J point of the QRS-ST segment (Fig. 11–1). The arrhythmia characteristically is abrupt in onset, has a rate of 140 to 160 beats/min, and is fairly well tolerated. Because the re-entry circuit consists largely of A-V nodal tissue, any maneuver that alters con-

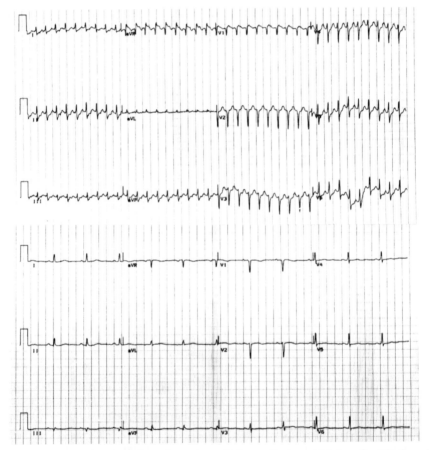

**Figure 11–1.** *Top panel*—Narrow complex tachycardia in a patient complaining of palpitations. Ret-rograde P waves can be seen in leads III, AVF, and $V_1$ immediately after the QRS (short RP), most consistent with A-V node reentrant tachycardia. *Bottom panel*—Sinus rhythm was restored after ter-mination of the tachycardia by adenosine.

duction and/or refractoriness in the A-V nodal pathways (the list is extensive) may be expected to be effective in terminating or preventing the tachycardia.[12]

## A-V Reciprocating Tachycardia

A-V reciprocating tachycardias represent a well-studied example of macro re-entry in which an accessory pathway between the atrium and ventricle participates in a circus-movement tachycardia. It is an arrhythmia that is generally diagnosed in younger individuals and usually is not of critical importance in the geriatric population. It is not clear why the arrhythmia is encountered so infrequently in the elderly but it may be attributable to either poor survival or to fibrotic degeneration of the accessory pathway occurring with age. Nevertheless, an occasional older patient will present with arrhythmias and a functioning accessory pathway.

The most common form of A-V reciprocating tachycardia is orthodromic, in which the impulse conducts antegrade over the A-V node and His-Purkinje system and retrograde over the bypass tract. This form of reciprocating tachycardia is characterized by a narrow complex QRS and a long RP interval. Because the A-V node is a requisite part of the re-entrant pathway, any intervention that increases refractoriness in the A-V node may be effective in terminating the tachycardia.[12] The post-termination ECG should reveal evidence of pre-excitation unless a retrograde-only (concealed) conducting bypass tract exists.

Antidromic A-V reciprocating tachycardia is characterized by a wide complex regular tachycardia that can be difficult to differentiate from ventricular tachycardia. Correct diagnosis is critical inasmuch as drugs such as digitalis and verapamil, which might be otherwise effective in altering A-V nodal conduction, have unpredictable effects on accessory pathway tissue, may facilitate antegrade A-V conduction of atrial fibrillation, and are useless for the treatment of ventricular tachycardia.

## Atrial Flutter

Atrial flutter is usually encountered in the setting of organic heart disease. It is characterized by the classic "saw-tooth" pattern of the baseline in the inferior leads, an atrial rate approximating 300 beats/min, and a proportionate ventricular response (usually 150 beats/min). Recent evidence has demonstrated that atrial flutter is a macro re-entrant arrhythmia located in part or totally within the right atrium.[18,19] Treatment consists of controlling the ventricular response followed by attempts to convert the rhythm to normal sinus. Conversion can usually be accomplished with class 1 antiarrhythmics, electrical cardioversion, or with rapid atrial pacing. A flutter rate slower than 300 beats/min or a ratio of atrial to ventricular impulses of greater than 2:1 in the absence of drug therapy implies a diseased conduction system with the risk of symptomatic bradycardia or heart block at the time of conversion.

## Atrial Fibrillation

Atrial fibrillation is extremely common in the elderly and is associated with a number of underlying diseases including coronary artery, hypertensive, valvular, and thyroid disease. Atrial fibrillation can also occur in the absence of overt struc-

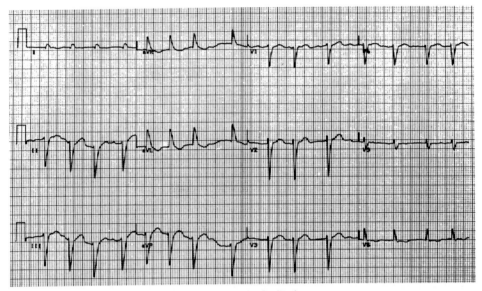

**Figure 11-2.** Atrial fibrillation.

tural heart disease and is then considered "lone" atrial fibrillation. The incidence of atrial fibrillation increases with age and is prevalent in 2% to 4% of patients older than the age of 60.[20-22] Mortality from atrial fibrillation is due in part to the underlying disease process and in part from systemic embolization, the risk of embolization being present regardless of the type of underlying disease process.[23-26]

Atrial fibrillation is relatively easy to diagnose with the ECG. It is characterized by an undulating baseline, lack of identifiable P wave, and irregular ventricular response (Fig. 11-2). Because the elderly frequently have underlying heart disease, the loss of the atrial contribution to ventricular filling is more likely to produce symptoms or cause deterioration of clinical status.

Treatment of atrial fibrillation can be divided into two stages—management of ventricular rate and conversion to sinus rhythm. Early management should consist of controlling the ventricular response with A-V nodal blocking drugs (digitalis, beta blockers, calcium channel blockers) and treating any reversible conditions (ischemia, heart failure, thyroid disease) that may have initiated the arrhythmia. Subsequent management should consist of reversion to sinus rhythm. Conversion can be accomplished with either drug therapy using type 1 antiarrhythmics or with electrical cardioversion. Maintenance of sinus rhythm has traditionally been accomplished by continued therapy with type 1 antiarrhythmics. Recent evidence, however, has shown that although quinidine therapy is better than no antiarrhythmic therapy in maintaining sinus rhythm, patients treated with quinidine may experience an increased total mortality.[27] Whether similar results can be expected with other class 1 antiarrhythmics is unclear but this data should be given careful consideration before initiating drug therapy. Consideration also should be given to anticoagulation before cardioversion in those cases in which atrial fibrillation has persisted for more than 3 days or if the time of onset is unknown. Atrial fibrillation that is associated with a slow ventricular response in the absence of drug therapy represents a special problem in the elderly. Slow conduction of atrial impulses implies a diseased conduction system that may manifest with a prolonged period of asystole or high grade A-V block after cardioversion. Once recognized, this risk can be reduced by provision for temporary pacing at the time of cardioversion.

## MULTIFOCAL ATRIAL TACHYCARDIA

Multifocal atrial tachycardia is a chaotic rhythm characterized by the presence of at least three distinct P-wave morphologies, often with different PR intervals, and an irregular ventricular response with an average rate greater than 100 beats/min. It is encountered most commonly in elderly patients with acute noncardiac illnesses such as an exacerbation of chronic obstructive lung disease.[28] Clinical differentiation from atrial fibrillation is essential because beta blockade, verapamil,[29] or magnesium[30] are effective therapies, whereas administration of digitalis may increase automaticity further and aggravate the arrhythmia.

## VENTRICULAR TACHYCARDIA

The diagnosis of ventricular arrhythmia in the elderly is founded on the same principles as in younger patients. That is, the finding of a wide complex premature beat without antecedent P wave, perhaps followed by a compensatory pause, strongly suggests that the impulse arises from within the ventricle. Ventricular premature depolarizations are relatively common in the elderly[5-7] and when associated with organic heart disease are associated with an increase in mortality, especially if the ectopy is complex (paired or multiform ventricular premature depolarizations) or in the form of nonsustained ventricular tachycardia.[9,10] Nonetheless, drug therapy for asymptomatic ventricular ectopy, even in the setting of organic heart disease, is controversial at present, with reports of benefit,[31] no benefit,[32-35] or an increased mortality in those patients randomized to drug therapy.[36] Treatment of symptomatic ectopy is probably best limited to beta-blocker therapy because it may provide symptom relief at relatively low risk. Insufficient evidence is available to justify treatment of asymptomatic nonsustained ventricular tachycardia with conventional antiarrhythmic drugs, although randomized trials to address this issue are being initiated. Symptomatic nonsustained ventricular tachycardia is approached at most centers with drug therapy guided by electrophysiologic study.

Sustained ventricular tachycardia is commonly associated with underlying structural heart disease. Although there are several distinct types of ventricular tachycardia,[37] the most common form in elderly patients is monomorphic tachycardia as a result of ischemic heart disease. The management of ventricular tachycardia begins with an attempt to control the arrhythmia with drug therapy, usually guided by serial electrophysiologic study. As with other arrhythmias, however, drug therapy is often complicated by concomitant medical problems and altered drug metabolism. If the tachycardia is not controlled with drug therapy, the next step is usually implantation of an automatic defibrillator (AICD). Although expensive and invasive, AICDs are extremely effective in preventing death from malignant ventricular arrhythmia[38,39] and preliminary data suggest that elderly patients are not at increased risk of death or complication as a result of the implant procedure.[40] In selected patients who have failed drug therapy and are not candidates for implantable defibrillators, consideration can be given to surgery, although this approach is associated with significant morbidity and mortality, especially in the elderly.[41]

## BRADYARRHYTHMIAS

Bradyarrhythmias may result from either a decrease in spontaneous automaticity or from conduction block. Sinus node automaticity,[42-44] heart rate variability,[45,46] and maximal heart rate achieved during exercise,[46] decline with age. In addition, the aged are likely to have atherosclerotic coronary disease, which can affect arteries that supply critical portions of the conduction system. The elderly are sensitive to drugs that are used to treat an assortment of medical problems common to the aged but which also slow the heart rate. Thus, it is not surprising that most symptomatic bradyarrhythmias are found in the elderly.

### SINOATRIAL BLOCK

This is a relatively frequent arrhythmia in the elderly and is the result of failure of a sinus node impulse to propagate to the atrium. Sinus exit block is characterized on the ECG as intermittent interruption of sinus rhythm either abruptly (type II) or in a decremental fashion (type I).[47] The latter can be difficult to distinguish from sinus arrhythmia but should be suspected if P waves are grouped. Transient sinoatrial block is most commonly the result of digitalis toxicity. Chronic sinoatrial block is often part of the sick sinus syndrome,[48] which is discussed in greater detail below. If several sinus impulses are blocked and there is concomitant failure of subsidiary pacemakers, patients may become symptomatic and require pacing. However, a detailed drug history should be obtained before any pacing therapy is considered.

### ATRIOVENTRICULAR BLOCK

Impulses that arise in the atrium may block in several locations as they travel to the ventricle. First degree A-V block is manifest on the ECG as PR-interval prolongation. Second-degree A-V block may be decremental with a progressively increased PR interval and periodic dropped beats (Wenckebach or Mobitz I A-V block) or intermittent and not associated with antecedent increases in the PR interval (Mobitz II). Third-degree A-V block can occur in either the A-V node or below. If it occurs in the A-V node, a narrow QRS complex escape rhythm can be expected to emerge with a rate sufficient to maintain an adequate blood pressure. A-V block resulting from disease in the more distal conduction system usually produces a wide QRS complex, slow ventricular escape rhythm that is frequently symptomatic.

Causes of high grade A-V block (Mobitz II second-degree block and third-degree block) that are encountered almost exclusively in the elderly include Lev's disease,[49] Lenegre's disease,[50] and calcific degeneration resulting from mitral annular calcification or aortic stenosis.[51] Other causes that are not unique to the elderly include drug effect, acute myocardial infarction,[52] myocarditis, collagen vascular disease, and amyloidosis.[53] All forms of symptomatic A-V block, except those caused by drug effect, are treated with permanent pacing.

It is essential to differentiate complete heart block from A-V dissociation. The latter may occur when the ventricular rate exceeds the atrial rate. Supraventricular capture will occur if atrial depolarization occurs when the A-V node and His-Purkinje system are not refractory. Thus, some irregularity of an escape rhythm should alert the clinician to the possibility that block is not complete. Instead of pacing, causes for atrial slowing or ventricular acceleration should be sought.

## Bundle Branch Block

Inasmuch as idiopathic fibrosis and other diseases that affect the conduction system are common in the elderly, bundle branch block is not an unexpected finding. Fascicular block as well as left and right bundle branch blocks are more common with advancing age.[54] Although isolated left anterior fascicular block and right bundle branch block are benign entities, there is some evidence that the combination of the two implies structural heart disease and is associated with a worse prognosis. Similarly, left bundle branch block is associated with an excess incidence of coronary artery disease, even when observed in isolation.[55] Consequently, although bifascicular block does not necessarily mandate special care, elderly patients who have it require careful follow-up, because they may eventually manifest clinically significant heart disease.[56]

## Sinus Node Dysfunction

Sinus node dysfunction most commonly occurs in the elderly[48,57] and manifests as marked sinus bradycardia, sinus pauses or exit block, alternating periods of bradyarrhythmias and tachyarrhythmias (brady-tachy syndrome, Fig 11–3), or as a failure of sinus rate to rise appropriately with exercise (chronotropic incompetence). A variety of conditions are thought to contribute to the development of sinus node dysfunction including coronary artery disease,[58,59] fibrosis associated with aging,[60,61] hypervagatonia,[62] hypothyroidism, and cardioactive drugs. Because many of the ECG manifestations of sinus node dysfunction are found in the asymptomatic elderly, extreme care is necessary before attributing a patient's symptoms to sinus node disease.

Sinus node dysfunction is often associated with diffuse conduction system disease and atrial arrhythmias.[48,63] A recent literature review found that 16% of patients who presented without A-V block, subsequently developed A-V block during a mean follow-up of 34 months.[63] Atrial fibrillation was found at the time of diagnosis in 8% of patients, and subsequently developed in an additional 16% dur-

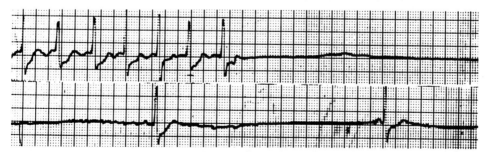

**Figure 11–3.** Episode of atrial fibrillation that terminates spontaneously and is followed by marked sinus bradycardia in a patient with brady-tachy syndrome.

ing 38 months of follow-up. Of particular importance in the management of these patients is evidence that permanent pacemakers that provide atrial demand pacing significantly diminish the incidence of atrial fibrillation—from 22% in patients with ventricular demand pacing, to 4% in patients with atrial demand pacing.[63] Atrial demand pacing appears to also diminish the incidence of systemic embolism compared with ventricular demand pacing,[63] probably as a result of the lower incidence of atrial fibrillation.

The presence of atrial tachyarrhythmias in patients with sinus node dysfunction often requires combination drug and pacemaker therapy. Indeed, in some patients who present with symptomatic tachyarrhythmias, bradyarrhythmias may not become manifest until antiarrhythmic therapy is initiated. Because of the evidence that patients with sinus node dysfunction have high incidences of atrial fibrillation and A-V block, and that atrial demand pacing diminishes the incidence of atrial fibrillation, we currently implant dual chamber pacemakers capable of independent atrial and ventricular demand pacing, that do not track atrial activity (DDI or DDIR mode) in these patients. The advantage of DDI pacing over standard dual chamber (DDD) pacing is that if (when) atrial fibrillation develops, the ventricular response is not excessive because the pacemaker does not track atrial activity. A more comprehensive description of cardiac pacemakers is available elsewhere.[64]

## ANTIARRHYTHMIC DRUG THERAPY

Antiarrhythmic drug therapy can be difficult in the geriatric patient. Low toxicity to therapeutic ratios for most agents results in narrow dosing ranges needed to achieve a desired effect without being either ineffective or causing adverse reactions related to excessive dosage. The importance of this small "margin of error" in dosing is magnified in the elderly by changes in vital organ function resulting from disease and aging that lead to altered pharmacokinetics and pharmacodynamics. Furthermore, the practice of polypharmacy in association with impairment of the patient's perceptive and cognitive abilities leads to an increased probability of adverse drug interactions, dosing errors, and noncompliance with therapy. This section will provide information pertaining to the use of antiarrhythmic drug therapy in the elderly in an attempt to assist the clinician in the management of serious or symptomatic arrhythmias while minimizing the probability of drug toxicity. Approved as well as investigational drugs will be discussed, with emphasis on specific adverse drug reactions likely to be encountered in the aged. A detailed description of the electrophysiologic actions, pharmacokinetics, specific indications, dosing recommendations, and side-effect profiles of each drug is available in more general references.[65,66]

### PHARMACOKINETIC ALTERATIONS

Pharmacokinetics deals with the study of the time course of drug bioavailability, distribution, metabolism, and elimination of the parent compound and its metabolites. These variables may be markedly influenced not only by specific disease states that are particularly prevalent in the elderly but also by normal age-related changes in physiology.

The amount of orally administered drug ultimately reaching the systemic circulation is determined by the amount absorbed from the gastrointestinal tract and the extent to which the drug undergoes first-pass hepatic metabolism. Orally administered antiarrhythmic drugs are primarily absorbed in the upper gastrointestinal tract. Absorption of most agents is virtually complete, except for amiodarone and sustained-release preparations of procainamide, quinidine, and disopyramide, with which as much as 50% of a dose may fail to be absorbed.[65] However, disease and age-related changes in gastrointestinal mucosal absorbing surface, blood flow, and motility may cause less efficient and unpredictable drug uptake. For example, aging has been associated with decreases in intestinal blood flow, the volume and acidity of gastric secretions, and gastrointestinal motility.[67] In addition, heart failure may result in decreased intestinal blood flow and mucosal edema secondary to systemic venous hypertension, which has been shown to decrease the absorption of quinidine[68] and probably affects the absorption of other medications.

The extent of hepatic first-pass metabolism also may markedly alter the bioavailability of some antiarrhythmic compounds. Lidocaine, propranolol, and verapamil undergo substantial degradation in the liver following absorption.[66,69,70] For verapamil, oral doses of up to 8 to 10 times the intravenous dose may be required to achieve equivalent plasma levels.[70]

Drug distribution is the movement of a drug from the systemic circulation to the tissues and is dependent on several factors including tissue perfusion, membrane permeability, and physiochemical properties of the drug, such as its lipid-water partition coefficient.[71] Antiarrhythmic drugs have their effect on specific target organs, and altered drug distribution may therefore markedly affect the elderly patient's responsiveness to a particular agent. Drug distribution is quantitatively expressed by its volume of distribution, which is the hypothetical volume into which a drug dose would have to be diluted to yield the observed plasma concentration.[66] This parameter is influenced by age-related changes in body composition, such as decreased total body weight with relative decreases in body muscle mass and water and relative increases in fat. Furthermore, distribution volume is inversely related to change in a drug's degree of plasma protein binding and directly related to the extent of tissue protein binding.[71]

Most antiarrhythmic drugs have large volumes of distribution, indicating that their tissue concentrations are higher than that of plasma.[66] Examples of altered volumes of distribution in the elderly are numerous. Age-related decreases in volume of distribution have been demonstrated for digoxin, lidocaine, and propranolol and have been attributed to decreases in body mass, particularly the percentage of muscle tissue.[71] Slight increases in the free fraction of phenytoin, which is highly bound to albumin, have been found to occur with age as a result of an increased volume of distribution.[72] In contrast, a marked decrease in the plasma-free fraction of disopyramide has been demonstrated to occur with aging because of increased binding to plasma alpha-1-acid glycoprotein, with a resultant reduction in volume of distribution.[73] Quinidine has been shown to increase plasma digoxin levels, in part as a result of its displacement of digoxin from tissue-binding sites, particularly in skeletal muscle, thus producing a decreased volume of distribution for digoxin.[66]

The liver is the major organ influencing antiarrhythmic drug metabolism. Changes in hepatic function with aging may have profound impact on the action and side effects of agents that undergo extensive hepatic degradation. Metabolites that are largely pharmacologically inactive (e.g., verapamil and lipid-soluble beta blockers) or active (e.g., lidocaine, quinidine, and encainide) may be produced.[65] Hepatic metabolism and clearance of drugs are directly influenced by liver blood flow, intrinsic liver enzyme activity, and the fraction of unbound drug in the plasma. Aging generally does not result in substantial declines in hepatic enzyme activity but may cause significant decreases in drug-plasma protein binding, which will lead to an increase in the fraction of circulating unbound drug available for hepatic metabolism. More importantly, substantial age-related declines in hepatic blood flow have been demonstrated.[71] Metabolism of drugs undergoing primarily function-limited hepatic clearance is markedly affected by change in intrinsic hepatic enzyme activity and the free fraction of drug in the plasma, but is minimally affected by liver blood flow. However, elimination of most antiarrhythmic drugs undergoing extensive hepatic clearance is not solely function limited because of marked affinities and large metabolizing capacities of the hepatic enzyme systems. An exception is phenytoin. Ninety percent of a dose of this drug undergoes hydroxylation in the liver by an enzyme system that frequently becomes saturated at plasma concentrations within the therapeutic range.[74] However, many antiarrhythmic agents (e.g., lidocaine, propranolol, and verapamil) are avidly metabolized by the liver as a result of extremely efficient enzyme activity and therefore have intrinsic hepatic clearances that far exceed hepatic blood flow. In these instances, drug clearance is strongly influenced by age-related and cardiac-disease–related reductions in hepatic blood flow.[71,75] Furthermore, agents such as propranolol may decrease their own hepatic clearance[76] and that of other agents whose clearances are flow limited by reducing cardiac output and hepatic blood flow. Between these two extremes are drugs whose hepatic clearance is importantly affected by all three factors (hepatic blood flow, intrinsic hepatic enzyme activity, and unbound plasma drug fraction), such as quinidine,[77] in which the effects of aging on drug clearance are more difficult to predict.

Antiarrhythmic drug elimination from the body is expressed in terms of total clearance, which represents the volume of blood completely cleared of drug per unit of time. Total drug clearance is primarily determined by the sum of renal and hepatic clearances. Most antiarrhythmic drugs at plasma concentrations in the therapeutic range are eliminated according to first-order kinetics. This means that the fraction of drug eliminated per unit of time remains constant. As a result, the elimination half-time (time required to halve the plasma concentration) remains constant and independent of the total body load. For drugs with first-order elimination kinetics, attainment of steady-state plasma concentrations with repetitive dosing and nearly complete elimination of drug from the body will occur within a time interval equal to four or five drug half-lives. Because the elimination half-life is directly dependent upon volume of distribution and is inversely proportional to total clearance, it can be readily appreciated how previously described age- and disease-related changes in these variables can markedly influence antiarrhythmic drug elimination.[66,71]

In contrast to intrinsic hepatic enzyme activity, renal function declines significantly in the elderly. Studies have demonstrated a 30% to 45% reduction in glomerular filtration rate and a 10% decline in renal blood flow per decade beginning, respectively, after the ages of 30 and 40 years.[76,77] Furthermore, this decrease in renal function may not be accurately reflected in the serum creatinine concentration because of age-related decreased muscle mass and creatinine production.[71] Virtually all antiarrhythmic agents rely on the kidney for elimination to some extent. However, when prescribing drugs for the elderly, particular care must be exercised when dosing with drugs that undergo primarily renal excretion, such as digoxin, procainamide, disopyramide, tocainide, bretylium, and lipid-insoluble beta blockers.[71] Although quinidine is primarily eliminated by the liver, up to 20% to 40% of a dose is excreted unchanged in the urine, which may result in dose-related side effects in the setting of severe renal dysfunction.[78] Furthermore, accumulation of antiarrhythmic drug metabolites undergoing renal excretion may be more apt to occur in the setting of age-related renal dysfunction, for example, N-acetylprocainamide metabolism.[79]

## PHARMACODYNAMIC ALTERATIONS

Alterations in organ function with aging may result in either increased or decreased sensitivity to an antiarrhythmic drug's biologic effect. In addition to the age-related changes in physiology described previously, adrenergic-receptor sensitivity is decreased, plasma norepinephrine levels are elevated,[80] baroreflex function is impaired,[81] and plasma renin activity decreases.[82] Cardiovascular disease resulting in decreased reserve is more prevalent,[65] as are other degenerative diseases related to aging that affect the central nervous, genitourinary, and gastrointestinal systems.

Examples of how these alterations in physiology may adversely influence antiarrhythmic drug pharmacodynamics in the aged are numerous. Verapamil, quinidine, and procainamide possess vasodilating activity and may be more likely to cause significant orthostatic hypotension. Agents that produce significant depression of myocardial contractility, such as disopyramide, beta blockers, verapamil, and flecainide, may precipitate symptomatic heart failure in elderly patients with depressed ventricular function and diminished cardiovascular reserve.[65,66] The increased prevalence of latent or overt sinus node and A-V conduction system abnormalities in elderly patients may result in significant bradyarrhythmias precipitated by agents such as digoxin, beta blockers, verapamil, amiodarone, and class I antiarrhythmic compounds.[65,83] Exacerbation or precipitation of ventricular tachyarrhythmias including torsade de pointes can result from therapy with class I agents, especially in the presence of hypokalemia and left ventricular dysfunction.[65,83] Older patients may be prone to obstructive uropathy, gastrointestinal hypomotility, and presbyopia when receiving agents possessing anticholinergic activity such as disopyramide.[83]

## ANTIARRHYTHMIC DRUG INTERACTIONS

Antiarrhythmic agents may interact with other drugs in ways that may potentiate or antagonize their biologic effects. This problem is particularly pronounced in elderly patients because of the increased incidence of concomitant diseases requiring therapy, polypharmacy, and age-related impairments in perception and cognition. Drug interactions may result from alterations in both pharmacokinetics and pharmacodynamics of the antiarrhythmic compound and other agents. Table 11–2 lists interactions occurring with commonly prescribed antiarrhythmic agents.[65,66,83]

In summary, it is clear that aging and associated diseases can influence antiarrhythmic drug pharmacology and increase the probability of untoward drug effects occurring primarily or resulting from interactions with other drugs. Once an arrhythmia has been identified and a decision made to treat, the metabolic and

**Table 11-2.** Drug Interactions Involving Major
Antiarrhythmic Agents

| Antiarrhythmic Drug | Interacting Agent | Interaction |
|---|---|---|
| Digoxin | Quinidine | Increased plasma digoxin concentration |
| | Amiodarone | Increased plasma digoxin concentration |
| | Verapamil | Increased plasma digoxin concentration |
| | Diuretics | Hypokalemia-induced potentiation of digitalis-induced arrhythmias |
| Verapamil | Beta blockers | Additive effects on depression of sinus node, A-V– conduction system, and left ventricular function |
| Amiodarone | Warfarin | Potentiation of warfarin anticoagulant effects |
| | Procainamide | Increased plasma procainamide concentration |
| | Quinidine | Increased plasma quinidine concentration |
| Lidocaine | Propranolol | Increased plasma lidocaine concentration |
| | Cimetidine | Increased plasma lidocaine concentration |
| | Phenobarbital | Decreased plasma lidocaine concentration |
| Quinidine | Warfarin | Potentiation of warfarin anticoagulant effects |
| | Phenobarbital | Decreased plasma quinidine concentration |
| | Phenytoin | Decreased plasma quinidine concentration |
| | Diuretics | Exacerbation of orthostatic hypotension: Potentiation of hypokalemia-induced arrhythmia, especially torsade de pointes |
| | Vasodilators | Exacerbation of orthostatic hypotension |
| | Tricyclic antidepressants | Exacerbation of orthostatic hypotension: Additive effects on depression of intraventricular conduction and proarrhythmia |
| Procainamide | Diuretics | Exacerbation of orthostatic hypotension: Potentiation of hypokalemia-induced arrhythmia, especially torsade de pointes |
| | Vasodilators | Exacerbation of orthostatic hypotension |
| | Tricyclic antidepressants | Exacerbation of orthostatic hypotension: Additive effects on depression of intraventricular conduction and proarrhythmia |
| Disopyramide | Anticholinergics | Additive anticholinergic side effects |
| | Diuretics | Potentiation of hypokalemia-induced arrhythmia, especially torsade de pointes |
| | Tricyclic antidepressants | Additive anticholinergic side effects; additive effects on depression of intraventricular conduction and proarrhythmia |
| | Verapamil, Beta-blockers | Exacerbation of heart failure |
| Flecainide | Verapamil, Beta-blockers | Exacerbation of heart failure |
| Bretylium | Vasodilators, diuretics | Exacerbation of orthostatic hypotension |
| Propranolol | Cimetidine | Increased plasma propranolol concentration |

*Source:* From Marinchak, RA, et al: Common Clinical Challenges in Geriatrics, WB Saunders, Philadelphia, 1988, pp 88–110, with permission.

physiologic status of the patient must be carefully assessed. As a general rule, it is prudent to initiate therapy at lower doses than those recommended for younger patients with gradual upward dose titration and careful monitoring of drug plasma levels and signs of the drug's biologic effects on the heart and other organ systems. In this manner, effective suppression of symptomatic or life-threatening arrhythmias will be facilitated while minimizing adverse reactions.

## PACEMAKER THERAPY

Cardiac pacemakers play an important role in the treatment of arrhythmias in elderly patients. Pacing can provide relief of symptoms such as syncope, presyncope, heart failure, and decreased exercise tolerance due to low cardiac output states. Furthermore, pacemaker therapy may be valuable in preventing bradycardia-related ventricular tachyarrhythmias (such as torsade de pointes) and in permitting the use of antiarrhythmic drug therapy that might otherwise exacerbate bradyarrhythmias. In selected instances, termination of supraventricular and ventricular tachyarrhythmias also may be accomplished with pacing techniques.[66] For a comprehensive review of cardiac pacing, the reader is referred elsewhere.[64]

Indications for cardiac pacing in the elderly do not differ from those in patients of younger age.[84] Although the anatomic site and cause of the cardiac abnormality leading to a bradyarrhythmia are important considerations, precise correlation of symptoms with a fall in heart rate is still of primary importance. Elderly patients may be more susceptible to symptoms resulting from bradyarrhythmias than are younger patients, because of diminished cardiovascular reserve and coexisting cerebrovascular disease. Furthermore, symptoms may be more subtle and easily overlooked because of noncardiac disease and age-related impairments in perception and cognition. An additional important consideration is the overall physical and mental state of the patient, including the presence of disease that may result in a poor long-term prognosis.

Cardiac pacing has been clearly documented to improve survival in patients with complete heart block and syncope.[85] Although symptoms related to bradycardia may be relieved, no similar improvements in survival with pacing have been conclusively demonstrated for patients suffering from sinus node dysfunction, bifascicular block in the absence of documented periods of complete heart block, advanced grades of A-V block associated with acute myocardial infarction, and carotid sinus hypersensitivity.[63,86-88] In these instances survival has been shown to be more strongly influenced by the presence of associated cardiac disease, particularly the extent of left ventricular dysfunction. Nevertheless, elderly patients with sinus node dysfunction are currently the most common group referred for cardiac pacing, with the intention of improving symptoms of bradycardia.[89]

The expansion of cardiac pacing technology also has resulted in more complex modalities of pacing. Single chamber ventricular demand units remain a mainstay of therapy. However, development of more sophisticated dual chamber units has permitted more hemodynamically advantageous pacing modalities to be prescribed for selected patients. Situations in which A-V synchronous pacing is clearly more appropriate include use in patients suffering from "pacemaker syndrome," defined as episodic weakness or syncope, inadequate cardiac output, and palpitations resulting from persistent A-V asynchrony or retrograde VA conduction during ventricular pacing. Another group of patients who might benefit from dual chamber pacing includes those patients with heart block and preserved sinus node function who manifest decreased exercise tolerance resulting from fixed-rate ventricular pacing. Recent improvements in design and programmability of dual chamber units and leads have greatly reduced the incidence of problems such as pacemaker-mediated tachycardia and atrial lead dislodgement. The presence of supraventricular tachycardias is a contraindication to DDD pacing. However, the development of the DDI mode of pacing has allowed the use of dual chamber pacing in those patients with transient supraventricular arrhythmias.[63] Development of single and dual chamber pacemakers that can appropriately increase pacing rate in response to sensed parameters that change with the need for alterations in cardiac output (e.g., body motion, minute ventilation, central venous temperature) has permitted rate-responsive pacing.[90]

Complications of cardiac pacing can result from failures of the pulse generator, pacing lead, or from patient-related factors. Pulse-generator malfunction is uncommon and present single chamber, fixed-rate units with lithium batteries have longevities of up to 10 years. A current problem with dual chamber, rate-responsive pacemakers, however, is decreased battery longevity. Lead failure is the most common problem encountered and can result from lead fracture, dislodgement, or insulation break. Patient-related factors include infection, pulse generator pocket migration or erosion, elevation of pacing threshold, transient loss of pacemaker sensing and capture, venous or intracardiac thrombosis and embolization, cardiac perforation, and inhibition of pacing due to sensing of external electromagnetic interference of skeletal myopotentials. "Twiddler's syndrome" also has been described in which manipulation of the implanted generator by the patient has resulted in lead fractures and pulse generator migration. An extensive review of complications related to cardiac pacing is available.[91]

## SUMMARY

The elderly patient is susceptible to a variety of cardiac rhythm disturbances that may or may not cause symptoms. It is incumbent on the physician who cares for geriatric patients to have a familiarity with the diagnostic criteria for each of these arrhythmias and with the drugs and devices that are used to treat them. This includes the potential adverse effects of therapy and methods to counter them. Even more important is a sense of when to intervene, which is based in part on a knowledge of "normal variation" in the aged.

## REFERENCES

1. Mihalic, MJ and Fisch, C: Electrocardiographic findings in the aged. Am Heart J 87:117, 1974.
2. Campbell, A, Caird, FI, and Jackson, TFM: Prevalence of abnormalities of electrocardiogram in old people. Br Heart J 36:1005, 1974.
3. Caird, FI, Campbell, A, Jackson, TFM: Significance of abnormalities of electrocardiogram in old people. Br Heart J 36:1012, 1974.
4. Rajala, S, Haavisto, M, Kaltiala, K, et al: ECG findings and survival in very old people. Eur Heart J 6:247, 1985.
5. Glasser, SP, Clark, PI, Applebaum, HJ: Occurrence of frequent complex arrhythmias detected by ambulatory monitoring: Findings in an apparently healthy asymptomatic elderly population. Chest 75:565, 1979.
6. Fleg, JL and Kennedy, HL: Cardiac arrhythmia in a healthy elderly population: Detection by 24-hour ambulatory electrocardiography. Chest 81:302, 1982.
7. Kanetlip, J, Sage, E, Duchene-Marullaz, P: Findings on ambulatory monitoring in subjects older than 80 years. Am J Cardiol 57:398, 1986.
8. Wajngarten, M, Grupi, C, Bellotti, GM, et al: Frequency and significance of cardiac rhythm disturbances in healthy elderly individuals. J Electrocardiol 23:171, 1990.
9. Aronow, WS, Epstein, S, Koenigsberg, M, et al: Usefulness of echocardiographic abnormal left ventricular ejection fraction, paroxysmal ventricular tachycardia, and complex ventricular arrhythmias in predicting new coronary events in patients over 62 years of age. Am J Cardiol 61:1349, 1988.
10. Aronow, WS, Epstein, S, Koenigsberg, M, et al: Usefulness of echocardiographic left ventricular

hypertrophy, ventricular tachycardia and complex ventricular arrhythmias in predicting ventricular fibrillation or sudden cardiac death in elderly patients. Am J Cardiol 62:1124, 1988.

11. Salerno, DM, Granrud, G, Hodges, H: Accuracy of commercial 24-hour electrocardiogram analyzers for quantitation of total and repetitive ventricular arrhythmias. Am J Cardiol 60:1299, 1987.

12. Marinchak, RA, Friehling, TD, Kowey, PR: A clinician's approach to diagnosing supraventricular tachycardia. Journal of Critical Illness 3:39, 1988.

13. Wellens, HJJ, Bar, FHM, Lie, KI: The value of the electrocardiogram in the differential diagnosis of a tachycardia with a widened QRS complex. Am J Med 64:27, 1978.

14. Massumi, RA, Tawakkol, AA, Kristin, AD: Reevaluation of electrocardiographic and bedside criteria for diagnosis of ventricular tachycardia. Circulation 36:628, 1967.

15. Dreifus, LS: Cardiac arrhythmias in the elderly. In Abrams, WB, Frohlich, ED (eds): Cardiology Clinics, Vol 4. Geriatric Cardiology. WB Saunders, Philadelphia, 1986, p 273.

16. Akhtar, M, Caracta, AR, Lau, SH, et al: Demonstration of intra-atrial conduction delay, block, gap and reentry: A report of two cases. Circulation 58:947, 1978.

17. Fisher, JD and Lehmann, MH: Marked intra-atrial conduction delay with split atrial electrograms: Substrate for reentrant supraventricular tachycardia. Am Heart J 111:781, 1986.

18. Waldo, AL: Mechanisms of atrial fibrillation, atrial flutter, and ectopic atrial tachycardia—A brief review. Circulation 75:III-37, 1987.

19. Olshansky, B, Okumura, K, Hess, PG, et al: Demonstration of an area of slow conduction in human atrial flutter. J Am Coll Cardiol 16:1639, 1990.

20. Ostrander, LD, Brandt, RL, Kjelsberg, MO, et al: Electrocardiographic findings among the adult population of a total natural community, Tecumseh, Michigan. Circulation 31:888, 1965.

21. Kannel, WB, Abbott, RD, Savage, DD, et al: Epidemiologic features of chronic atrial fibrillation: The Framingham Study. N Engl J Med 306:1018, 1982.

22. Lake, FR, McCall, MG, Cullen, KJ, et al: Atrial fibrillation and mortality in an elderly population. Aust NZ J Med 19:321, 1989.

23. Hinton, RC, Kistler, JP, Fallon, JT, et al: Influence of etiology of atrial fibrillation on incidence of systemic embolism. Am J Cardiol 40:509, 1977.

24. Brand, FN, Abbott, RD, Kannel, WP, et al: Characteristics and prognosis of lone atrial fibrillation: 30 year follow-up in the Framingham Study. JAMA 254:3449, 1985.

25. Treseder, AS, Sastry, BSD, Thomas TPL, et al: Atrial fibrillation and stroke in elderly hospitalized patients. Age Ageing 15:89, 1986.

26. Peterson, P and Godtfredsen, J: Atrial fibrillation—A review of course and prognosis. Acta Med Scand 216:5, 1984.

27. Coplen, SE, Antman, EM, Berlin, JA, et al: Efficacy and safety of quinidine therapy for maintenance of sinus rhythm after cardioversion: A meta-analysis of randomized control trials. Circulation 82:1106, 1990.

28. Shine, KI, Kastor, JA, Yurchak, PM: Multifocal atrial tachycardia: Clinical and electrocardiographic features in 32 patients. N Engl J Med 27:344, 1968.

29. Levine, JT, Michael, JR, Guarnieri, T: Treatment of multifocal atrial tachycardia with verapamil. N Engl J Med 312:21, 1985.

30. Iseri, LT, Fairshter, RD, Hardemann, JL, et al: Magnesium and potassium therapy in multifocal atrial tachycardia. Am Heart J 110:789, 1985.

31. Burkart, F, Pfisterer, M, Kiowski, W, et al: Effect of antiarrhythmic drug therapy on mortality in survivors of myocardial infarction with asymptomatic complex ventricular arrhythmias: Basel antiarrhythmic study of infarct survival (BASIS). J Am Coll Cardiol 16:1711, 1990.

32. Aronow, WS, Mercando, AD, Epstein, S, et al: Effect of quinidine or procainamide versus no antiarrhythmic drug on sudden cardiac death, total cardiac death, and total death in elderly patients with heart disease and complex ventricular arrhythmias. Am J Cardiol 66:423, 1990.

33. Furberg, CD: Effect of antiarrhythmic drugs on mortality after myocardial infarction. Am J Cardiol 32C-6C, 1983.

34. IMPACT Research Group: International mexiletine and placebo antiarrhythmic coronary trial: I. Report on arrhythmia and other findings. J Am Coll Cardiol 4:1148, 1984.

35. Gottlieb, SH, Achuff, SC, Mellits, D, et al: Prophylactic antiarrhythmic therapy of high-risk survivors of myocardial infarction: Lower mortality at 1 month but not at 1 year. Circulation 75:792, 1987.

36. Cardiac Arrhythmia Suppression Trial Investigators: Preliminary report: Effect of encainide and

flecainide on mortality in a randomized trial of arrhythmia suppression after myocardial infarction. N Engl J Med 321:406, 1989.

37. Akhtar, M: Clinical spectrum of ventricular tachycardia. Circulation 82:1561, 1990.

38. Mirowski, M: The automatic implantable cardioverter-defibrillator: An overview. J Am Coll Cardiol 6:461, 1985.

39. Guarnieri, T, Levine, JH, Griffith, LSC, et al: When "sudden cardiac death" is not so sudden: Lessons learned from the automatic implantable defibrillator. Am Heart J 115:205, 1988.

40. Thakur, RK, Tresch, DT, Troup, PJ, et al: Are automatic internal cardiac defibrillators justified in the elderly. Clinical Research 36:830A, 1988.

41. Cox, JL: Patient selection criteria and results of surgery for refractory ischemic ventricular tachycardia. Circulation 79:I-163, 1989.

42. Gelfand, ML: The octogenarian electrocardiogram. Geriatrics 12:156, 1957.

43. Agruss, NS, Rosin, EY, Adolph, RJ, et al: Significance of chronic sinus bradycardia in elderly people. Circulation 46:924, 1972.

44. Kirk, JE and Kvorning, SA: Sinus bradycardia: A clinical study of 518 consecutive cases. Acta Med Scand 266 (Suppl):625, 1952.

45. Camm, AJ, Evans, KE, Ward, DE, et al: The rhythm of the heart in active elderly subjects. Am Heart J 99:598, 1980.

46. Kostis, JB, Moreyra, AE, Amendo, MT, et al: The effect of age on heart rate in subjects free of heart disease. Circulation 65:141, 1982.

47. Chou, T: Electrocardiography in Clinical Practice, ed 2. WB Saunders, Philadelphia, 1986, pp 349–366.

48. Rubenstein, JJ, Schulman, CL, Yurchak, PM, et al: Clinical spectrum of the sick sinus syndrome. Circulation 46:5, 1972.

49. Lev, M: The pathology of complete atrioventricular block. Prog Cardiovasc Dis 6:317, 1964.

50. Lenegre, J: Etiology and pathology of bilateral bundle block in relation to complete heart block. Prog Cardiovasc Dis 6:409, 1964.

51. Nair, CK, Runco, V, Everson, GT, et al: Conduction defects and mitral annulus calcification. Br Heart J 44:162, 1980.

52. Norris, RM: Heart block in posterior and anterior myocardial infarction. Br Heart J 31:352, 1969.

53. Davies, MI, Anderson, RH, and Becker, AE: The Conduction System of the Heart. Butterworth & Co, London, 1983.

54. Ostrander, LD: Bundle branch block—An epidemiologic study. Circulation 30:872, 1964.

55. McAnulty, JH, Rahimtoola, SH, Murphy, E, et al: Natural history of "high risk" bundle branch block. N Engl J Med 307:138, 1982.

56. Edmonds, RE: An epidemiologic assessment of bundle branch block. Circulation 34:1081, 1966.

57. Hartel, G, and Talvensaari, T: Treatment of sinoatrial syndrome with permanent cardiac pacing in 90 patients. Acta Med Scand 198:341, 1975.

58. Bigger, JT, Jr and Reiffel, JA: Sick sinus syndrome. Annu Rev Med 30:91, 1979.

59. Chung, EK: Sick sinus syndrome: Current views. Mod Concepts Cardiovasc Dis 49:61, 1980.

60. Kaplan, BM, Langendorf, R, Lev, M, et al: Tachycardia-bradycardia syndrome (so called "sick sinus syndrome"). Am J Cardiol 26:497, 1973.

61. Rasmussen, K: Chronic sinus node disease: Natural course and indications for pacing. Eur Heart J 2:1455, 1981.

62. Jordan, JL, Yamaguchi, I, Mandel, WJ: Studies on the mechanism of sinus node dysfunction in the sick sinus syndrome. Circulation 57:217, 1978.

63. Sutton, R and Kenny, R: The natural history of sick sinus syndrome. PACE 9:1110, 1986.

64. Furman, S, Hayes, DL, Holmes, DR, Jr: A practice of Cardiac Pacing. Futura Publishing Co, Inc, Mount Kisco, NY, 1989.

65. Nestico, PF and Morganroth, J: Cardiac arrhythmias in the elderly: Antiarrhythmic drug treatment. In Abrams, WB and Frohlich, ED (eds): Cardiology Clinics, Vol 4. Geriatric Cardiology. WB Saunders, Philadelphia, 1986, p 285.

66. Zipes, DP: Management of cardiac arrhythmias: Pharmacological, electrical, and surgical techniques. In Braunwald, E (ed): Heart Disease: A Textbook of Cardiovascular Medicine, ed 3. WB Saunders, Philadelphia, 1988, p 621.

67. Crooks, J, O'Malley, K, and Stevenson, IH: Pharmacokinetics in the elderly. Clin Pharmacokinet 1:280, 1976.

68. Crouthamel, WG: The effect of congestive heart failure on quinidine pharmacokinetics. Am Heart J 90:335, 1975.

69. Evans, GH and Shand, DG: Disposition of propranolol. V. Drug accumulation and steady state concentrations during chronic oral administration in man. Clin Pharmacol Ther 14:487, 1973.
70. Schomerus, M, Spiegelhalder, B, Stieren, B, et al: The physiological disposition of verapamil in man. Cardiovasc Res 10:605, 1976.
71. Rocci, ML, Vlasses, PH, Abrams, WB: Geriatric clinical pharmacology. In Abrams, WB and Frohlich, ED (eds): Cardiology Clinics, Vol 4. Geriatric Cardiology. WB Saunders, Philadelphia, 1986, p 213.
72. Patterson, M, Heazelwood, R, Smithurst, B, et al: Plasma protein binding of phenytoin in the aged: In vivo studies. Br J Pharmacol 13:1321, 1984.
73. Hayler, AM and Holt, DW: Effect of age on plasma protein binding of disopyramide. In Proceedings of the BPS. January 5-7, 1983, p 605 P.
74. Bigger, JT, Jr: Management of arrhythmias: In Braunwald, E (ed): Heart Disease: A Textbook of Cardiovascular Medicine. WB Saunders, Philadelphia, 1980, p 717.
75. Castledon, CM and George, CF: The effect of aging on the hepatic clearance of propranolol. Br J Clin Pharmacol 7:49, 1979.
76. Rowe, JW, Andres, R, Tobin, JD, et al: The effect of age on creatinine clearance in man: A cross-sectional and longitudinal study. J Gerontol 31:155, 1976.
77. Wesson, LG, Jr: Renal hemodynamics in physiological states. In Wesson, LG (ed): Physiology of the Human Kidney. Grune & Stratton, New York, 1969, p 96.
78. Harrison, DC, Meffin, PJ, Winkle, RA: Clinical pharmacokinetics of antiarrhythmic drugs. Prog Cardiovasc Dis 20:217, 1977.
79. Drayer, DE, Lowenthal, DT, Woosley, RL, et al: Cumulation of N-acetyl-procainamide, an active metabolite of procainamide in patients with impaired renal function. Clin Pharmacol Ther 22:63, 1977.
80. Vestal, RE, Wood, AJJ, Shand, DG: Reduced beta-adrenoreceptor sensitivity in the elderly. Clin Pharmacol Ther 26:181, 1979.
81. Gribben, B, Pickering, TG, Sleight, P, et al: Effect of and high blood pressure on baroreflex sensitivity in man. Circ Res 29:424, 1971.
82. Weidmann, P, De Myttenaere-Bursztein, A, Maxwell, MH, et al: Effect of age on plasma renin and aldosterone in normal man. Kidney Int 8:325, 1975.
83. Harris, R: Cardiac arrhythmias. Clinical Geriatric Cardiology, ed 2. JB Lippincott, Philadelphia, 1986, p 408.
84. Frye, RI, Collins, JJ, De Sanctis, RW, et al: Guidelines for permanent cardiac pacemaker implantation. J Am Coll Cardiol 4:434, 1984.
85. Edhag, O and Swann, A: Prognosis of patients with complete heart block or arrhythmic syncope who were not treated with artificial pacemakers: A long-term follow-up study of 101 patients. Acta Med Scand 200:457, 1976.
86. Hindman, MC, Wagner, GS, JoRo, M, et al: The clinical significance of bundle branch block complicating acute myocardial infarction. 2. Indications for temporary and permanent pacemaker insertion. Circulation 58:689, 1978.
87. Peters, RW, Scheinman, MM, Modin, G, et al: Prophylactic permanent pacemakers for patients with chronic bundle branch block. Am J Med 66:978, 1979.
88. Ritter, WS, Atkins, JM, Blomqvist, CG, et al: Permanent pacing in patients with transient trifascicular block during acute myocardial infarction. Am J Cardiol 38:205, 1976.
89. Parsonnet, V, Crawford, C, and Bernstein, A: The 1981 United States survey of cardiac pacing practices. J Am Coll Cardiol 3:1321, 1984.
90. Humen, D, Kostuk, W, Klein, G: Activity-sensing rate-responsive pacing: Improvement in myocardial performance with exercise. PACE 8:52, 1985.
91. Mond, HG: Pacemaker Malfunction. Part II. The Cardiac Pacemaker, Function and Malfunction. Grune & Stratton, New York, 1983, p 259.

# PART 3

# Therapy Considerations

# CHAPTER 12

# Cardiovascular Drugs in the Elderly

*Stephen E. Borst, PhD*
*David T. Lowenthal, MD, PhD*

It is well known that the elderly population is rapidly increasing in developed countries (see Chapter 1, Demographics of Aging). In 1900, persons older than 65 years of age made up 4% of the U.S. population; currently, they comprise 12% of the population and this incidence is expected to reach 17% by the year 2020. Because the elderly have a large number of acute and chronic illnesses, they use a disproportionate share of drugs and medical services. The 12% of our population older than age 65 accounts for at least 25% of all drug expenditures.[1]

Cardiovascular disease is by far the greatest cause of morbidity and mortality in the elderly, and drugs with cardiovascular actions are the most widely prescribed. Of the 100 drugs most commonly prescribed for the elderly, 40 (including diuretics) are prescribed for their cardiovascular effects. The wise use of these agents in the elderly requires greater individualization of therapy than is usually needed in a younger population as well as knowledge of the effects of age and underlying disease on the pharmacokinetics, pharmacodynamics, and toxicity of these agents.

The incidence of adverse drug reactions is much higher in the elderly than in young adults.[2] *A number of factors contribute to this problem. Physiologic changes* that are part of normal aging result in altered distribution and disposition of many drugs. This in turn results in altered, usually, higher, plasma drug concentrations than for an equivalent dosage given to a 35-year-old patient. *Greater interindividual variability* in almost all physiologic parameters is a hallmark of aging. Therefore, even when the pharmacokinetics of a given drug are not significantly altered for the elderly population as a whole, certain individuals may be a greater risk for altered pharmacodynamic responses. *Polypharmacy* contributes to altered kinetic and dynamic effects. Elderly patients frequently receive a large number of medications, and thus the potential for drug interaction is increased. In addition, it is often more difficult in the elderly to identify the adverse effects of a drug because of the interaction of the underlying acute disease and the coexistence of multiple chronic diseases. A consequence of polypharmacy, expense of drugs, and multiple disease states is that *compliance* is often a major problem for the elderly. The elderly patient is, in general, more susceptible to adverse drug reactions because of *lower physiologic reserves.* Finally, a paucity of data exists regarding cardiovascular drugs in the elderly, more so from the lack of developmental research on pharmacodynamics than on pharmacokinetics.

## PHYSIOLOGIC CHANGES OCCURRING IN AGING

### CHANGES AFFECTING PHARMACOKINETICS

Pharmacokinetics may be defined as the sum total of what the body does to a drug, including absorption, distribution, metabolism, and elimination. A number of physiologic changes that occur as a part of normal aging result in altered drug kinetics. These changes have been well studied and the most important are summarized in Table 12–1. There is a decrease in lean body mass and an increase in fat. These changes result in an increased volume of distribution and lower initial plasma concentrations for lipophilic drugs (central alpha-agonists, antihypertensives, most beta blockers, tricyclic antidepressants). Conversely, because of a decrease in volume of distribution, higher initial plasma concentrations are encountered with hydrophilic drugs (aminoglycoside antibiotics, digoxin, angiotensin converting enzyme (ACE) inhibitors). An important example is the increased plasma levels of digoxin that occur because of a decrease in skeletal muscle, to which digoxin is avidly bound.[3]

There is a gradual decrease over the adult lifespan in glomerular filtration, renal plasma flow, and the total number of functioning nephrons.[4] Blood flow to the kidney is reduced 40% to 45% between the ages of 25 and 65.[5] As a result, the clearance of many drugs excreted by the kidney is impaired in the elderly patient. The major classes of these drugs are listed in Table 12–2. Reduced renal function in the elderly is not always reflected in an elevated serum creatinine because creatinine production from skeletal muscle is also reduced with age. A reasonable estimate of creatinine clearance may be made from the serum creatinine level using the following algorithm.[6] In women, multiply clearance by 0.85 to account for decreased body size.

$$\text{creatinine clearance in ml/min} = \frac{(140 - \text{age}) \times (\text{body weight in kg})}{72 \times \text{serum creatinine in mg/dl}}$$

**Table 12–1.** Physiologic Changes in Aging That Affect Drug Action

| Altered Parameter | Consequence |
|---|---|
| Decreased lean body mass | Decreased distribution of hydrophilic drugs |
| Increased body fat | Increased distribution of lipophilic drugs |
| Decreased renal function | Accumulation of renally cleared drugs |
| Decreased serum albumin | Decreased binding and increased free concentration of acidic drugs |
| Increased serum alpha-1 acid glycoprotein | Increased binding and decreased free concentration of basic drugs |
| Decreased liver metabolism | Accumulation of hepatically cleared drugs |
| Decreased cardiac reserve | Risk of heart failure |
| Decreased autonomic and baroreceptor function | Risk of postural hypotension |
| Multiple disease states | Risks associated with polypharmacy |

**Table 12–2.** Elimination of
Cardiovascular Drugs

| Primarily Renal | |
|---|---|
| digoxin | diuretics |
| disopyramide | procainamide |
| | ACE inhibitors |
| | (except |
| tocainide | fosinopril) |
| atenolol | nadolol |

| Primarily Hepatic | |
|---|---|
| lidocaine | propranolol |
| prazosin | verapamil |
| diltiazem | mexiletine |

| Mixed Renal and Hepatic | |
|---|---|
| quinidine | |

Changes in plasma protein binding of drugs are attributable to a decreased concentration or altered drug-binding affinity for plasma albumin or to an increased concentration of the actue phase reactant alpha-1 acid glycoprotein. Weak acids, such as salicylates, barbiturates, phenytoin, and theophylline, bind extensively to albumin. Reduced binding of these drugs in the elderly results in higher free-drug concentrations. Weak bases, such as propranolol, lidocaine, and disopyramide, bind to alpha-1 acid glycoprotein. In these cases, the free-drug concentrations may be reduced in the elderly.

In the liver, there is a decrease in hepatic blood flow with age and, in general, there is a decrease in the rate of many drug oxidation reactions (phase 1) with little change in drug conjugation reactions (phase 2). Commonly prescribed drugs that undergo hepatic excretion are listed in Table 12–2. A number of drugs can alter the metabolism of other drugs by inducing the hepatic cytochrome P450 drug oxidizing enzyme system. The major examples are listed in Table 12–3. The bioavailability of drugs showing high first pass extraction by the liver (propranolol, labetalol, lidocaine) is somewhat greater in the elderly. This occurs as a result of a

**Table 12–3.** Drugs Affecting Liver Metabolism

| Drug | Effect | Consequence |
|---|---|---|
| Rifampin | Induction of liver oxidizing | Decreased plasma concentrations |
| Barbiturates | enzymes | of hepatically metabolized |
| Phenytoin | | drugs |
| Disopyramide | | |
| Tobacco | | |
| Phenylbutazone | Inhibition of liver | Increased plasma concentrations |
| Cimetidine | oxidizing enzymes | of hepatically metabolized |
| Metronidazole | | drugs |
| Chloramphenicol | | |

reduction in their metabolism by the liver and does not appear to have long-term clinical significance.

### CHANGES AFFECTING PHARMACODYNAMICS

Pharmacodynamics may be defined as what the drug does to the body, that is, the action of a drug at its principal target(s). Compared with pharmacokinetic studies, there are far fewer examples on the effect of normal aging on pharmacodynamics, mainly because these changes are more difficult to study. Nevertheless, several significant changes have been identified.

There is, with age, a gradual loss in the elasticity of the arteries. The arterial tree becomes more like a system of rigid pipes in which the same cardiac output would result in higher systolic and lower diastolic pressure. This effect occurs principally in the inhabitants of developed nations and is manifested as hypertension (see Chapter 5, Hypertension in the Elderly) that is primarily systolic in type.[7,8] Inelasticity of the carotid sinuses and aortic arch arteries combine independently with hypertension to reduce the sensitivity of baroreceptors.[9,10] This change, together with documented reductions in sympathetic autonomic responsiveness, combine to put the older patient at greater risk for postural hypotension. Because a number of cardiovascular drugs can cause postural hypotension (see Table 12–4; prazosin, terazosin, nifedipine, methyldopa, diuretics) and because the elderly are predisposed to this condition for a variety of other reasons, the decision of whether to treat mild-to-moderate hypertension in an elderly patient must be made carefully. Postural hypotension produces increased incidence of falls in the elderly, resulting in morbidity and mortality[11] secondary to the complications of falling (e.g., hip fracture and subdural hematoma).

Reduced beta-adrenergic responsiveness is a general phenomenon of aging. In the heart, reductions occur in the inotropic and chronotropic responses to both circulating catecholamines and to norepinephrine released from sympathetic nerve terminals. The density of beta receptors in the heart is unchanged with age, but there is a reduction in the ability of beta-agonists to stimulate cyclic adenosine monophosphate generation, due both to reduced affinity of the receptor for the agonist and impairment of the catalytic subunit of adenylate cyclase.[12] The loss of beta-adrenergic responsiveness contributes to reduced cardiac reserve in the elderly. Beta receptors contribute to the normal postural hemodynamic response by

**Table 12–4.**
Drugs Causing
Postural
Hypotension

---

Beta blockers
Alpha blockers
   Prazosin, terazosin, doxazosin
Diuretics
Phenothiazines
Nifedipine
Methyldopa, l-dopa
Monoamine oxidase inhibitors
Quinidine

---

increasing cardiac output to counteract the fall in blood pressure that occurs after assuming upright posture. Thus, the reduced beta-adrenergic responsiveness in the elderly puts this group at further risk of postural hypotension. Finally, it would be predicted that if beta-adrenergic responsiveness is reduced with age, so should be the efficacy of beta-agonists and antagonists. However, the clinical significance of this contention remains controversial.[13,14]

The impairment that occurs with age in renal sympathetic innervation results in reduced activation of the renin-angiotensin system in response to the sensing of low blood pressure by the baroreceptor system or the sensing of volume contraction by the kidney or heart. The resulting increases in plasma renin activity and aldosterone concentrations are therefore blunted. The impaired secretion of aldosterone in the elderly results in potassium retention and can increase the vulnerability of the patient to hyperkalemia caused by beta blockers and ACE inhibitors.

## ADVERSE DRUG REACTIONS

Adverse drug reactions occur in 10% to 20% of the hospitalized elderly and account for 10% of medical admissions in this age group. The incidence of adverse drug reactions in the elderly is two to three times that observed in young adults.[15] Even this figure may be an underestimate, as adverse reactions are more difficult to distinguish from underlying disease in the elderly. Whether age, per se, contributes to adverse reactions is controversial. However, many of the major predictors of adverse reactions are closely associated with age including polypharmacy, greater severity of disease, reduced drug clearance, and previous drug reactions.

Postural hypotension (PH) is an important problem in the elderly and may be exacerbated by a number of cardiovascular drugs. Drugs commonly causing PH are listed in Table 12–4. These include alpha- and beta-blockers, diuretics, vasodilators, and calcium channel blockers.[16] Postural hypertension is present in 20% of the population aged 65 years or older (PH being defined as a drop, upon standing, in systolic blood pressure to 20 to 30 mmHg that is sustained for at least 1 to 2 minutes).[8] In those older than 75, the prevalence is 30% to 45%.[17,18] PH is an important cause of falls in the elderly, resulting in a serious morbidity. Contributing factors to PH include dehydration, diabetes and other diseases causing peripheral neuropathy as well as a number of drugs with cardiovascular indications.[19] Upright posture produces a pooling of blood in the lower body, which, if unopposed by autonomic responses, will result in hypotension. Increased heart rate and contraction of capacitance vessels in the lower body are major components of the postural hemodynamic response. These responses result from catecholamines released at sympathetic nerve terminals, mediated by beta-adrenergic receptors in the case of heart rate and alpha$_1$ adrenergic receptors in the case of contraction of capacitance vessels. Beta-adrenergic responses are decreased with age.[12] The resulting impairment of beta-adrenergically mediated reflex tachycardia is a contributing factor to PH. It is not clear whether decreased alpha$_1$ responsiveness contributes to the increased occurrence of PH in the elderly. This reduced responsiveness has been found to occur in some tissues and species, but not in others. However, Williams and coworkers[20] found that 83% of elderly subjects with PH experienced a fall in total peripheral resistance following upright tilting, indicating a probable decline in autonomic responsiveness. In either case, drugs that block alpha receptors have the potential to cause PH. Volume depletion as a result of diuretic therapy can be another mechanism of PH.

## CONSIDERATIONS FOR SPECIFIC CLASSES OF
## CARDIOVASCULAR DRUGS

Table 12–5 lists various cardiovascular drugs that exhibit age-related alterations in disposition or response.

### BETA-BLOCKERS

Beta blockers are chosen less frequently as a first-line drug for hypertension in the elderly[21] because of the belief that they are less efficacious in this group of patients. Their usefulness, at low dosages, as antianginal agents remains unchallenged. The rationale for a presumed reduction in the efficacy of beta-blockers is that beta-adrenergic responsiveness is reduced with aging and therefore there is less action for the beta-blocker to antagonize. Whether or not beta-blockers are actually less efficacious in the clinical setting is controversial.[22] Some studies have shown a reduced response[13] and others have shown no change.[14] Reduced clearance of beta-blockers in the elderly results in higher plasma concentrations, and this may offset the reduced efficacy. Clearance of the more hydrophilic beta-blockers (atenolol, nadolol) is less when glomerular filtration is reduced.[23] Clearance of the more lipophilic beta-blockers (propranolol) is less when liver function is reduced.[24] Plasma levels of propranolol following administration of the same dose are approximately double in the elderly population as compared with a young population (see Tables).

### CENTRAL ALPHA-AGONISTS

Central alpha-agonists (clonidine, methyldopa, guanfacine, and guanabenz) are used almost exclusively for treating hypertension (see Chapter 5, Hypertension in the Elderly). Methyldopa and guanabenz are eliminated primarily in the liver, clonidine by both the liver (30%) and kidney (70%), and guanfacine is mainly eliminated unchanged by the kidney.

As a class, these drugs are safe when given to the elderly, but drowsiness, dry mouth, and rapid return to baseline hypertension on cessation of clonidine may cause problems in the elderly. Transdermal clonidine lessens the likelihood for the rebound rise in blood pressure because of the residual depot of drug within the dermis. The central nervous system effects of central alpha-agonists may become exaggerated in a demented patient and, therefore, these highly lipid-soluble drugs need to be given with great caution to the elderly.

### ANGIOTENSIN CONVERTING ENZYME INHIBITORS

All ACE inhibitors are eliminated unchanged by the kidney. Lisinopril clearance is reduced with age as well as in cardiac failure.[25] Cilazapril is rapidly metabolized by nonspecific esterases to form the active metabolite cilazaprilat. Peak plasma concentrations of cilazaprilat following single-dose administration of cilazapril are only slightly elevated in the elderly compared with the young.[26] Plasma concentrations of cilazaprilat required for 90% inhibition of plasma ACE activity are the same in the young and the elderly.[26] Benazepril is metabolized somewhat more slowly to benazaprilat, so that both compounds contribute to ACE inhibition following benazepril administration. The clearance of benazepril is unaffected by

**Table 12–5.** Cardiovascular Drugs Exhibiting Age-Related Alterations in Disposition or Response

| Drug | Age-Related Factor | $V_d$ | $t_{1/2}$* | Cl | Comment |
|---|---|---|---|---|---|
| Digoxin | Renal clearance | ↓ | ↑ | ↓ | Reduce dosage and lengthen dosing interval. |
| Diuretics | Renal site of action<br>Renal clearance<br>Reduced effect | ND | ND | ND | Volume depletion, electrolyte imbalance ($K^+$↓, $Na^+$↓, $Mg^{++}$↓). |
| Lidocaine | Liver clearance | ↓ | ↑ | ↑ | Reduce dosage to avoid CNS toxicity. |
| Procainamide | Renal clearance | ND | ND | ↓ | Reduce dosage and lengthen dosage interval. |
| Quinidine | Liver and renal | ↑ | ↑ | ↓ | Individualize dosage based on need to convert atrial fibrillation or suppress ventricular ectopy. Watch for widening Q-T interval and increased intraocular pressure. Can precipitate digitalis toxicity. |
| Disopyramide | Renal clearance<br>Anticholinergic | ND | ↑ | ↓ | Reduce dosage. Check bowel and bladder function. Watch for increased intraocular pressure. |
| ACE inhibitors | Renal clearance | ND | ND | ↓ | Watch for cough, azotemia, and ↑$K^+$ |
| Diltiazem | Liver clearance<br>Increased efficacy | ↑ | ↑ | ↓ | Watch for SA node dysfunction. |
| Lipophilic beta blockers | Liver clearance<br>Decreased efficacy | ↑ | ↑ | ↓ | Watch for CNS toxicity. |
| Hydrophilic beta blockers | Renal clearance<br>Decreased response | ND | ↑ | ↓ | Watch for CNS toxicity. |
| Prazosin | Liver clearance<br>Reduced bioavailability | ↓ | ↑ | ↑ | Useful for benign prostatic hypertrophy, but can precipitate orthostatic hypotension. Same is true for terazosin, a once daily, longer-acting drug. |
| Verapamil | Liver clearance | ↑ | ↑ | ↓ | Slowed conduction at SA and A-V nodes. Left ventricular dysfunction can be precipitated with beta-blocker. |

*$t_{1/2}$ is derived from clearance according to the formula $t_{1/2} = 0.693\ V_d/Cl$; Cl = clearance; CNS = central nervous system; ND = no data available; SA = sinoatrial node; $V_d$ = volume of distribution.

age and that of benazaprilat is only slightly reduced.[27] Hyperkalemia and cough are the major concerns with ACE inhibitors.

## CALCIUM ENTRY BLOCKERS

Nicita-Mauro[28] has studied nifedipine, verapamil, and nitrendipine as monotherapy in the elderly for the treatment of stable hypertension and of paroxysmal hypertensive crisis. Adequate reduction in systolic pressure was accomplished, although minor side effects were observed (heat sensation, lower limb edema, headache, dyspepsia). No data exist for the treatment of angina with calcium entry blockers (CEBs) in the elderly. To date, no studies have examined age-related responses to CEBs. All CEBs are metabolized by the liver and there is no apparent alteration in their elimination kinetics with age.

## DIURETICS

Diuretics are eliminated by the kidney, and because renal function is reduced with age, drug accumulation may occur. Both *volume contraction* and *water retention* with clinically significant hyponatremia ($Na^+ < 125$ mEq/l) may result. The former condition is superimposed on age-related reductions in total body water and intracellular water and the latter condition is superimposed on tubular resistance to elevated concentrations of vasopressin.

Additionally, hypokalemia and hypomagnesemia, both of which are arrhythmogenic states, are complications of diuretics to which the elderly may be exquisitely sensitive. Thiazide diuretics reduce urinary excretion of calcium, and hypercalcemia may result. However, this renal physiologic action has been employed in some patients with osteoporosis on the rationale that senile osteoporosis is a calcium deficiency condition. Whether the lipid elevations that occur as a result of diuretic therapy in the elderly are of significance has not been determined.

In the elderly, low-dosage thiazide therapy for hypertension and/or edema is best for initiating treatment. The dose of hydrochlorothiazide (12.5 to 25 mg once daily) should be half that used for a young patient. Due to tubular resistance, furosemide dosage may need to be increased for a diuretic and natriuretic response.

## ANTIARRHYTHMICS

Both hepatic metabolism of quinidine and renal excretion of quinidine metabolites are decreased with age,[29] especially beyond age 60. Although quinidine metabolites are known to be active in rats and mice,[30] this has not yet been demonstrated for humans. In addition, the tubular reabsorption of quinidine is increased by drugs that alkalinize the urine.[31] Among these, hydrochlorothiazide, antacids, and carbonic anhydrase inhibitors prescribed for glaucoma are commonly taken by elderly patients. Chronic infection of the urinary tract with urea-splitting organisms produces an alkaline urine, which conceivably can potentiate quinidine toxicity. Elevated quinidine levels may predispose the patient to digitalis toxicity and vice versa.[32,33] The studies of Doering[32] and Leahey[33] did not address usage in the elderly when the interaction was described.

Procainamide is predominantly eliminated unchanged by the kidneys, with tubular secretion playing an important role. Procainamide clearance is reduced in elderly patients to an even greater degree than is glomerular filtration.[34] For the elderly patient, the dose should be reduced by 50% and the dosage interval widened.[35] Procainamide clearance is also inhibited by cimetidine, which can result in procainamide toxicity in elderly patients.[34] Procainamide is acetylated by the liver to form the active metabolite n-acetyl-procainamide, which is avidly tissue-bound and which can have lasting effects for a protracted period. Acetylation, as is typical of liver/drug conjugation reactions, is not compromised in the elderly. A slower acetylation phenotype results not only in elevated plasma procainamide concentrations, but also in positive antinuclear antibodies (80%) and drug-induced systemic lupus erythematosus.[36]

Lidocaine is frequently used for control of ventricular arrhythmia and has the potential for serious toxicity. Dosing guidelines have been based on factors known to change lidocaine distribution or clearance.[37] Clearance is reduced (and dosage should be reduced) in heart failure and when propranolol is used concomitantly. Abernathy and Greenblatt[38] found that lidocaine clearance after single-dose IV administration is reduced in elderly males, but not in females. They recommend that the same loading dose should be used in elderly males as in young males, but that the maintenance dose should be reduced 35% in male patients older than 65 years of age. Lidocaine toxicity is more common in the elderly, and this population should be monitored for confusion, paresthesia, respiratory depression, hypotension, and seizures. The metabolites of lidocaine, glycinexylidine and monoethylglycinexylidine, are active and can contribute to toxicity.

Disopyramide is also handled by renal elimination and the dose should be lowered once creatinine clearance falls below 50 ml/min. The major problem with disopyramide is that it has strong negative inotropic actions as well as potent anticholinergic activity. Thus, left ventricular dysfunction, urinary tract obstruction, and glaucoma can be aggravated.

Phenytoin is eliminated by hepatic biotransformation. It may be used to treat digitalis toxicity, particularly in the elderly.[3] Phenytoin can increase the metabolism of other drugs by inducing liver microsomal enzymes (cytochrome P450 drug-oxidizing enzymes) and is itself metabolized by these enzymes. Coadministration of phenobarbital, which also induces microsomal enzymes, produces a variable effect on phenytoin action. Low doses of phenobarbital induce increased phenytoin metabolism by enzyme induction. High doses of phenobarbital produce a competitive-substrate inhibition of phenytoin metabolism.[39] The plasma protein binding of phenytoin is reduced from 90% in the young to 70% in the elderly, resulting in higher free-drug concentrations in the elderly. Because the elderly receive multiple forms of medications, the potential for lack of effect or toxicity through its narrow therapeutic window necessitates careful monitoring of phenytoin levels.

Mexiletine, unlike quinidine, does not potentiate digitalis toxicity. Mexiletine is eliminated almost completely by hepatic metabolism, involving oxidation followed by conjugation (sulphation and glucuronidation). Although liver function is reduced with age and gastrointestinal absorption of mexiletine is slowed in the elderly,[40] these changes do not result in altered plasma concentrations in the elderly.[40,41] Grech-Belanger and associates[40] have stated that there is no pharmacologic basis for altering mexiletine dosage in the elderly.

## DIGITALIS

Digoxin is the seventh most commonly prescribed drug in the United States.[42] It is used for conditions that are more common in the elderly, including heart failure and atrial tachyarrhythmias. Digoxin is used in approximately 20% to 30% of hospitalized patients.[43] Digoxin toxicity is a common problem because of the narrow therapeutic window (0.8 to 2.0 ng/ml is desirable; toxicity begins in the range of 2.0 to 3.0 ng/ml). Taggart and McDevitt[44] suggest that digoxin may be overused in the elderly and that patients with left ventricular failure and sinus rhythm should be put on digitalis only if their symptoms cannot be controlled by diuretics alone. Elimination of digoxin is primarily by the kidney and is proportional to creatinine clearance. Digoxin does not bind appreciably to plasma proteins but does bind to tissues, especially skeletal muscle.[45] Steady-state serum digoxin levels in patients on a maintenance dose regimen are about double in patients aged 70 years or older compared with younger patients.[46] This effect is due to a combination of a smaller volume of distribution owing to a reduction in lean body mass and reduced clearance. As a result, if a loading dose is not given, the elderly patient may take 2 weeks to reach steady state rather than the usual 1 week.[47] A number of factors predispose the elderly to digoxin toxicity including diuretic-induced potassium deficiency and increased number of medication errors.[48] In addition, digitalis toxicity in the elderly may not be recognized because it produces different symptoms in the old than it does in the young.[49] Whereas the younger patient develops nausea and vomiting, the older patient often develops anorexia, cognitive changes, hazy vision, or arrhythmias. Earlier ischemic events may have left scars that can serve as ectopic foci. As a result, ventricular fibrillation as a manifestation of digitalis toxicity is much more common in the elderly. Digitalis toxicity may be increased by other drugs including quinidine, verapamil, nefedipine, diltiazem, and flecainide. It is suggested that the mechanism for these drug interactions is reduced digitalis clearance by the liver and kidney.

The combination of slower and variable elimination with the narrow therapeutic window for digoxin requires that digoxin dosage be individualized in the elderly patient. Digoxin is preferred for the elderly because of its shorter duration of action and greater safety margin.[50] Digitoxin, in contrast to digoxin, is highly (90%) bound to plasma proteins. Slower elimination of digitoxin in the elderly may result in higher plasma concentrations with the same administered dose.[51] The half time for elimination is 73 hours in the elderly, compared with 15 hours in the young.[46] Because of the potential for the prolonged retention of digitoxin, its use in the elderly is negligible.

## CHOLESTEROL-LOWERING AGENTS

The Framingham Study indicates that elevated low density lipoprotein (LDL) and depressed high density lipoprotein (HDL) are predictive of coronary disease, but that the importance of these factors is less in the elderly than in the middle-aged population.[52] In fact, there are at present no data linking reduced serum cholesterol in the elderly to improvement in such clinical endpoints as fatal myocardial infarction, need for bypass surgery, or exercise-induced angina. This consideration and the difficulty in patient compliance with bile-acid–sequestering resins, such as cholestyramine, have effectively confined the use of the resins to the patient younger than 65 years of age.[53] With the advent of the more efficacious and better tolerated hydroxymethylglutaryl coenzyme A (HMG CoA) reductase inhibitors, this advice needs to be reconsidered.[53] However, only limited drug trials have been performed in the elderly with these agents. Two groups[54,55] have studied simvastatin in elderly subjects with hypercholesterolemia. Both found this agent to be effective in reducing serum LDL by about 30% and both found the drug to be relatively well tolerated, with a low incidence of gastritis. However, the use of HMG CoA reductase inhibitors should be carefully monitored inasmuch as these agents can cause liver damage, as evidenced by elevation of serum liver transaminases. Cataract formation increases with age and whether HMG CoA reductase inhibitors raise this incidence is unknown.

## NITRATES

The organic nitrates are potent smooth muscle relaxants with specificity for vascular smooth muscle. At low doses, they have a greater effect on venous than on arterial smooth muscle. Several investigators have noted increased response to nitrates in the elderly patients. This is true whether the endpoint measured is decreased arterial pressure[56] or decreased mean left ventricular filling pressure.[57] Animal studies have shown that nitrate-induced relaxation of vascular smooth muscle *in vitro* is unaltered in aging.[58] The mechanism of the increased sensitivity is thought to involve reduced liver metabolism (resulting in higher plasma drug concentrations) and dampened baroreceptor responsiveness (resulting in a lowered ability to counteract nitrate-induced hypotension).[56] Nitrates cause a number of adverse reactions for which the elderly are at particular risk. These agents can cause shunting of blood in the lung, resulting in reduced oxygenation of the blood, presenting a problem for those with chronic obstructive pulmonary disease. Nitrates also can cause resting and postural hypotension and bradycardia. These adverse effects are more common in elderly patients.[59] The elderly can benefit from nitrate therapy, but they should be started on lower doses than young patients. The dose may be increased cautiously, once the sensitivity of the given individual has been established.

## CONCLUSIONS

It is clear that the wise use of cardiovascular drugs in the elderly population presents a challenge to the physician. The potential for untoward effects due to overmedication is created by physiologic changes that occur during aging. In general, these changes tend to decrease drug clearance, with a resulting increase in plasma drug concentrations following administration of a given dose. The potential for adverse drug reactions is also increased dramatically by a number of other factors related to age, including the polypharmacy that is associated with multiple disease states and reduced physiologic reserves in the elderly. Physicians should consider treating the elderly less aggressively or even not treating some conditions that they would treat in the younger patient, for example, mild or isolated systolic hypertension. Some general recommendations have been developed regarding dosing regimens for specific agents in the elderly. However, it should be stressed that interindividual variation is great in the elderly. For this reason, individualization of therapy and careful monitoring of results is very important.

## REFERENCES

1. Vestal, RE: Pharmacology and aging. J Am Geriatr Soc 30:191–200, 1982.
2. Lowenthal, DT: In Abrams, WB and Berkow, R (eds): The Merck Manual of Geriatrics. Merck, Sharp and Dohme, Rahway, NJ, 1990, pp 181–193.

3. Hoffman, BF and Bigger JT: In Goodman, AG, Gilman, LS, Rall, TW, et al (eds): The Pharmacological Basis of Therapeutics, ed 7. Macmillan, New York, 1985, pp 716–747.

4. Weg, RB: In Woodruff, D and Birren, J (eds): Changing physiology of aging: Normal and Pathological. Aging: Scientific Perspectives and Social Issues. D. Van Nostrand Co, Inc, New York, 1975, pp 229–256.

5. Richey, DP: Effects of human aging on drug absorption and metabolism. In Goldman, R and Rockstein, M (eds): The Physiology and Pathology of Human Aging. Academic Press, New York, 1975.

6. Cockcroft, DW and Gault, MH: Prediction of creatinine clearance from serum creatinine. Nephron 16:31–41, 1976.

7. Kannel, WB: Blood pressure and the development of cardiovascular disease in the aged. In Caird, FL, Dahl, JLC, and Kennedy, RD (eds): Cardiology in old age. Plenum Press, New York, 1976, pp 143–175.

8. Amery, A, Wasir, H, Bulpitt, C, et al: Aging and the cardiovascular system. Acta Cardiol (Brux) 6:443, 1978.

9. Lipsitz, LA: Abnormalities in blood pressure homeostasis that contribute to falls in the elderly. Clin Geriatr Med 1:637–648, 1985.

10. Lowenthal, DT, Kim, DI, Affrime, MB, et al: Overview of physiology in senescence. Chest 83(2):408–409, 1983.

11. Rubenstein, LZ and Robbins, AS: Falls in the elderly: A clinical perspective. Geriatrics 39:67–78, 1984.

12. Scarpace, PJ and Armbrecht, HJ: Adenylate cyclase in senescence: Catecholamine and parathyroid hormone pathways. Rev Clin Basic Pharmacol 6:105–118, 1987.

13. Buhler, FR, Burkart, F, Lutold, BE, et al: Anti-hypertensive beta blocking action as related to renin and ages: A pharmacologic tool to identify pathogenetic mechanisms in essential hypertension. Am J Cardiol 36:653–668, 1975.

14. Andersen, GS: Atenolol versus bendroflumethiazide in middle-aged and elderly hypertensives. Acta Med Scand 218:165–172, 1985.

15. Nolan, L and O'Malley, K: Prescribing for the elderly. Part 1. Sensitivity of the elderly to adverse drug reactions. J Am Geriatr Soc 36:142–149, 1988.

16. Berkow, R (ed): Merck Manual, ed 14. Merck and Co, Rahway, NJ, 1982, pp 402–404.

17. Caird, FI, Andrews, GB, and Kennedy, RD: The effect of posture on blood pressure. Br Heart J 35:527–530, 1973.

18. MacLennan, WJ, Hall, MR, Timothy, JI: Postural hypotension in old age: Is it a disorder of the nervous system or of the blood vessels? Age Aging 9:25–32, 1980.

19. Mader, SL: Aging and postural hypotension. J Am Geriatric Soc 37:129–137, 1989.

20. Williams, BO, Caird, FL, Lennox, IM: Hemodynamic response to postural stress in the elderly with and without postural hypotension. Age Aging 14:193–201, 1985.

21. Ray, WA, Schaffner, W, Oates, JA: Therapeutic choice in the treatment of hypertension. Initial treatment of newly diagnosed hypertension and secular trends in the prescribing of anti-hypertensive medications for medical patients. Am J Med 81(6C):9–16, 1986.

22. Fitzgerald, JD: Age-related effects of $\beta$-blockers and hypertension. J Cardiovasc Pharmacol 12:S83–S92, 1988.

23. Rigby, JW, Scott, AK, Hawksworth, GM, et al: A comparison of the kinetics of atenolol, metoprolol, exprenolol and propranolol in elderly hypertensive and young healthy subjects. Br J Clin Pharmacol 20:327–331, 1985.

24. Castleden, CN and George, CG: The effects of aging on the hepatic clearance of propranolol. Br J Clin Pharmacol 7:49–54, 1979.

25. Thomson, AH, Kelly, JG, Whiting, B: Lisinopril population pharmacokinetics in elderly and renal disease patients with hypertension. Br J Clin Pharmacol 27:57–65, 1989.

26. Williams, PEO, Brown, AN, Rajaguru, S, et al: A pharmacokinetic study of cilazapril in elderly and young volunteers. Br J Clin Pharmacol 27:211S–215S, 1989.

27. Kaiser, G, Ackerman, R, Dieterle, W, et al: Pharmacokinetics and pharmacodynamics of the ace inhibitor benazepril hydrochloride in the elderly. Eur J Clin Pharmacol 38:379–385, 1990.

28. Nicita-Mauro, V: Calcium antagonists in the treatment of arterial hypertension in the elderly. Am J Nephrol 6(Suppl)1:115–119, 1986.

29. Ochs, HR, Greenblatt, DJ, Woo, E, et al: Reduced quinidine clearance in elderly patients. Am J Cardiol 42:481–485, 1978.

30. Drayer, DE, Lowenthal, DT, Restivo, KM, et al: Steady state serum levels of quinidine and active quinidine metabolites in cardiac patients in varying degrees of renal function. Clin Pharmacol Ther 24:31–39, 1978.

31. Gerhardt, RE, Knous, RF, Thyrum, PT, et al: Quinidine excretion in aciduria and alkaluria. Ann Intern Med 71(5)927–933, 1969.

32. Doering, W: Quinidine-digoxin interaction: Pharmacokinetics, underlying mechanism and clinical implications. N Engl J Med 301:400–404, 1979.

33. Leahey, EB: Digoxin-quinidine interaction: Current status. Ann Intern Med 93:775–776, 1980.

34. Bauer, LA, Black, D, Gensler, A: Procainamide-cimetidine drug interaction in elderly male patients. J Am Geriatr Soc 38:467–469, 1990.

35. Lowenthal, DT and Affrime, MB: Cardiovascular drugs for the geriatric patient. Cardiology 36(8):65–74, 1981.

36. LaDu, BN: Pharmacogenetics: Defective enzymes in relation to drugs. Annu Rev Med 23:453–468, 1972.

37. Greenblatt, DJ, Bolognini, V, Koch-Weser, J, et al: Pharmacokinetic approach to the clinical use of lidocaine intravenously. JAMA 236:273–277, 1976.

38. Abernathy, DR and Greenblatt, DJ: Impairment of lidocaine clearance in elderly male subjects. J Cardiovas Pharmacol 5(6):1093–1096, 1983.

39. Hansten, PD: Drug Interactions, ed 4. Lea & Febiger, Philadelphia, 1979, p 74.

40. Grech-Belanger, O, Barbeau, G, Kishka, P, et al: Pharmacokinetics of mexiletine in the elderly. J Clin Pharmacol 29:311–315, 1989.

41. El Alaf, D, Carlier, J, Dresse, A: Effects of age on the pharmacokinetics of mexiletine. Int J Clin Pharmacol Res VI(4):303–307, 1986.

42. Rubin, I: 1980: The top 200 drugs. Pharmacv Times 47(April):17, 1981, pp 17–25.

43. Whiting, B, Lawrence, JR, Sumner, CJ: Digoxin pharmacokinetics in the elderly. In Crooks, J and Stevenson, IH (eds): Drugs and the Elderly, September 1979.

44. Taggart, AJ and McDevitt, DG: Digitalis: Its place in modern therapy. Drugs 20:398–404, 1980.

45. Caird, FI: Metabolism of digoxin in relation to therapy in the elderly. Geront Clin 16:68–74, 1972.

46. Cusack, B, Kelly, J, O'Malley, K, et al: Digoxin in the elderly: Pharmacokinetic consequences of old age. Clin Pharmacol Ther 25:772–776, 1979.

47. Stults, BM: Digoxin use in the elderly. J Am Geriatr Soc 30(3):158–164, 1986.

48. Tweedale, MG: Diruretic drugs. In Dukes, MNG (ed): Meyler's Side Effects on Drugs, ed 9, Excerpta Medica, Amsterdam, 1980, pp 337–367.

49. Goldberg, PB, and Roberts, J: Pharmacology. In Weisfeldt, ML (ed): The Aging Heart. Raven Press, New York, 1980, pp 215–246.

50. Davison, W: Unwanted drug effects in the elderly. In: Meyler, L and Peck, M (ed): Drug-induced diseases. Excerpta Medica, Amsterdam, 1972, pp 307–321.

51. Ewy, GA, Kapadia, GG, Ylao, L, et al: Digoxin metabolism in the elderly. Circulation 39:449–453, 1969.

52. Kannel, WB, Castelli, WP Gordon, T: Cholesterol in the prediction of atherosclerotic disease: New perspectives based on the Framingham study. Ann Intern Med 90:85–91, 1979.

53. Tikkanen, MJ: Hypercholesterolemia in the elderly: Is drug treatment justified? Eur Heart J 9:79–82, 1988.

54. Bach, LA, Cooper, ME, O'Brien, RC, et al: The use of simvastatin, an HMG CoA reductase inhibitor, in older patients with hypercholesterolemia and atherosclerosis. J Am Geriatr Soc 38:10–14, 1990.

55. Antonicelli, R, Onorato, G, Pagelli, P, et al: Simvastatin in the treatment of hypercholesterolemia in elderly patients. Clin Ther 12:2, 165–171, 1990.

56. Marchionni, N, Ferrucci, L, Boncinelli, L, et al: Age-related changes in the pharmacodynamics of intravenous glyceryl trinitrate. Aging 1990 2(1):59–64.

57. Alpert, JS: Nitrate therapy in the elderly. Am J Cardiol 65:23J–27J, 1990.

58. Fleisch, JH and Hooker, CS: The relationship between age and relaxation of vascular smooth muscle in the rabbit and rat. Circ Res 38:243–249, 1976.

59. Come, PC and Pitt, B: Nitroglycerin-induced severe hypotension and bradycardia in patients with acute myocardial infarction. Circulation 54:624–628, 1976.

# CHAPTER 13

# Intervention Therapy for Coronary Artery Disease in the Elderly

*Carl J. Pepine, MD*
*Anne Pepine, BS*

It has been well documented that there is an increase in the number of elderly patients with coronary artery disease (CAD) undergoing coronary bypass operations. Recently, an increase in the number of elderly patients undergoing nonsurgical intervention therapy also has been occurring. One reason for these trends is the large increase in the number of elderly patients in our population. The Census Bureau found that in 1985 there were approximately 30 million people in the United States aged 55 or older. It is estimated that this number will increase to approximately 35 million by the year 2030. Also, the average life expectancy in our country continues to increase. Inasmuch as age is a major risk factor for CAD, as the population of the United States ages, an increasing number of elderly patients will present with signs and symptoms of CAD.

The purpose of this chapter is to critically examine the results of intervention therapy for CAD applied to the elderly to determine in which elderly patients such therapy can be justified. This is particularly pertinent given the fact that there is a high mortality among elderly patients with CAD. Treatment of patients with interventional therapy has been promising. But unfortunately, just as CAD incidence and mortality rates increase with age so does the frequency of other co-morbid conditions that influence the outcome of both CAD and intervention procedures. It is also important to note that, as yet, no large randomized controlled trials specifically focusing on the elderly have been conducted. So the information obtained must be based upon analysis of relatively small subgroups or from observations drawn from clinical experiences that are uncontrolled.

## DEFINITION OF TERMS

Before proceeding, it is appropriate to review some terminology. There is no standard definition of "elderly" and its definition has changed over the years as the population in the United States has increased in age. There is no doubt that any absolute chronologic definition will continue to change in a direction toward the older years. Even at this point in time, elderly is considered by some to represent patients 60 years of age and older whereas to others elderly is considered to represent septuagenarians. For the purposes of this review, elderly will be considered to represent patients 65 years of age or older. When we refer to other subsets of aged people we will specifically note their age. Unfortunately, this is a major limitation to the data available. It is important to mention that a simple chronologic definition in not completely adequate because some physiologic qualifications are also needed. There are the infirm elderly and those who are 75 and lead the active life style of a 60 year old.

Likewise, terms like long-term outcome and life expectancy in the elderly take on different meanings. Clearly, life expectancy for the elderly patient with CAD will not be as long as it is for a younger patient regardless of the intervention used. Thus, the outcome estimates from any intervention require some adjustment of expectations for the possible benefit relative to the elderly. At the age of 75 in the United States one has an average expectation of approximately 10 more years of life. So for the purposes of intervention therapy in the elderly it would seem appropriate that approximately 10 years of life represents an excellent long-term outcome and is the reference standard that should guide intervention therapy. Similarly, it would be more undesirable for an elderly patient with only 10 years of life expectancy to invest considerable time in an intervention procedure that has a high risk for needed additional procedures. On the other hand, this may be well worth the time and discomfort for a younger patient who is waiting for the proper timing to have a more definitive procedure.

Another concept that requires attention is intervention therapy for CAD. In its broad sense, the term "intervention cardiology" is applied to both noninvasive pharmacologic and invasive therapeutic interventions that are directed to intervene in the pathologic processes associated with CAD. For the purposes of this review, our discussion of intervention therapy will be restricted to two major areas of activity in elderly patients: *intravenous thrombolytic therapy for acute thrombolytic intervention* in patients with known or suspected acute myocardial infarction and *mechanical intervention with percutaneous transluminal coronary angioplasty* (PTCA) for revascularization of patients with acute or chronic manifestations of CAD. This should by no means be considered the scope of intervention therapy but simply areas in which there are sufficient data to permit some reliable estimate of the potential risks and benefits for elderly patients.

## THROMBOLYTIC THERAPY FOR SUSPECTED ACUTE MYOCARDIAL INFARCTION

Unfortunately, aggressive intervention management of elderly patients with acute myocardial infarction is often avoided or considered contraindicated by some. Many of the large, controlled trials of thrombolytic therapy specifically excluded patients who were older than 75 years of age. Thus, only limited data for the very elderly are available. Furthermore, most of what is available relates to those patients between 65 and 75 years of age. One reason for exclusion of the older patients may have been the well known age-related progressive rise in frequency of major hemorrhagic and other complications.[1,2] However, elderly patients also have a much higher mortality rate after myocardial infarction than younger patients. For this reason, they have the potential to derive the most benefit provided the benefit is not offset by a rise in morbidity.

Some limited data are available for the elderly from subgroup analysis of several large controlled trials. No predetermined upper age limit for enrollment was used in the International Study of Infarct Survival (ISIS-2).[3] Here intervention with the combination of intravenous streptokinase and chewable aspirin resulted in > 43% mortality reduction (16.1% to 9.1%) in those 60 to 69 years old. But only about a 40% reduction (6.2% to 3.7%) was observed in patients younger than 60 years of age. Stated another way, these results represent a potential gain of about 7 lives per 100 younger patients treated. For those 70 and older, the savings of lives was about 8 per 100 patients (Fig. 13–1). Also in this trial there were no excess bleeding or hypotension events among the 401 patients who were 80 years of age or older. One recent reanalysis has suggested that the savings of lives in those 80 and older was even more spectacular and averaged 17 lives per 100 octogenarians treated.[4]

In the Anglo-Scandinavian Study of Early Thrombolysis (ASSET), patients older than 75 years of age were excluded; however, the subgroup of patients who

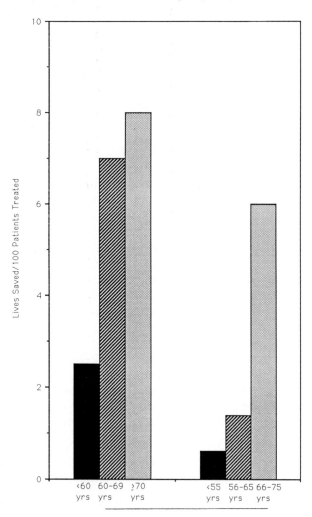

**Figure 13–1.** Saving of lives in elderly patients compared with younger patients based on data from the ISIS-2,[3] using streptokinase plus aspirin *(left),* and the ASSET,[5] using tPA *(right).* Note the progressive increase in the number of lives saved by thrombolytic intervention as age increases. This beneficial effect of intervention in the elderly was present with both thrombolytic treatments.

were 66 to 75 years of age derived greater benefit from therapy with tissue plasminogen activator (t-PA) than the younger patients. Mortality in this elderly group was reduced more than 34% (from 16.4% to 10.8%). In patients who were 56 to 65 years of age, there was an 18% reduction in mortality (7.9% to 6.5%) and, in those younger than 55 years of age, there was only a 14% reduction in mortality (from 4.4% to 3.8%).[5] This represents a potential of almost 6 lives saved per 100 elderly patients treated compared with less than one life saved per 100 younger patients treated (Fig. 13–1).

Based on the aforementioned considerations, it is highly likely that elderly patients have the potential to derive considerable benefit from intervention with thrombolytic therapy for suspected acute myocardial infarction. This is because the elderly have a higher infarction-related mortality and the potential to save lives does not seem to be offset by an important increase in lethal complications.

## PTCA FOR ACUTE OR CHRONIC MANIFESTATIONS OF CAD

Before dealing with the applications and results of PTCA in the elderly, several factors important in the selection of patients for coronary bypass surgery (CABG) must be considered inasmuch as bypass surgery represents the alternate revascularization procedure and produces very satisfactory palliation of symptoms. First is the motivation and desire of the elderly individual to return to an active life style and the patient's willingness to accept the 3 to 4 months of rehabilitation needed after CABG. For many elderly patients with CABG, this comes with the prospect for an increase in debilitating complications. Secondly, the elderly patient's overall general condition, including physiologic status and mental status, must be evaluated in detail.

Certain specific co-morbid factors also effect the outcome of CABG, and these also must be examined critically in each elderly case. Most important are diabetes, cerebral and peripheral vascular diseases, systemic hypertension, renal insufficiency, pulmonary disease, and obesity. These factors all substantially increase the risks in the early and late postoperative periods and also influence survival. Another very important factor is gender. Females have a considerably higher risk of death and complications than male patients of comparable age within the elderly group.[6] All of these issues have an important influence on the choice of revascularization therapy in the elderly patient (Table 13–1). When these factors are present to further increase the risks of bypass surgery or limit its potential benefits, a more conservative approach in favor of PTCA may be warranted. Percutaneous transluminal coronary angioplasty, in general, is an attractive nonsurgical alternative that can be performed under most circumstances with an acceptable low morbidity and mortality compared with bypass surgery. Unfortunately, there is an impressive relationship between advancing age and increasing operative and early and late postoperative risks. We will next examine the results of reports employing PTCA in elderly patients to determine whether the low morbidity and mortality observed in younger patients also applies to the elderly patients.

## RESULTS OF PTCA IN ELDERLY PATIENTS COMPARED
## WITH YOUNGER PATIENTS

Grüntzig and colleagues[7] initially excluded from consideration for PTCA patients older than 60 years of age. However, their attitudes changed when

**Table 13–1.**
Clinical
Characteristics
Favoring Choice
of PTCA for
Revascularization
in Elderly
Patients

Female gender
Prior CABG
Class III or IV angina
Angina at rest
Heart failure or left ventricular dysfunction
Co-morbid diseases
  Diabetes
  Cerebral vascular disease
  Peripheral vascular disease
  Renal insufficiency
  Chronic obstructive pulmonary disease
  Obesity
Intolerance to medications

increased morbidity and mortality from bypass surgery in the elderly patients became well documented and experience with PTCA became extensive.[8] Thus, by the mid 1980s PTCA was attempted as an alternative revascularization procedure in an increasing proportion of older patients with appropriate lesions (Table 13–2). The largest early analysis of these attempts was presented in the first National

**Table 13–2.** Single- and Multi-Center Series Showing Initial Results of PTCA in Elderly Patients*

| Series/Last Year of Series | | n | Success | % of Patients | | |
| | | | | Death | EM-CABG | MI |
|---|---|---|---|---|---|---|
| *Single Center* | | | | | | |
| Jones & Grüntzig†[8] | 1982 | 159 | 84 | 0 | 6.8 | 5.6 |
| Hust et al[10] | 1983 | 121 | 81 | 0.8 | 4.1 | 1.7 |
| Raizner[13] | 1984 | 119 | 81 | 0.8 | 4.1 | 2.5 |
| Dorros et al[12] | 1984 | 71 | 88 | 1.2 | 1.2 | 4.8 |
| Zaidi et al[11] | 1984 | 169 | 91 | 0 | 6.0 | 7.7 |
| Holt et al[15] | 1985 | 54 | 80 | 0 | 5.6 | 5.6 |
| *Multi-Center* | | | | | | |
| NHLBI PTCA Registry[9] | 1981 | 370 | 53 | 2.2 | 6.8 | 5.6 |
| NHLBI PTCA Registry[14] | 1986 | 486 | 80 | 3.1 | 5.4 | 5.3 |

EM-CABG = Emergency coronary artery bypass graft; MI = myocardial infarction; NHLBI = National Heart, Lung, and Blood Institute; PTCA = percutaneous transluminal coronary angioplasty; N = number of elderly patients.
†Unstable AP.

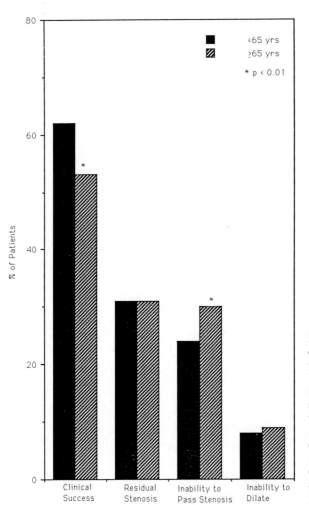

**Figure 13–2.** Results of PTCA in elderly patients compared with younger patients from the 1977–81 NHLBI PTCA Registry.[9] The reduced success rate *(left column)* appears due to the inability to pass the catheter through the stenosis *(third column from left)* in the elderly compared with the younger patients. This probably relates to the equipment limitations of that time and the tortuosity of elderly patient's coronary arteries.

Heart, Lung, and Blood Institute PTCA registry in which we participated.[9] At that point in time (1977 to 1981), only about 12% of the patients undergoing PTCA were elderly. In that report 2709 patients younger than 65 years of age were compared with 370 patients aged 65 years or older. The baseline characteristics of these two patient groups were different. The elderly patient group included a larger percentage of females (38%) compared with the younger group (21%) and a larger percentage of patients with prior CABG (12%) compared with the younger group (9%). These findings suggested that the increased risks of bypass graft surgery in elderly patients who were either female or had previous bypass surgery were taken into account in the type of subsequent revascularization procedure chosen. Relative to other cardiovascular risk factors, some additional differences were noted. A history of either cigarette smoking or previous myocardial infarction was less frequent in the elderly group compared with the younger patients (50% vs. 73% and 21% vs. 26%). But the proportion of patients with either a cholesterol > 250 mg/dl or diabetes were similar in each group. Also, the proportions with unstable angina and

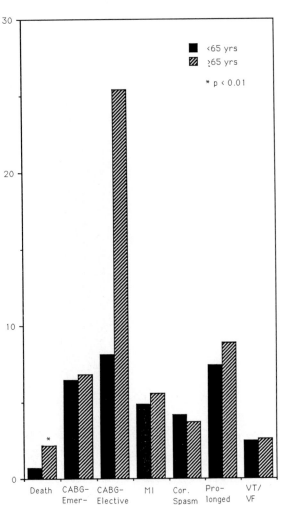

**Figure 13-3.** In-hospital complications comparing elderly and younger patients from the 1977–81 NHLBI PTCA Registry.[9] Note the increased death rate and need for elective coronary bypass graft surgery (CABG) in the elderly compared with younger patients. MI = myocardial infarction; Cor. = coronary artery; VT/VF = ventricular tachycardia or ventricular fibrillation.

severe angina, classed as either angina at rest or Canadian class III or IV, was higher in the elderly age group (75% and 56% vs. 61% and 45%) compared with the younger group. The coronary angiographic characteristics of both the stenoses dilated and the nondilated vessels were similar. But there was a greater percentage of patients with an ejection fraction $< 30\%$ in the elderly age group (2.2%) compared with the younger age group (0.4%).

The results of PTCA, comparing the elderly and younger patient groups, are summarized in Figure 13-2. It is apparent the clinical success rate was significantly lower than that routinely achieved in the younger aged patients. This difference was largely the result of the inability to pass the catheter through the stenosis. Success rates were low by current standards, and they relate to limited operator experience, case selection, and the limited equipment available between 1977 and 1981. The complication rates were higher in the elderly patients, as is also apparent from Figure 13-3. The death rate and need for elective CABG were significantly greater in the elderly patient group. Also the major clinical events in the first year after PTCA

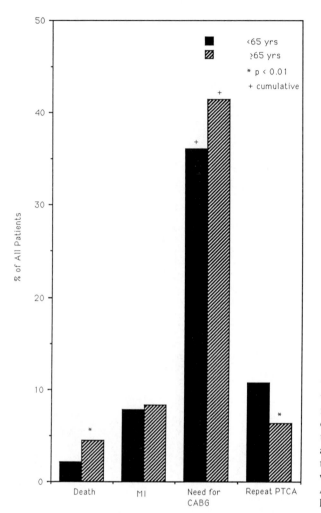

**Figure 13–4a.** Major events in the first year after PTCA from the 1977–81 NHLBI PTCA Registry.[9] Data for all patients are in Figure 4a and for only successfully dilated patients in Figure 4b. Note that the death rate and need for CABG were higher in the elderly. But the increased need for CABG and death rate appeared related to the unsuccessful procedures inasmuch as this trend was not observed in the subgroup of elderly patients with successful PTCA *(Figure 4b).* Abbreviations are the same as for Figure 13–3.

were different in the two patient groups (Fig. 13–4a). Late death occurred more frequently in the patients 65 years of age or older and the need for late CABG also occurred more frequently than in younger patients. This was related to inclusion of the unsuccessful cases as these differences in death and elective CABG rate were not present in the subgroup with successful PTCA (see Fig. 13–4b). However, the need for a repeat PTCA procedure was less in the elderly patients compared with the younger patients. The latter was true for all elderly patients and also for the elderly patients who had had successful PTCA procedures.

These early multicenter results were generally acceptable given that the alternative was CABG, and they indicated that PTCA could be done in the elderly. However, the longer-term results are needed. In addition, a more objective evaluation of the relative merits of alternate therapy, that is, continued pharmacologic treatment and coronary bypass surgery, are awaited.

A number of single center reports were very positive relative to results of PTCA in the elderly. Grüntzig and his colleagues[8] reviewed their experience from

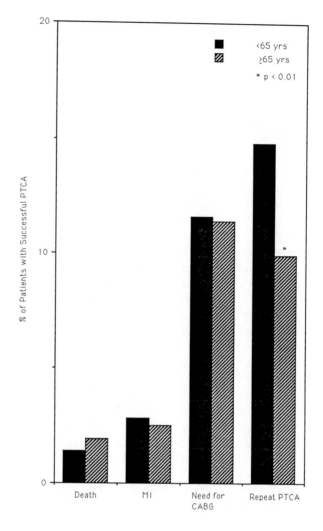

**Figure 13–4b.**

a single institution with patients who were older than 65 years of age.[8] They compared 159 patients aged 65 years or older with 971 patients younger than 65 years of age. They also found that there was a larger percentage of females in the elderly patient group. Smoking history and family history of diabetes as well as a history of hypercholesterolemia occurred significantly less frequently in the elderly patients. From the angiographic standpoint, there was a higher frequency of calcification noted at cinefluoroscopy at the site of the lesion in the elderly patient group. Although there was a trend toward a greater percentage of patients with a low ejection fraction in the elderly group, this trend did not achieve statistical significance. The percent of patients aged 65 years or older with ejection fractions < 30% was more than double that of the patients who were younger than 65 years of age. Grüntzig and his colleagues[8] found no significant difference in the results of PTCA comparing the younger with the older patients. The success rates were 87.7% in the younger patients compared with 85.7% in the older patients. There was a significant difference in results when the patients were divided by the presence of either single-vessel or multi-vessel disease. The success rate in patients with multi-vessel disease was significantly greater in the younger patient group compared with the elderly patient group. This disparity was largely attributed to failure to cross the stenosis in a high percentage of the elderly patients with multi-vessel disease. This finding helped explain the lower success rate observed in the elderly patients and may relate to the increased tortuosity of coronary arteries in elderly patients. Grüntzig and his colleagues[8] found no significant difference in either the major or minor complications comparing the elderly and the younger patient groups.

A number of other workers reported results of smaller numbers of elderly patients undergoing PTCA (see Table 13-2). Hust and coworkers[10] examined the results of 121 elderly patients who underwent PTCA and their primary success rate was 81%. Zaidi and associates[11] reported the results of 169 patients with a primary success rate of 91%. Dorros and coworkers[12] reported results on 71 patients, in whom the primary success rate was 88%. Most recently Raizner et al[13] reported data from 119 elderly patients and their success rate was 81%.

The results of the second National Heart, Lung, and Blood Institute PTCA registry, which was based upon data accumulated from 1985 to 1986, are the most recent.[14] These data are based upon a series of 486 patients aged 65 years or older which were obtained from a larger cohort of patients numbering 1801. By the end of 1986, approximately 27% of patients undergoing PTCA were elderly compared with only 12% in the registry that closed in 1981. In general, a greater fraction of elderly patients had a history of hypertension and congestive heart failure, again supporting the previous results. Although the elderly group had more patients with multi-vessel disease, the number of lesions in the vessels approached with PTCA were similar in the younger and older patient groups. The angiographic success rates were also similar in both groups and by 1986 averaged approximately 80% for the elderly compared with 53% in 1981. Although the type of complications in the catheterization laboratory did not differ, the elderly group appeared more likely to require emergency CABG (5.4%) compared with the younger group (2.8%). The elderly also were more likely to need elective bypass surgery (3.9%) compared with the younger group (1.6%) (Fig. 13-5). The in-hospital mortality rate was significantly higher in the elderly patients (3.1%) compared with the younger group (0.2%).

Interestingly, the 2-year follow-up of the symptom status with cumulative rates of myocardial infarction, need for CABG, and repeat PTCA were not significantly different in the elderly and younger patients. The death rate after 2 years, however, was significantly higher among the elderly patients (8.8% compared with 2.9%). When the relative risk for death among the elderly was adjusted for factors more prevalent among those patients who were elderly, for example, history of congestive heart failure, multi-vessel coronary disease, unstable angina, hypertension, and female gender, the relative risk was substantially reduced (3.3% reduced to 2.4%) but remained significantly greater for the elderly than the younger patients.

The two large multi-center series show a lower success rate and higher mortality rate than any other single center study. The last National Heart, Lung, and Blood Institute registry report probably reflects most closely the practice today.

There are few data about results of PTCA in elderly patients with unstable angina. Recently, Holt and associates[15] reported results of 54 patients aged older than 70 years who underwent PTCA for unstable angina. Unstable angina was defined as either recent onset ($< 1$ month) or accelerating class III or IV angina,

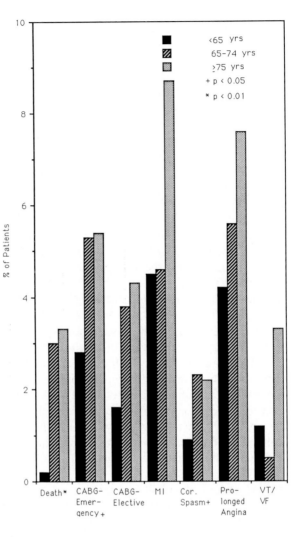

**Figure 13–5.** In-hospital complications comparing two elderly patient groups with the younger patients from the 1985–86 NHLBI PTCA Registry.[13] Note the trend for all complications to increase in frequency with increasing age. Abbreviations are the same as for Figure 13–3.

or new onset of rest angina (> 2 episodes). There were 20 men and 34 women and 37% had multi-vessel disease. PTCA was successful in 80%. In the 11 unsuccessful cases, emergency CABG was needed in three. There were no deaths; three patients had acute myocardial infarction, of which two were Q wave and one non Q wave. After a mean follow-up of approximately 3 years of the 43 successfully dilated patients, four had died, one had a non–Q-wave myocardial infarction, and eight had symptomatic restenosis. Six of the latter cases needed repeat revascularization procedures. Of these patients, 72% were angina free at last follow-up. Comparing these results with PTCA to those with CABG or medical therapy is difficult without controlled clinical trials. Nevertheless, these results are very encouraging for elderly patients with unstable angina.

It is important to recognize that all of these reports are uncontrolled cohort or registry-type observations. Given the high success rates and the low rates of non-fatal complications, PTCA is emerging as an extremely attractive alternative therapy for the elderly individual. The controlled, randomized trials currently under way will provide objective data to determine the relative value of PTCA compared with other revascularization procedures.

## SUMMARY AND CONCLUSION

The central aim of this review was to examine the application of intervention therapy for CAD in the elderly population. The data reviewed indicates that it is no longer appropriate to use age 70 or 75 as the upper limit of eligibility for thrombolytic intervention in patients with acute myocardial infarction. Elderly who are physiologically active without contraindications to thrombolytic therapy should be considered eligible. Additional controlled trials specifically targeted at the elderly population are needed to better define the precise dosing regimen and the magnitude and extent of bleeding complications in this group. Nevertheless, it appears appropriate to recommend thrombolytic intervention for most eligible elderly patients presenting with acute myocardial infarction. This recommendation is based on the fact that the higher mortality in the elderly results in more lives saved per patient treated than for younger patients. It is important to reemphasize that this recommendation is for treating elderly patients with acute infarction as suggested by ST-segment elevation and/or Q waves, without contraindications to thrombolytic therapy. Those with non–Q-wave infarctions, hypertension, recent stroke, history of bleeding, or other contraindications are not candidates.

Regarding intervention therapy in other elderly patients with acute and chronic manifestations of coronary disease, results also appear very encouraging. Elderly patients appearing to tolerate PTCA include those with all forms of angina from chronic stable angina to unstable angina. Although only observational data are on hand at present, our review suggests these elderly patients tolerate PTCA well and indeed may benefit. The elderly patients who have co-morbid factors that adversely influence the application of CABG for revascularization may be the best candidates for PTCA.

At present, the challenge for the physician is to carefully assess each elderly patient on an individual basis for intervention therapy. This evaluation should be aimed at identifying factors that may permit application of intervention treatment to the elderly patients who are most likely to receive the greatest benefit.

## REFERENCES

1. Lew, AS, Hod, H, Cercek, B, et al: Mortality and morbidity rates of patients older and younger than 75 years with acute myocardial infarction treated with intravenous streptokinase. Am J Cardiol 59(1):1–5, 1987.
2. Chaitman, BR, Thompson, B, Wittry, MD, et al, for the TIMI Investigators: The use of tissue-type plasminogen activator for acute myocardial infarction in the elderly: Results from thrombolysis in myocardial infarction Phase I, open label studies and the thrombolysis in myocardial infarction Phase II pilot study. J Am Coll Cardiol 14(5):1159–1165, 1989.
3. ISIS-2 (Second International Study of Infarct Survival) Collaborative Group: Randomised trial of intravenous streptokinase, oral aspirin, both, or neither among 17,187 cases of suspected acute myocardial infarction: ISIS-2. Lancet 2:349–360, 1988.
4. Muller, DWM and Topol, EJ: Selection of patients with acute myocardial infarction for thrombolytic therapy. Ann Intern Med 113(12):949–960, 1990.
5. Wilcos, RG, von der Lippe, G, Olsson, CG, et al, for the ASSET Study Group. Trial of tissue plasminogen activator for mortality reduction in acute myocardial infarction. Anglo-Scandinavian study of early thrombolysis (ASSET). Lancet 2:525–530, 1988.

6. Faro, RS, Golden, MD, Javid, H, et al: Coronary revascularization in septuagenarians. J Thorac Cardiovasc Surg 86(4):616–620, 1983.
7. Grüntzig, AR, Senning, A, Siegenthaler, WE: Nonoperative dilatation of coronary-artery stenosis, percutaneous transluminal coronary angioplasty. N Engl J Med 301(2):61–68, 1979.
8. Jones EL, Abi-Mansour, P, Grüntzig, AR: Coronary artery bypass surgery and percutaneous transluminal coronary angioplasty in the elderly patient. Cardiology 73:223–234, 1986.
9. Mock, MB, Holmes, DR, Jr, Vlietstra, RE, et al: Percutaneous transluminal coronary angioplasty (PTCA) in the elderly patient: Experience in the National Heart, Lung, and Blood Institute PTCA Registry. Am J Cardiol 53:89C–91C, 1984.
10. Hust, RG, Raizner, AE, Lewis, JM, et al: Transluminal coronary angioplasty in the elderly: An important therapeutic option. Circulation 70:II-36, 1984.
11. Zaidi, AR, Hollman, J, Franco, I, et al: Coronary angioplasty: Can you refer older patients? Geriatrics 40(3):38–44, 1985.
12. Dorros, G, King, JF, Manley, JC, et al: The high risk coronary bypass patient: Coronary angioplasty in geriatric patients (≥70 years). J Am Coll Cardiol 5(2):446, 1985.
13. Raizner, AE, Hust, RG, Lewis, JM, et al: Transluminal coronary angioplasty in the elderly. Am J Cardiol 57:29–32, 1986.
14. Kelsey, SF, Miller, DP, Holubkov, R, et al, and Investigators from the NHLBI PTCA Registry: Am J Cardiol 66:1033–1038, 1990.
15. Holt, GW, Sugrue, DD, Bresnahan, JF, et al: Results of percutaneous transluminal coronary angioplasty for unstable angina pectoris in patients 70 years of age and older. Am J Cardiol 61:994–997, 1988.

# CHAPTER 14

# Cardiac Surgery in the Elderly Patient

*John D. Mannion, MD*
*Frederick R. Armenti, MD*
*Richard N. Edie, MD*

A meaningful and comprehensive definition of "the elderly" is difficult. Webster's dictionary describes the elderly as "past middle age." Bernard Baruch once said "to me old age is always 15 years older than I am." In the early 1970s, reviews on cardiac surgery defined 65 years as the elderly. During the past two decades, however, there has been an increasingly large series of successful cardiac surgeries in septuagenarians and octogenarians. It is well known that the use of numeric age categorizations may be arbitrary and even misleading as the aging process is not strictly a function of chronologic age. Sir William Olser long ago emphasized that physiologic age, as manifested by the extent of vascular disease, was more relevant than chronologic age. In an attempt to differentiate between the elderly and the aged, the World Health Organization in 1963 concluded that the needs of the elderly, namely occupation, interests, and hobbies as well as the use of acquired skills and knowledge, were different from those of the aged who required care, help, and services.[1]

In recent years, the growth of the geriatric population in the United States has been exponential. Whereas 26.8 million people in the United States (11.6%) were older than the age of 65 in 1982, this number is expected to increase to 65 million (21%) in 2030.[2] In 1990, 7.4 million Americans were older than 80 and this number is anticipated to increase to 12 million (4.3%) by 2010.[1] The 1980 U.S. Census revealed that the life expectancy of a 70 year old was greater than 10 years and an 80 year old, 7 years.[3] Forty-three percent of Americans will reach the age of 80, and, of these, 40% will have symptomatic cardiovascular disease.[4] Dr. Robert Dripps, Professor of Anesthesia at the University of Pennsylvania, envisioned this trend as he wrote in 1948, "Until comparatively recently the aged were so few that little thought was given to them as a group. They were just old people: wise or childish, feeble or well preserved. By the inescapable statistics of the census takers, however, we are forced now to study the process of aging as well as economic and social problems of the aged. Surgery has much to offer the aged and the few facts presented . . . suggest that this offer can be made with considerable confidence."

Chronologic age has been known as an incremental risk factor for surgery, as the aging process progressively reduces the physiologic reserve of all organ systems. In addition, the elderly often do not have the mental fortitude and determination to endure both the physical and psychologic stress associated with a surgical procedure. On the other hand, during the past few years, the risks of operation have progressively declined due to improved preoperative evaluation, anesthetic management, surgical technology, postoperative intensive care, and rehabilitation support services. Consequently, large numbers of patients in their seventh and eighth decades of life have demonstrated dramatic functional improvement following cardiac surgery and have returned to a meaningful life style.

Given that the major goal of geriatric medicine is to enable the patient to continue an independent and productive existence, it then follows that it is the quality of life, and not its absolute longevity, that is of paramount importance to these elderly people. Maurice Chevalier is reported to have said "old age is not so bad when you consider the alternative." Oliver Wendell Holmes stated on his 91st birthday on March 8, 1882: "The riders in a race do not stop short when they reach the goal. There is a little finishing canter before coming to a standstill. . . . There is time to hear the kind voices of friends and to say to oneself, 'the work is done.'" It is in this light that the elderly patient with cardiac disease should be evaluated.

This chapter will be divided into three aspects: first, a general discussion of the preoperative evaluation, the surgical procedure, and postoperative care; second, a review of the recent results of myocardial revascularization; and third, valvular surgery in the elderly.

## GENERAL DISCUSSION

### PREOPERATIVE EVALUATION

The preoperative evaluation in the elderly is comparable with that used for younger individuals, but the risk-benefit ratio of surgery versus medical management must be more sharply defined in this patient population. First, thorough consideration must be given to the patient's general overall condition with special emphasis on the mental status and physiologic makeup. Significant noncardiac conditions, even though they may be overshadowed by the severity of the cardiac disease, should be fully evaluated. Finally, an assessment must be made of the support system available to the patient.

### General Condition

The elderly patient more often than not is referred for cardiac surgery late in the course of the disease. By this time, medical management has been exhausted and often the symptoms are end-stage and life-threatening. The body has suffered the ravages of the disease process as the patient has been inactive, malnourished, and frequently has developed cardiac cachexia. Even though the hemodynamic or ischemic cardiac problem may be correctable surgically, the patient often does not have the strength, stamina, or caloric reserve to withstand the stress of a major operation. It is unfortunate that the severity of the cardiac disease usually precludes any attempt at maximizing the patient's nutritional status preoperatively.

Both the organic mental status and psychologic framework of the elderly patient are of paramount importance. The patient must be able to think clearly and

to understand the effects and consequences of both the operation and the postoperative recovery. A history of recent memory loss, transient ischemic attack, stroke, or other neurologic disorder must enter into the evaluation. Psychologically, the patient must be determined to face the discomforts that accompany a surgical procedure in exchange for the relief of symptoms and the opportunity for improved quality of life. Although it is usually impossible to perform an in-depth evaluation before operation, it is often worthwhile for the physician to discuss with the patient, family, and friends the importance of motivation and the will to get well. Specific questions regarding how vigorous a patient was before the onset of the cardiac illness or how the patient had reacted to previous medical or surgical stress are appropriate. Finally, before making a final recommendation, the physician should evaluate both available support structures and the environment to which the patient will return.

Once the overall general condition has been assessed, each specific organ system then should be screened systematically.

**Cardiovascular System**

The evaluation of the cardiovascular system in the elderly should be carried out whenever possible by noninvasive methods and cardiac catheterization reserved for obtaining information not available by other means. First, it is of the utmost importance to determine as accurately as possible the status of the patient's ventricular function. This can be done by history, physical examination, chest x-ray, electrocardiogram (ECG), and other noninvasive techniques. The history will establish whether the patient's symptoms have been chronic or of more recent onset. Cardiomegaly, ventricular gallop, significant murmurs, or evidence of pulmonary hypertension and congestive heart failure can be elicited on physical examination. The chest x-ray will reveal cardiomegaly, congestive heart failure, valvular calcification, or dilatation of the ascending aorta. The ECG may indicate old myocardial infarction, new ischemia, or a conduction delay. Echocardiography or radionuclide wall-motion studies are quite accurate for determining overall ventricular ejection fraction. In addition, these techniques are most useful in differentiating local segmental wall abnormalities from inoperable generalized global ventricular dysfunction.

In a patient with symptomatic calcific aortic stenosis, most of the significant information can be gathered by noninvasive methods, including Doppler flow measurement of the transvalvular pressure gradient. Caution must be used, however, in interpreting this information inasmuch as a pressure gradient of only 30 to 50 mm Hg may represent a critical stenosis in a patient with a low cardiac output state. Cardiac catheterization is used to measure right heart and pulmonary artery pressures, and in selected instances, to confirm the pressure gradient across the aortic valve. Angiography should be limited to defining the coronary anatomy as it is usually not necessary to perform ventriculography. Finally, it is helpful to assess the size of the aortic valve annulus for aid in planning the type of prosthesis to be inserted. Calcification or aneurysmal dilatation of the ascending aorta and evidence of mitral insufficiency also should be identified because these factors may influence the conduct of the operation.

Similarly, in a patient with mitral valvular disease, both the clinical evaluation and noninvasive data are of paramount importance. A patient with calcific mitral stenosis, a normal left ventricle, and moderate pulmonary hypertension clearly has

a different surgical risk than one with a dilated ischemic left ventricle and resulting mitral regurgitation. In either situation, echocardiography is the noninvasive procedure of choice to demonstrate the mitral valve pathology, evaluate left ventricular function, and measure the size of the right heart chambers. Transesophageal echocardiography is especially helpful for delineating the functional anatomy of the regurgitant mitral valve whether it be due to annular dilatation, leaflet prolapse, chordal elongation, or rupture. In addition, calcification of the mitral annulus should be noted preoperatively inasmuch as this may be a crucial risk factor for surgery.

In the elderly patient with ischemic heart disease, standard ECG stress testing is often difficult or dangerous to perform. The patient may have unstable symptoms, a lack of stamina, or the inability to cooperate, thus making the data inconclusive. A delayed thallium scan may be useful in differentiating a reversible ischemic area from a fixed transmural scar. Radionuclide wall-motion studies can accurately measure ventricular function. Angiography is essential to define the coronary anatomy, assess the quality of the obstructed vessels, and estimate the territory of the myocardium supplied by each coronary artery. All these factors must be considered when one is deciding between percutaneous transluminal coronary angioplasty and surgical revascularization. Specifically, the physician must evaluate how a patient would tolerate an acute angioplasty failure and the resulting surgical emergency.

As previously mentioned, cardiac catheterization should be used judiciously in the elderly patient. Both the timing and the information gained from this procedure are important. Clearly it is prudent, but often not possible, to optimize the patient's congestive heart failure or unstable ischemia before performing the catheterization. It is imperative therefore to plan what information is necessary and then to perform the procedure as expeditiously as possible. Because many elderly patients have borderline renal function, discretion must be used in administering radiographic dye.

## Pulmonary System

The elderly patient often has a lack of pulmonary reserve even though the basic lung function is relatively normal. Respiratory failure is the most frequent postoperative noncardiac complication encountered after open heart surgery. Preoperatively, it is not only important to evaluate but to optimize the patient's pulmonary status if needed with bronchodilators, antibiotics, and pulmonary physiotherapy. Meaningful laboratory pulmonary function studies are difficult to obtain but, if possible, may help differentiate restrictive from obstructive pulmonary disease and may guide the physician toward the appropriate medical therapy.

## Renal System

The elderly patient has a natural decline in glomerular filtration rate as reflected by urea retention and decreased creatinine clearance. Electrolyte metabolism may be altered owing to intrinsic renal disease and/or chronic diuretic therapy. Coexisting, longstanding hypertension may affect renal blood flow.

It is not unusual for an elderly patient with chronic congestive heart failure on high-dose diuretic therapy to present with azotemia, either prerenal and/or renal in origin. If prerenal, gentle fluid administration and/or a dilute dopamine infusion will increase renal blood flow and improve the azotemia. In a patient with borderline renal function, the use of radiopaque dye must be kept to a minimum to minimize the development of acute renal failure.

## Central Nervous System

It is not unusual for the elderly patient to have coexisting extracranial and intracranial vascular disease. One of the most devastating postoperative complications of cardiac surgery is an irreversible central nervous system catastrophe. A history of temporary mental confusion, transient ischemic attack, or stroke should be thoroughly investigated by conducting a history, physical examination, and non-invasive studies such as a computed tomography scan of the brain and Doppler flow studies of the carotid arteries. If significant coexisting vascular disease is found, such as an internal carotid artery stenosis, carotid endarterectomy and a cardiac procedure can be performed at the same time.

## Gastrointestinal System

There is an increased incidence of asymptomatic peptic ulcer disease, cholelithiasis, and diverticulosis in the elderly. These conditions may be exacerbated after cardiac surgery. In addition, the elderly patient is susceptible to the development of postoperative gastric stress ulcers. Prophylactic control of gastric pH using antacids and acid-reducing agents should be obtained. Liver dysfunction, often secondary to chronic congestive heart failure, may cause alteration in the coagulation profile. Thus, bleeding and prothrombin times and platelet and fibrinogen levels should be measured, and any abnormalities corrected preoperatively.

## Cancer Screening and Other Conditions

Undetected neoplasms are not unusual in the elderly. Index of suspicion must be high in the patient with fatigue, anemia, weight loss, or unexplained lymphadenopathy. If a malignancy is detected, a full evaluation should be performed to determine the presence or absence of metastatic disease. With this knowledge, the treatment course can be appropriately planned. For example, a patient with mitral regurgitation and an obstructing colon carcinoma should undergo the abdominal procedure with inotropic or intra-aortic balloon support as necessary before the mitral valve replacement. The reasons for this sequence of operations here are twofold. First, there are excellent means of treating the abnormal cardiac physiology of mitral regurgitation. Secondly, by performing the bowel surgery first, the risk of contamination of a newly placed prosthetic heart valve is reduced. On the other hand, a patient with unstable angina pectoris due to left main coronary artery obstruction and a colon carcinoma should undergo myocardial revascularization procedure first because there would be a substantial risk of myocardial infarction if the abdominal procedure took precedence.

The aforementioned evaluation should extend to the elderly patient with other coexisting vascular disease, especially an enlarging abdominal aneurysm or significant peripheral arterial occlusive disease. The patient should have his or her cardiac condition fully evaluated preoperatively and then the surgical procedures staged depending upon the findings.

Diabetes mellitus, although not an incremental risk factor in cardiac surgery in the elderly, may become difficult to control in the perioperative period. Often, an insulin infusion is required to control blood sugar postoperatively. The diabetic patient may have altered wound healing and a poor resistance to infection.

Careful attention must be given to the medications planned for the patient, especially narcotics and sedatives. Consideration should be given to discontinuing aspirin and all antiplatelet agents at least 5 days prior to surgery; however, cardio-

tonic and antianginal medications along with antiarrhythmics should be continued up to the time of operation.

## Summary of Preoperative Evaluation

After completion of the aforementioned evaluation, a clear recommendation can be made for cardiac surgery in the elderly patient. The cardiologist and surgeon should discuss their approach with both the patient and the family. The final decision, however, must be made by the patient, preferably without any persuasion by either physicians or family. In an analysis of 100 consecutive octogenarians who underwent cardiac surgery, Edmunds and coworkers[5] concluded that the preoperative selection of patients was the most important determinant for overall mortality even though they identified emergency operation, preoperative cachexia, previous myocardial infarction, and New York Heart Association (NYHA) class IV disease as independent risk factors for early death.

## SURGICAL PROCEDURE

Once cardiac surgery has been decided upon, the focus is shifted to anesthetic management, the planning of the operation, and the technical aspects of the procedure including cardiopulmonary bypass.

Special attention must be given to the anesthetic requirement in the elderly patient. Appropriate preoperative monitoring with arterial and pulmonary artery catheters is mandatory. Induction of anesthesia should be as smooth as possible to avoid hypoxia and the resultant arrhythmias. Older people may require less and also react inappropriately to anesthetic agents. The use of short-acting inhalation agents and minimal narcotics is preferable. Fluid replacement should be judicious inasmuch as it is very easy to overload such a patient, with resultant pulmonary congestion and congestive heart failure.

The planning of the surgical procedure is critical. The operation should be conservative and aimed at correcting only the necessary defects. For example, it is usually prudent to bypass only the large, critically obstructed coronary arteries rather than attempt to achieve complete myocardial revascularization. Expeditious valve replacement may be preferable to attempting a difficult valve repair with its inherent chance for failure and longer cardiopulmonary bypass time.

Meticulous attention must be made to the technical aspects of the operation. The elderly patient often has very friable or calcified tissue, and thus its handling must be done with utmost care. Calcified plaques in the ascending aorta may cause extreme difficulty in both aortic cannulation and proximal saphenous vein bypass anastomoses. Clamping of the aorta in these instances may be hazardous and cause calcium embolization or aortic dissection. Generalized "egg shell" calcification of the aorta may make handling of the aorta, including aortic valve replacement, prohibitive. Eccentric calcified plaques in the coronary arteries may cause technical difficulties in the distal anastomoses. The right atrial appendage is often small and quite friable and should be avoided during venous cannulation. Vigorous retraction of the heart may cause avulsion of the epicardium or possible cardiac disruption in the atrioventricular groove. This latter complication is not uncommon in a patient with a calcified mitral annulus. Venting the left ventricle is important inasmuch as ventricular distention is not well tolerated, but the use of a vent must be judicious to prevent ventricular perforation. With the retrograde cardioplegic technique,

proper placement of the balloon-tip catheter in the coronary sinus and careful measurement of back pressure during the instillation of the cardioplegic solution are essential. In patients with low cardiac output, it is often preferable to use afterload reduction and/or intra-aortic balloon counterpulsation rather than high-dose inotropic pressure support to reduce the work of the left ventricle. If intra-aortic balloon counterpulsation is necessary, special attention must be given to its insertion. It is often preferable to cannulate the femoral artery under direct vision and then to pass the intra-aortic balloon into the descending aorta over a guide wire to minimize the risk of aortic dissection or perforation.

Hemostasis in the elderly patient may be difficult to achieve, and thus attention should be paid throughout the operation to this concern. Heparinization and the effect of cardiopulmonary bypass on the platelets and other clotting factors may lead to coagulopathy that often is difficult to control.

Cardiopulmonary bypass plays an important role in the overall success of the operation. The elderly patient does not tolerate long periods of bypass well. Tsai and associates[6] in their series reported that there was increased morbidity and mortality in those patients who had perfusion time of more than 150 minutes and aortic cross-clamp time of greater than 100 minutes. Often, the elderly patient has hypertension or coexisting cerebral vascular disease and then it is essential to keep the nonpulsatile perfusion pressure higher than usual to maintain adequate cerebral blood flow. Hypothermia should be used judiciously and periods of circulatory arrest kept to a minimum for the same reasons. Renal function must be carefully monitored and diuretics given as necessary for fluid mobilization. The blood conserving measures and the administration of packed red blood cells in lieu of excessive crystalloid should be used throughout the procedure to minimize the level of dilutional anemia.

## POSTOPERATIVE CARE

Once in the postoperative surgical intensive care unit (ICU), the goal should be to normalize the patient as quickly as possible. Often, the patient is confused and unable to cooperate owing to the stress of the operation and the unfamiliarity with the ICU setting. As a result, a higher nurse-patient ratio may be required. Early reoperation for bleeding should be undertaken rather than treating this condition conservatively, to minimize the risk of multiple blood transfusions and the development of cardiac tamponade. Respiratory complications and subsequent ventilatory dependency become the focus for other organ complications; thus, all efforts must be made toward early extubation and mobilization.

When the ICU setting is no longer necessary, the patient should be promptly transferred to a step-down unit where vigorous physical and occupational rehabilitation should be undertaken. During this time in the recovery period, specific plans should be made for further convalescent care after hospital discharge. A team comprised of physicians, nurses, and paraprofessional personnel should coordinate the patient's ultimate rehabilitation.

## MYOCARDIAL REVASCULARIZATION IN THE ELDERLY

The risk of any intervention therapy must be carefully weighed and compared with the expected benefits. This is especially true for coronary bypass surgery in the elderly patient, in whom the risk, in terms of both morbidity and mortality, is elevated in comparison with a younger counterpart. Fortunately, there is now an increasing volume of literature analyzing the results of coronary artery bypass graft (CABG) surgery in older patients, enabling a more accurate prediction of operative results. Several years ago, bypass surgery in the population older than 80 years of age was anecdotal and considered heroic; today, many cardiac surgery centers have a significant personal experience with the oldest of the elderly patients.

As the average life span has increased, so has the age of the patient undergoing coronary bypass surgery. In 1979, 23% of bypass procedures were performed in patients older than 65; in 1986, the percentage rose to 41.[7] The median age of coronary bypass patients at the Cleveland Clinic rose from 50 to 62 from 1972 to 1986.[8] In fact, the average age of bypass patients in some centers is older than 68 years.[9] This rise leads many physicians now to consider age 70, and not 65, as the onset of old age. Thus, the elderly represent a significant and increasing percentage of the population who receive cardiac surgery and who, consequently, consume a large percentage of our total healthcare costs.[10] It is not unreasonable to ask if bypass surgery, the most common form of heart surgery in the elderly, is a wise investment, not only in terms of national expense, but also in terms of the physical and emotional cost to the patient.

## LITERATURE REVIEW

There are several difficulties in evaluating the results of coronary bypass surgery in the elderly. First, there have been no prospective, randomized trials that include this age group; both the Coronary Artery Surgery Study (CASS) and the European Coronary Surgery Study excluded patients older than 65. All series of bypass surgery in elderly patients are inherently biased by a very careful patient selection. Second, most reviews retrospectively analyzed data to determine an association between independent risk factors and morbidity and mortality, relief of angina, or patient survival. Few reviews emphasized all three. Third, preoperative status, complications, and long-term results are reported in different ways, making direct comparison among reports difficult. Finally, there are relatively few series that compare the results of elderly patients with younger ones during the same period at the same institution.[9,11,12]

**Table 14–1.** Operative Mortality of
Patients Older Than 70 Years of Age

| Author | Year | Age | Number | Deaths | Mortality (%) |
|---|---|---|---|---|---|
| Acinapura et al[9] | 1990 | 70 | 1385 | 111 | 8.0 |
| Azariades et al[13] | 1990 | 70 | 1081 | 65 | 6.0 |
| Gardner et al[14] | 1990 | 70 | 723 | 48 | 6.6 |
| McIntyre et al[15] | 1990 | 70 | 250 | 9 | 3.6 |
| Ivert et al[16] | 1989 | 70 | 45 | 5 | 12.0 |
| Tsai et al[17] | 1989 | 70 | 649 | 42 | 6.5 |
| Horneffer et al[11] | 1987 | 70 | 228 | 21 | 9.3 |
| Montague et al[18] | 1985 | 70 | 581 | 14 | 2.4 |
| Gersh et al[19] | 1983 | 70 | 241 | 16 | 6.6 |
| Total | | | 5183 | 331 | 6.4 |

**Table 14–2.** Operative Mortality of Patients Older Than 75 Years of Age

| Author | Year | Age | Number | Deaths | Mortality (%) |
|---|---|---|---|---|---|
| Horvath et al[20] | 1990 | 75 | 222 | 24 | 10.8 |
| Loop et al[8] | 1988 | 75 | 467 | 22 | 4.7 |
| Rich et al[21] | 1988 | 75 | 60 | 2 | 3.3 |
| Rahimtoola et al[12] | 1986 | 75 | 178 | 5 | 2.8 |
| Gersh et al[19] | 1983 | 75 | 42 | 4 | 9.5 |
| Total | | | 969 | 57 | 5.9 |

To compare the data from different series, preoperative status, operative mortality, and postoperative complications were tabulated. Many series contained information on patients with bypass alone and bypass plus valve surgery. For this review, only patients older than 70 who had undergone revascularization alone were included. In all series, the operative mortality rates of patients with revascularization alone could be separated from the other patients, but often not the preoperative status and complications. Consequently, the operative mortality rates were taken from all series, whereas the risk factors, complications, and results were taken only from series when available. Although this method of presenting data introduces an obvious bias in analyzing the results of the clinical series, it maximizes the number of patients in each category, and therefore minimizes errors from small numbers.

## OPERATIVE MORTALITY

In Tables 14–1 to 14–3, the operative mortality of patients older than 70, 75, and 80 are presented. Not surprisingly, the elderly as a group have a higher operative mortality than that reported in younger patients. Patients older than 80 have the highest mortality of all. It is surprising, however, that the average mortality in 80 year olds is only 10.8%. It might be postulated that generally only superior results are reported and that the 10.8% represents an underestimation of the true mortality. However, a recent tabulation of results in The Society of Thoracic Surgeons database discussed at the 1991 Surgical Thoracic Society meeting revealed an operative mortality of 11.9% in 704 patients aged 80 or older. These results

**Table 14–3.** Operative Mortality of Patients Older Than 80 Years of Age

| Author | Year | Age | Number | Deaths | Mortality (%) |
|---|---|---|---|---|---|
| Dixon et al[22] | 1990 | 80 | 13 | 0 | 0.0 |
| Mullany et al[23] | 1990 | 80 | 159 | 17 | 10.7 |
| Naunheim et al[24] | 1990 | 80 | 71 | 9 | 13.0 |
| Tsai et al[17] | 1989 | 80 | 64 | 2 | 3.1 |
| Edmunds et al[5] | 1988 | 80 | 41 | 10 | 24.0 |
| Montague et al[18] | 1985 | 80 | 16 | 2 | 13.0 |
| Rich et al[25] | 1985 | 80 | 7 | 0 | 0.0 |
| Total | | | 371 | 40 | 10.8 |

suggest that in properly selected patients, CABG surgery can be done with an elevated, but acceptable mortality.

PREOPERATIVE STATUS OF ELDERLY PATIENTS

### Patient Selection and Preoperative Risk Factors

The role preoperative selection has on postoperative results cannot be overemphasized. Edmunds and colleagues[5] have pointed out the paradox that the operative mortality of some series of 80 year olds is lower than that of 70 year olds.[19,25,27] In addition, both one of the lowest and highest operative mortalities for elderly patients was reported by the same surgeons at the same institution.[5,28]

Risk factors can be separated into noncardiac and cardiac. The noncardiac risk factors can be further subdivided into those that are vascular and nonvascular in origin. The noncardiac vascular and the cardiac risk factors appear to be the most important.

### Noncardiac Risk Factors

A comparison of the preoperative status of elderly patients with younger patients at the same institution during the same period is shown in Table 14–4. The incidence of the risk factors is shown in Table 14–5. Few noncardiac risk factors can be assessed. However, elderly patients are more apt to be female, and probably have a higher incidence of chronic diseases of the pulmonary, renal, and neurologic systems. Gersh and coworkers[29] did note that significant pulmonary disease was equal in patients older and younger than 65, but the decrease in pulmonary reserve was not specifically measured. The same was true for renal disease.

Older patients, however, have an increased incidence of noncardiac vascular disease due, for example, to diabetes, hypertension, and peripheral vascular atherosclerosis. The exact role that noncardiac risk factors exert on operative mortality is not certain although peripheral vascular disease has been shown to correlate with an increase in mortality. Moreover, it seems logical that the nonvascular and vascular problems would tend to increase the operative mortality.[29,30]

### Cardiac Risk Factors

The increased incidence of noncardiac vascular risk factors is paralleled by primary risk factors, which include both the extent of anatomic disease and the severity of clinical syndromes. The 22% incidence of left main coronary stenosis noted in Table 14–5 is higher than the 15% noted in the CASS registry.[26] The like-

**Table 14–4.** Comparison of Risk Factors in Younger and Older Patients

| | Male | Peripheral Vascular Disease | Diabetes Mellitus | Prior Myocardial Infarct | Unstable Angina | Left Ventricular Function | Left Main Stenosis |
|---|---|---|---|---|---|---|---|
| Acinapura et al[9] | L | NR | H | H | H | L | H |
| Loop et al[8] | L | H | H | NR | NR | ND | H |
| Horneffer et al[11] | L | H | ND | ND | H | ND | NR |
| Rahimtoola et al[12] | L | NR | ND | ND | ND | ND | ND |

L = lower; H = higher; NR = not recorded; ND = no difference.

**Table 14–5.** Percentages of Risk Factors from Selected Series

| | Male (%) | Peripheral Vascular Disease | Diabetes Mellitus | Prior Myocardial Infarct | Unstable Angina | Left Main Stenosis |
|---|---|---|---|---|---|---|
| Average | 0.66 | 0.24 | 0.23 | 0.60 | 0.66 | 0.22 |
| n | 13.00 | 6.00 | 9.00 | 10.00 | 9.00 | 7.00 |
| SD | 0.06 | 0.06 | 0.14 | 0.11 | 0.14 | 0.11 |

n = number; SD = standard deviation.

lihood of triple-vessel disease is also increased.[23] Preoperative myocardial infarction appears higher in the elderly. It is unclear but conceivable that ventricular function in the elderly is worse than that in younger age groups. For instance, in the CASS study, the incidence of left ventricular dysfunction was approximately 60% in both 80 year olds and in younger groups; however, the eldest as a group had more severe disease.[19] Mullany and associates[23] found that the single most important factor that predicted operative mortality in octogenarians was poor left ventricular function.

The disabling symptoms that bring patients to the attention of the intervention cardiologists and surgeons are reflected in the high incidence of unstable, rest, and postinfarction angina. These clinical situations result in more frequent need for intra-aortic balloon use preoperatively,[23] and a greater likelihood of urgent or emergency surgery.[20,24]

## POSTOPERATIVE COMPLICATIONS

An assessment of the likelihood of postoperative complications is of equal importance in the treatment of the elderly as is the expected operative mortality. Many elderly patients, and their families, tend to avoid any treatment that involves significant postoperative morbidity. More than the risk to life itself, the elderly often fear that an unsuccessful operation will be associated with long periods of discomfort, disorientation, and isolation from their families.

The majority of the elderly will have at least one postoperative complication. In fact, if transient arrhythmias are considered, 92% of the patients in one series had complications. Even with the exclusion of arrhythmias, the complication rate in the elderly was higher than in the younger population (Table 14–6).

**Table 14–6.** Comparison of Postoperative Complications in Younger and Older Patients

| | Stroke | Reoperation for Bleeding | Prolonged Pulmonary Dysfunction | Sternal Infection | Renal Failure or Dialysis | Perioperative Myocardial Infarction |
|---|---|---|---|---|---|---|
| Acinapura et al[9] | H | NR | H | NR | H | H |
| Loop et al[8] | H | H | H | ND | H | ND |
| Horneffer et al[11] | H | H | H | H | H | NR |
| Rahimtoola et al[12] | NR | NR | NR | NR | NR | NR |

H = higher; NR = not recorded; ND = no difference.

**Table 14-7.** Percentages with Complications From Selected
Series

| | Stroke | Reoperation for Bleeding | Prolonged Pulmonary Dysfunction | Sternal Infection | Renal Failure or Dialysis | Perioperative Myocardial Infarction | Major Complications |
|---|---|---|---|---|---|---|---|
| Average | 0.04 | 0.05 | 0.08 | 0.02 | 0.04 | 0.05 | 0.32 |
| n | 11.00 | 9.00 | 8.00 | 5.00 | 6.00 | 8.00 | 5.00 |
| SD | 0.03 | 0.01 | 0.04 | 0.01 | 0.04 | 0.04 | 0.19 |

n = number; SD = standard deviation.

## Major Complications

Major complications from selected series are listed in Table 14-7. There is a higher incidence of stroke, bleeding, prolonged mechanical ventilation or respiratory distress, renal failure, or the need for dialysis. Postoperative disorientation or psychosis is also more prevalent.

By multivariate analysis, Montague and colleagues[18] noted that the presence of peripheral vascular disease or emergent surgery correlated with postoperative complications. Low body weight[21] and cachexia[5] have been correlated with postoperative complications and eventual poor outcomes. On the other hand, a higher rate of sternal infections or sepsis was not evident in the elderly.

The incidence of postoperative myocardial infarctions in the elderly is not greater than in younger patients, implying that the primary cardiac disease is as effectively treated in both patient cohorts. In fact, the percentage of patients that succumb for a cardiac reason postoperatively appears to be decreased in the elderly in comparison with younger patients.[8,9]

## Postoperative Atrial Fibrillation

Exclusion of postoperative atrial fibrillation after revascularization from the list of major complications does not imply an entirely benign course for patients with this arrhythmia. Atrial fibrillation increases with age,[8,31] usually prolongs hospitalization, and may be temporarily associated with strokes. Although the postoperative incidence of arrhythmias may be reduced with beta blockers, this therapy is often contraindicated in the elderly because of pulmonary dysfunction.

### USE OF THE INTERNAL MAMMARY ARTERY

The use of the internal mammary artery in older patients has increased progressively and the recent results have been gratifying.[13,14] Gardner and associates[14] reported its use in more than 90% of elderly patients. In comparison with patients who received only saphenous vein bypasses, those who had mammary artery grafts showed no increase in postoperative complications and had a low (2.8% to 4.9%) operative mortality. Moreover, it appears that the survival in this group is prolonged. Thus, the consensus at present is that old age itself in not a contraindication of the use of the internal mammary artery as a bypass conduit.

### POSTOPERATIVE STAY

The elderly have a longer postoperative hospital stay mainly due to the increase in postoperative complications. As Rahimtoola and coworkers[12] noted, however, this may not necessarily translate into a significant increase in overall hospital cost.

## SHORT-TERM AND LONG-TERM OUTCOME

### Functional Recovery

The expectation of an active life in elderly patients without disabling coronary syndromes is surprisingly good. Katz and associates[32] noted that persons aged 70 to 74, 75 to 79, or 80 to 84 could expect an independent life for an additional time span of 8.1, 6.8, or 4.7 years respectively. A most gratifying aspect of bypass surgery in the elderly is that the majority of patients are relieved of angina. The pooled results from several series reflects an angina-free rate that approaches 80% and in fact may be better than those in younger patients. Despite the increased operative risks in terms of morbidity and mortality, the relief of symptoms and return to active life are dramatic.

### Life Expectancy

Both Loop[8] and Rahimtoola[12] and their colleagues have noted that the life expectancy after successful bypass surgery is no different from an age-matched general population. In most series, the observed mortality is equal or better than the U.S. population, adjusted for age and gender.[12,23,24]

## SUMMARY

Coronary bypass surgery in the elderly, including 80 year olds, can be done with an acceptable mortality. The increased incidence of postoperative complications is counterbalanced by the excellent relief of symptoms. Inasmuch as patients do return to an active life and enjoy years of independent living, bypass surgery does not appear to be inappropriate use of medical resources. However, there have been no prospective, randomized trials, and thus it is important to recognize that these excellent results have occurred in selected patients. Continued careful patient selection and astute clinical judgment will remain the cornerstone for successful surgical outcomes in the future.

## RESULTS OF VALVE SURGERY IN THE ELDERLY

The overall operative mortality for cardiac valve surgery has been reported to be between 5% and 12%.[33] Before the age of 60, the age per se does not increase the risk of operation.[34] Recently, several large series have reported favorable results for valve replacement in septuagenarians and octogenarians.[5,35-42] In an attempt to determine whether age was an independent predictor of major morbidity and mortality, many authors have reported their results on valvular surgery in patients older than 70 years. Fremes and the group from Toronto[43] showed that older patients have more frequent left ventricular dysfunction, coronary artery disease, and more often require urgent surgery, thus concluding that older age itself was a risk factor. In Lytle's[44] large series from the Cleveland Clinic there was an adverse effect of old age in aortic valve replacement, but not in mitral valve surgery. Sethi and coworkers,[33] reporting on the experience in the Veterans Administration Cooperative Study, showed an increased risk for those undergoing mitral surgery but not aortic valve surgery. Scott and colleagues[45,46] from Stanford showed an increased risk in their elderly patients having either mitral or aortic valve surgery.

As the population ages, more elderly patients are presenting with symptomatic valvular disease from calcific aortic stenosis and ischemic mitral regurgitation. Most reports of valvular surgery in this population corroborate the relative success of valve replacement and demonstrate that, although there is an increase in the perioperative morbidity and mortality, the majority of the long-term survivors return to an active and productive existence.[5,35,40,42,47] In this era, which concerns itself with both the quality of life and the escalating cost of healthcare, consideration must be given both to the surgical approach and to alternative therapies in dealing with the elderly patient with valvular heart disease.

## AORTIC VALVE SURGERY

Calcific aortic stenosis is the most prominent pathologic valvular condition encountered in the elderly, and aortic valve replacement is the most commonly performed valve procedure.[48] Once symptoms of syncope, angina, or congestive heart failure develop in patients with aortic stenosis, life expectancy without operation is 1.5 to 3 years.[49] Medical therapy does little to improve the quality of life in these end-stage patients, and the risk of sudden death is high. Conversely, aortic valve replacement usually allows these patients to return to an active and independent life style.

Recent reports of aortic valve replacement in the elderly are numerous. Bessone and coworkers[50] analyzed 219 consecutive patients operated on between 1972 and 1986 who were older than the age of 70. They found that there was a 12.1% mortality rate for aortic valve replacement alone in this cohort of patients as compared with a 5.7% reported mortality rate for younger patients. In patients who had associated coronary artery disease, the operative mortality was 8.9%. Some degree of perioperative morbidity occurred in 35% of the patients and included reoperation for bleeding, low cardiac output, congestive heart failure, arrhythmias, and respiratory insufficiency. Late complications of the hospital survivors were infrequent, with 95% of the patients having none. These complications included neurologic events, bleeding secondary to anticoagulation, and valve dysfunction. The long-term survival in this cohort was 77.2% ± 5.5%, which is significantly better than the expected survival of the general population at the age of 75. Of the survivors in this series, 98% returned to NYHA functional class I or II. Blakeman and the group[51] from Loyola reported similar results in 100 patients older than the age of 75, with 68 of 71 long-term survivors (96%) being in NYHA classification I or II.

Many patients with calcific aortic stenosis have critical coronary artery disease that is unexpected and asymptomatic. Although the combination of myocardial revascularization with aortic valve replacement complicates and lengthens the operative procedure, the results support performance of the combined procedure.[6,52-56] It is important, however, to modify the operation so that only the most critical vessels are bypassed to minimize operative time. Often it is difficult to mobilize the hypertrophied left ventricle to visualize the arteries on the posterior surface of the heart. In addition, it is usually wiser to use saphenous vein as the conduit because it shortens the operative time and supplies a greater initial blood flow to the hypertrophied muscle.

The type of valve prosthesis selected is of importance. Borkon and associates[57] from Johns Hopkins analyzed 141 patients with both mechanical and bioprosthetic aortic valves. They showed that those with bioprosthetic valves experienced fewer valve-related complications. Specifically, there was a reduced incidence of antico-agulant-related hemorrhage in the patients who received bioprosthetic valves. Therefore, they favor a bioprosthetic valve in all of their patients older than 70 years of age. Akins and coworkers[58] reported that the freedom from structural valve deterioration in their patients with heterograft porcine valves was 91% for all patients at 10 years and almost 100% in those patients older than the age of 70. Jamieson and colleagues,[37] reporting on 635 patients who underwent aortic valve replacement with a porcine bioprosthesis, showed that structural valve deteriora-tion was virtually nonexistent at 10 and 12 years in patients 70 years of age or older. For these reasons, bioprosthetic valves in the aortic position often are favored for the elderly patient.

Finally, alternative procedures to valve replacement must be considered. To date, the results of valve debridement and decalcification have been disappointing. Craver[59] reported on 11 patients who underwent ultrasonic debridement of the aor-tic valve and annulus. Although there were excellent immediate hemodynamic results, five patients showed new valvular regurgitation and three required reoper-ation. He concluded that the early occurrence of aortic regurgitation in a higher percentage of patients makes it an unacceptable alternative to valve replacement. Likewise, balloon dilatation for aortic stenosis has resulted in minimal short-term benefit with a high incidence of restenosis.[60] There are selected patients, however, who are in need of an urgent noncardiac operation and in these instances, balloon dilatation of a stenotic valve could result in a safer operation.[61-63]

As the proportion of elderly in the population grows, there will be an increase in the number of patients with critical aortic valvular dysfunction. Although the operative mortality and perioperative complication rate in these patients is higher than in younger patients, the benefits of aortic valve replacement with or without myocardial revascularization are substantial, and an aggressive surgical attitude is warranted even in patients with left ventricular dysfunction.

## MITRAL VALVE REPLACEMENT

Isolated mitral valvular disease is less common in the elderly. Calcification of the mitral valve apparatus secondary to rheumatic disease can result in either mitral regurgitation or, less commonly, stenosis in older patients. On the other hand, mitral regurgitation resulting from myxomatous degeneration or ischemia occurs with increasing frequency in the elderly. Usually, the clinical presentation and sub-sequent risk of surgery depends on the etiology and duration of the mitral disease process. The patient with calcific mitral stenosis, moderate pulmonary hyperten-sion, and normal left ventricular function is markedly different from one with a dilated ischemic cardiomyopathy and mitral regurgitation. The latter group of patients presents the highest surgical risk owing to left ventricular dysfunction. When severe disease exists, mitral valve repair or replacement is usually recom-mended. Recently, there has been a trend in the elderly, as with younger patients, to preserve and repair the native mitral valve whenever possible. Duran and coworkers[64] showed a decrease in operative mortality from 11.4% to 1.9% when mitral valve repair was possible rather than replacement. Although other reports have also shown a decrease in the operative mortality with valve repair, fewer older patients are candidates for this approach because of the degree of calcification present and, in these instances, valve replacement is preferred. Because removal of the native valve and division of the chordal attachments may have a detrimental effect on left ventricular function, preservation of the posterior chordal attachments is recommended if possible. David and colleagues[65-67] demonstrated this by finding a decrease in the resting and systolic volume index when the chordae tendineae were preserved.

In general, risks of mitral valve surgery in the elderly exceed those of aortic valve surgery. As with younger patients, the risk of surgery on the mitral valve is multifactorial, with preoperative left ventricular function, degree of pulmonary hypertension, presence of endocarditis, extent of associated coronary artery disease, and urgency of the surgery all being important. In good-risk patients older than 70 years of age, mitral valve replacement can be performed with an operative mortality of 5% to 10%.[68] As more risk factors are present, the mortality increases. The highest risk is predicted in elderly patients with associated coronary artery disease and poor left ventricular function who require urgent surgery. The operative mortality in this group may exceed 50%.[6]

Scott and associates[45] confirmed the finding that an elevation in the serum bilirubin, indicating hepatic dysfunction, is also a significant predictor of operative mortality in mitral valve replacement. Hyperbilirubinemia usually indicates right heart failure with severe tricuspid regurgitation. These patients should be identified preoperatively as individuals having a considerable operative risk with mitral valve surgery. In good-risk elderly patients, mitral valve repair or replacement can be recommended with a reasonable operative risk. As the risk factors increase in the elderly patient and the predicted operative mortality climbs, serious consideration should be given to nonsurgical treatment of seriously ill patients.[6]

The majority of patients who undergo mitral valve replacement have a clear indication for long-term anticoagulation, whether it be a history of atrial fibrillation or an embolic event, a large left atrium, or low cardiac output. As a result, a mechanical prosthesis usually is recommended in this patient population.

## DOUBLE VALVE REPLACEMENT

Although the numbers are small in most series dealing with the elderly, combined aortic and mitral valve replacement can be performed in patients older than 70 years of age. Besides age, the predictive factors of mortality seem to be urgency of surgery, preoperative ventricular function, and tricuspid valve disease.[68] Operative mortalities in these patients range from 20% to 50%. Although most patients considered for double-valve replacement have less severe disease as measured by gradients or valve area than those operated upon for single-valve replacement, the magnitude of the operation dictates that the patient be in a good-risk category if a successful result is to be anticipated.[69]

## COMPLICATIONS

Clearly there is an increased incidence of complications after valvular surgery in the elderly as compared with the younger population. Up to 30% of the patients older than 70 years of age suffer a neurologic problem, either temporarily or permanently. It is thought that this complication most often is due to calcium emboli, either from the ascending aorta or the diseased valve. The surgical technique demands careful removal of the valve and debridement of the annulus to minimize the risk of calcium embolization and to properly seat the valve prosthesis.

Other immediate complications in decreasing order of frequency are pulmonary, renal, and peripheral vascular. Long-term complications are related to infection, thromboembolism, and anticoagulation-related hemorrhage. These latter risks, however, are quite similar to younger patients undergoing valve replacement.

### Summary

The decision to proceed with cardiac valve surgery in patients older than 70 years must be made with careful deliberation. Clearly, the risks of surgery are increased, but the potential benefits in rehabilitating the individual back to a productive and full life are real. An aggressive surgical approach should be taken in patients with aortic stenosis. More caution should be used in advocating mitral valve or double-valve replacement in the elderly, especially when other factors place these individuals in a high-risk category. Both patients and their families should be fully aware of the potential risks and benefits in weighing their decision to proceed with surgical therapy.

## REFERENCES

1. Anderson, WF: Transactions and Studies of the College of Physicians of Philadelphia: Medical and History; series V, vol VI, No. 4, December, 1984.
2. Bureau of Census: Projections of the population of the United States by age, sex and race: 1983–2080. Current population reports, series P-25, no 952. Government Printing Office, Washington, DC, 1984.
3. National Center for Health Statistics: United States life tables: U.S. decennial life tables for 1979–1981, vol 1, no 1. Government Printing Office, Washington, DC, 1985 (DHHS Publication No. (PHS) 85-1150-1).
4. National health interview survey 1983–85. National Center for Health Statistics, Hyattsville, Md., 1986.
5. Edmunds, LH, Stephenson, LW, Edie, RN, et al: Open-heart surgery in octogenarians. N Engl J Med 319 (3):131–136, 1988.
6. Tsai, TP, Matloff, JM, Chaux, A, et al: Combined valve and coronary artery bypass procedures in septuagenarians and octogenarians: Results in 120 patients. Ann Thorac Surg 42:681–684, 1986.
7. Feinlab, M, Havlik, RJ, Gillum, RF, et al: Coronary heart disease and related procedures. Circulation 79(suppl I):I13–18, 1989.
8. Loop, FD, Lytle, BW, Cosgrove, DM, et al: Coronary artery bypass graft surgery in the elderly. Cleve Clin J Med 55:23–34, 1988.
9. Acinapura, AJ, Jacobowitz, IJ, Kramer, MD, et al: Demographic changes in coronary artery bypass surgery and its effect on mortality and morbidity. Eur J Cardio-thorac Surg 1:175–181, 1990.
10. Baker, BS: Consumer nemesis of the 80's: Rising health care costs. Health Values 10:19–22, 1986.
11. Horneffer, PJ, Gardner, TJ, Manolio, TA, et al: The effects of age on outcome after coronary bypass surgery. Circulation 76(V):V6–12, 1987.
12. Rahimtoola, SH, Grunkemeier, GL, Starr, A: Ten year survival after coronary artery bypass surgery for angina in patients aged 65 years and older. Circulation 74(3):509–517, 1986.
13. Azariades, M, Fessler, CL, Floten, HS, et al: Five-year results of coronary bypass grafting for patients older than 70 years: Role of internal mammary artery. Ann Thorac Surg 50:940–945, 1990.
14. Gardner, TJ, Greene, PS, Rykiel, MF, et al: Routine use of the left internal mammary artery graft in the elderly. Ann Thorac Surg 49:188–194, 1990.

15. McIntyre, AB, Ballenger, JF, King, AT: Coronary artery bypass surgery in the elderly. South Caro-
    lina Medical Association 86(8):435–439, 1990.
16. Ivert, T, Lindblom, D, Welti, R: Coronary artery bypass grafting in patients 70 years of age and
    older. Eur J Cardio-thorac Surg 3:52–57, 1989.
17. Tsai, TP, Chaux, A, Kass, RM, et al: Aortocoronary bypass surgery in septuagenarians and octo-
    genarian. J Cardiovasc Surg 30:364–368, 1989.
18. Montague, NT, Kouchoukos, NT, Wilson, TA, et al: Morbidity and mortality of coronary bypass
    grafting in patients 70 years of age and older. Ann Thorac Surg 39(6):552–557, 1985.
19. Gersh, BJ, Phil, D, Kronmal, RA, et al: Coronary arteriography and coronary artery bypass surgery:
    Morbidity and mortality in patients ages 65 years or older. Circulation 67(3):483–490, 1983.
20. Horvath, KA, DiSea, VJ, Peigh, PS, et al: Favorable results of coronary artery bypass grafting in
    patients older than 75 years. J Thorac Cardiovasc Surg 99:92–96, 1990.
21. Rich, MW, Keller, AJ, Schectman, KB, et al: Morbidity and mortality of coronary bypass surgery
    in patients 75 years of age or older. Ann Thorac Surg 46:638–644, 1988.
22. Dixon, AC, Ito, L, Fukuyama, O: Outcome following open-heart surgery in an oriental octagenarian
    population in Hawaii. Hawaii Med J 49(8):303–307, 1990.
23. Mullany, CJ, Darling, GE, Pluth, JR, et al: Early and late results after isolated coronary artery
    bypass surgery in 159 patients age 80 years and older. Circulation 82(5):IV229–236, 1990.
24. Nauheim, KS, Dean, PA, Fiore, AC, et al: Cardiac surgery in the octogenarian. Eur J Cardio-thorac
    Surg 4:130–135, 1990.
25. Rich, MW, Sandza, JG, Kleiger, RE, et al: Cardiac operations in patients over 80 years of age. J
    Thorac Cardiovasc Surg 90:56–60, 1985.
26. Myers, WO, Davis, K, Foster, ED, et al: Surgical survival in the coronary artery surgery study
    (CASS) registry. Ann Thorac Surg 40:245–260, 1985.
27. Silvay, G, Feinberg, B, Jurado, R, et al: Open heart surgery in patients in the eighth and ninth
    decades of life. In Proceedings of the Eighth Annual Meeting, Society of Cardiovascular Anes-
    thesiologists, April 27–30, 1986, Montreal, Canada. Society of Cardiovascular Anesthesiolo-
    gists, Richmond, Va, 1986, p. 152.
28. Stephenson, LW, McVaugh, HM, Edmunds, HL: Surgery using cardiopulmonary bypass in the
    elderly. Circulation 58(2):250–254, 1978.
29. Gersh, BJ, Kronmal, RA, Schaff, HV, et al: Comparison of coronary artery bypass surgery and
    medical therapy in patients 65 years of age or older. N Engl J Med 13:217–224, 1985.
30. Gersh, BJ, Kronmal, RA, Schaff, HV, et al: Long-term 5-year results of coronary bypass surgery in
    patients 65 years old or older. Circulation 68(Suppl)II:II190–199, 1983.
31. Fuller, JA, Adams, GG, Buxton, B: Atrial fibrillation after coronary artery bypass grafting. J Thorac
    Cardiovasc Surg 97:821–825, 1989.
32. Katz, S, Branch, LG, Branson, MH, et al: Active life expectancy. N Engl J Med 309:1218, 1983.
33. Sethi, GK, Miller, CD, Souchek, J, et al: Clinical, hemodynamic, and angiographic predictors of
    operative mortality in patients undergoing single valve replacement. J Thorac Cardiovasc Surg
    93:884, 1987.
34. Elder, AT and Cameron, EWJ: Cardiac surgery in the elderly. Br Med J 229:140–141, 1989.
35. Galloway, AC, Colvin, SB, Grossi, EA, et al: Ten-year experience with aortic valve replacement in
    482 patients 70 years of age or older: Operative risk and long-term results. Ann Thorac Surg
    49:84–93, 1990.
36. Jamieson, WR, Dooner, J, Munro, AL, et al: Cardiac valve replacement in the elderly: A review of
    320 consecutive cases. Circulation 64(Suppl II):177, 1981.
37. Jamieson, WR, Burr, LH, Munroe, AL, et al: Cardiac valve replacement in the elderly: Clinical
    performance of biological prosthesis. Ann Thorac Surg 48:173–185, 1989.
38. Mullany, VJ, Clarebough, JK, White, AL: Open heart surgery in the elderly. Aust NZ J Surg
    57:733–737, 1987.
39. Naunheim, KS, Dean, PA, Fiove, AC: Cardiac surgery in the octogenarian. Eur J Cardio-thorac
    Surg 4:130–135, 1990.
40. Houser, SL, Hashmi, FH, Lehman, TJ, et al: Cardiac surgery in octogenarians: Are the risks too
    high? Connecticut Medicine 52(10):579–581, 1988.
41. Fiove, AC, Naunheim, KS, Barner, HB, et al: Valve replacement in the octogenarian. Ann Thorac
    Surg 47:104–108, 1989.
42. Arom, KV, Nicoloff, DM, Lindsay, WG, et al: Should valve replacement and related procedures be
    performed in elderly patient? Ann Thorac Surg 38:466, 1984.

43. Fremes, SE, Goldman, BS, Ivanov, J, et al: Valvular surgery in the elderly. Circulation (Suppl I) 80(3):I-77, 1989.
44. Lytle, BW, Cosgrove, DM, Loop, FD, et al: Replacements of aortic valve combined with myocardial revascularization: Determinants of early and late risk for 500 patients, 1967–1981. Circulation 68:1149, 1983.
45. Scott, WC, Miller, DC, Haverich, A, et al: Operative risks of mitral valve replacement: Discriminate analysis of 1329 procedures. Circulation (Suppl II)72:II-108, 1985.
46. Scott, WC, Miller, DC, Haverick, A: Determinants of operative mortality for patients undergoing aortic valve replacement. JTCVS 89:400–413, 1985.
47. Katz, NM, Ahmed, SW, Clark, BK, et al: Predictors of length of hospitalization after cardiac surgery. Ann Thorac Surg 45:656–660, 1988.
48. Ross, J, and Braunwald, E: Aortic stenosis. Circulation 38(Suppl 5):61, 1968.
49. Rappaport, E: Natural history of aortic and mitral valve replacement. Am J Cardiol 35:221, 1975.
50. Bessone, LN, Pupello, DF, Hiro, SP: Surgical management of aortic valve disease in the elderly: A longitudinal analysis. Ann Thorac Surg 46:264–269, 1988.
51. Blakeman, BM, Pifarre, R, Sullivan, HJ, et al: Aortic valve replacement in patients 75 years and older. Ann Thorac Surg 44:637–639, 1987.
52. Hochberg, MS: Aortic valve replacement in the elderly: Encouraging postoperative clinical and hemodynamic results. Arch Surg 112:1475–1480, 1977.
53. Kouchoukos, NT, Lell, WA, Rogers, WJ: Combined aortic valve replacement and myocardial revascularization. Ann Surg 197:721, 1983.
54. Nunley, DL, Grunkemeier, GL, Starr, A: Aortic valve replacement with coronary bypass grafting. J Thorac Cardiovasc Surg 85:705, 1983.
55. McGovern, JA, Pennock, JL, Campbell, DB, et al: Aortic valve replacement and combined aortic valve replacement and coronary artery bypass grafting; predicting high risk group. J Am Coll Cardiol 9:38, 1987.
56. Matloff, JM and Czer, LSC: Cardiac valve replacement in the presence of coronary atherosclerosis. In Matloff, JM (ed): Cardiac Valve Replacement—Current Status. Martinus Nijhoff, Hingham, Mass., pp 111–112, 1985.
57. Borkon, AM, Soule, LM, Baughman, KL, et al: Aortic valve selection in the elderly patient. Ann Thorac Surg 46:270–277, 1988.
58. Akins, CW, Beckley, MJ, Daggett, WM, et al: Myocardial revascularization with combined aortic and mitral valve replacements. J Thorac Cardiovasc Surg 90:272, 1985.
59. Craver, JM: Aortic valve debridement by ultrasonic surgical aspirator: A word of caution. Am Thorac Surg 49:746, 1990.
60. Robicsek, F: Balloon valvuloplasty in calcified aortic stenosis: A cause for caution and alarm. Ann Thorac Surg 45:515–525, 1988.
61. Letac, B: Balloon aortic valvuloplasty in patients aged 80 or older: The treatment of choice. Circulation 76(Suppl IV):IV-187, 1987.
62. Block, PC: Aortic valvuloplasty—A valid alternative? N Engl J Med 319:169–171, 1988.
63. McKay, RG, Safian, RD, Lock, JE, et al: Balloon dilatation of calcific aortic stenosis in elderly patients: Postmortem, intraoperative and percutaneous valvuloplasty studies. Circulation 74:119, 1986.
64. Duran, CG, Pomar, JL, Revuelta, JM, et al: Conservative operation for mitral insufficiency—Critical analysis supported by postoperative hemodynamic studies in 72 patients. JTCVS 79:326–337, 1980.
65. David, TE, Stauss, DH, Mesher, E, et al: Is it important to preserve the chordae tendineae and papillary muscles during mitral valve replacement? Can J Surg 24:236–239, 1981.
66. David, TE, Burns, RJ, Bacchus, CM, et al: Mitral valve replacement for mitral regurgitation with and without preservation of chordae tendineae. J Thorac Cardiovas Surg 88:718–725, 1984.
67. David, TE, Uden, DE, Strauss, HD: The importance of the mitral apparatus in left ventricular function after correction of mitral regurgitation. Circulation 68(Suppl II):76–82, 1983.
68. Christakis, GT, Weisel, RD, David, TE, et al: Predictors of operative survival after valve replacement. Circulation 78(Suppl I):I25–34, 1988.
69. Stephenson, LW, Edie, RN, Harken, AH, et al: Combined aortic and mitral valve replacement: Changes in practice and prognosis. Circulation 69:640, 1984.

# CHAPTER 15

# Rehabilitation and Life-style Modification in the Elderly

*Joan F. Carroll, MA*
*Michael L. Pollock, PhD*

The population of the United States is growing older. In 1980, 11% of the population was older than the age of 65, and this proportion is expected to increase to 20% by the year 2030.[1] Since 1980, the population in the 65 to 74 year age range has increased by 11% while the 75- to 84-year-old group has increased by 17.1%. The fastest-growing segment of the population is the group older than age 85, which increased 24.8% during the past decade. In absolute numbers, there are expected to be 34.9 million elderly by the year 2000, an increase of 17.1% over 1987.[2] From the point of view of health, well-being, quality of life and economics, maintaining functional independence and an active life style are important to the individual and to society. Coronary heart disease (CHD) is of particular concern since it is the most common cause of morbidity and mortality in the elderly[3] and is a major factor affecting escalating healthcare costs.[4] This need for an enhanced quality of life emphasizes the importance of both primary and secondary prevention of CHD and other debilitating diseases. Risk factor modification and cardiac and other types of rehabilitation are an integral part of such programs.

Cardiac rehabilitation is the "process by which the person with cardiovascular disease . . . is restored to and maintained at his or her optimal physiologic, psychologic, social, vocational, and emotional status."[5] As such, it should include measures to prevent progression of disease and reduce the risk of new coronary events. Preventive measures encompass the concept of risk factor modification.

The risk factor concept in cardiovascular disease is derived from a variety of epidemiologic studies and prospective investigations. Kannel and coworkers[6] stated that a factor is considered to be causal for CHD if the following criteria are met: the presence of the proposed risk factor must precede the disease; there must be a dose-related relationship between the factor and CHD; the factor must be predictive of disease in different population samples and be predictive of disease independently of other risk factors. In addition, the association between the proposed risk factor and CHD must be pathogenetically plausible and must be supported by clin-

209

ical and animal experiments. Presently, smoking, hypertension, and elevated cholesterol levels are identified as primary risk factors, that is, factors that have been firmly linked to the development of atherosclerosis. Obesity, stress, inactivity, and diabetes mellitus have been called secondary or contributing risk factors, that is, those factors that seem to be associated with the genesis of CHD but need additional research to prove an independent causal relationship.[7,8]

In the 1960s, more than 50% of the deaths in the United States were due to diseases of the heart and blood vessels. Since then, there has been a decrease in mortality from cardiovascular diseases in the United States.[6,8] Between 1972 and 1985, mortality from stroke and heart disease decreased by 50.2% and 34.6%, respectively.[9] It is believed that positive changes in diet, smoking, cholesterol levels, physical activity, and control of hypertension as well as improved medical and surgical care played an important role in this decline.[4,6,9-12]

Physical activity has been shown to be an important factor in the primary and secondary prevention of CHD. In addition, physical activity for middle-age and elderly persons is important in the development and/or maintenance of functional capacity and independence. Retrospective and prospective observational studies of sedentary and active populations have linked an active life style with a decreased incidence of CHD[13-20] and increased longevity.[21] Caspersen[22] has emphasized the importance of physical activity in preventing CHD, in light of the large proportion of the population that leads a sedentary life style. With regard to secondary prevention of recurrent myocardial infarction (MI), although the results of individual studies often do not show significant differences between cardiac rehabilitation and control groups, when the data from several studies are pooled, cardiac rehabilitation intervention produces a significant reduction in mortality (but not morbidity) from CHD.[23-25] In view of the important role of physical activity in both primary and secondary prevention, the purpose of this chapter is to review exercise training standards for the healthy adult participant and the modifications necessary for the elderly and cardiac populations. The importance of risk factors in the elderly population will be discussed along with the concept of risk factor modification.

## EXERCISE TRAINING STANDARDS FOR THE HEALTHY ADULT

The American College of Sports Medicine (ACSM) has formulated training standards for the promotion of cardiovascular and muscular fitness in healthy adults (Table 15–1).[26] Improvement in aerobic capacity ($\dot{V}O_2$max) is dependent on the frequency, intensity, and duration of training as well as on the mode of activity and the initial level of fitness. Intensity and duration are inversely related with the total amount of work accomplished being an important factor in fitness development.[27-33] Activities performed at a lower intensity for a longer duration will provide the same benefits as activities performed at a higher intensity and a shorter duration provided the energy requirements of the activities are equivalent. A frequency of 3 d/wk with a day of rest between workouts is recommended when a training program is initiated to avoid problems with muscle soreness, fatigue, and injury. Pollock and coworkers[34] found twice the injury rate in those training 30 minutes, 5 d/wk compared with those training for 45 minutes, 3 d/wk. Frequency of training can be increased to 5 d/wk after several weeks or months of conditioning depending on age, fitness level, training intensity, and absence of injury. Based on

**Table 15–1.** Exercise Training Standards for the Healthy Adult[26]

| | |
|---|---|
| Frequency: | 3–5 d/wk. |
| Intensity: | 60%–90% maximum heart rate ($HR_{max}$) or 50%–85% of maximal oxygen uptake ($\dot{V}O_2max$), or $HR_{max}$ reserve. |
| Duration: | 20–60 min of continuous aerobic activity. |
| Mode: | Any activity that uses large muscle groups, can be maintained continuously, and is rhythmic and aerobic in nature. |
| Resistance training: | A minimum of one set of 8–12 repetitions of eight to ten exercises that condition the major muscle groups performed at least 2 d/wk. |

the standards recommended in Table 15–1, the average improvements expected from a 6- to 12-month training program include a 15% to 30% increase in $\dot{V}O_2max$, a 1 to 2 kg loss in weight (or a 1% to 3% body fat loss), and a 20% to 30% increase in strength.[31–33,35–48] Training for fewer than 3 d/wk usually results in less than a 15% improvement in $\dot{V}O_2max$[32,39,41,44,49] and no reduction in body weight and fat.[50]

The American Heart Association (AHA) has also promulgated exercise standards for the development of health and fitness.[51] The chief difference between these standards and those of the ACSM[26] lies in the fact that the AHA specifies only minimum standards (i.e., a frequency of 3 d/wk, a duration of 20 to 30 minutes per exercise session, and an intensity of 50% to 60% $\dot{V}O_2max$) whereas the ACSM provides a range of values that can accommodate persons of varying fitness levels.

When the total energy expenditure is equivalent, training adaptations appear to be independent of the mode of training.[52,53] For example, running, walking, and stationary cycling programs resulted in equivalent improvements in aerobic capacity and body composition when intensity, frequency, and duration were held constant.[53] However, when walking is used as a mode of training, the intensity is generally less than in jogging programs; the duration or frequency of training must then be increased to compensate. A variety of endurance activities can be used in training; the choice of activity should be tailored to the needs, goals, and preferences of the individual. Possible activities include jogging, swimming, rope skipping, aerobic dancing, walking, cycling, cross-country skiing, rowing, stair climbing, skating, and various endurance game activities.

A participant's initial level of fitness is an important consideration when designing an exercise program. Persons of low initial fitness, such as the elderly and cardiac patients, can make substantial improvements in aerobic fitness at intensities less than 50% to 60% $HRR_{max}$ (maximal heart rate reserve).[31,54] In contrast, persons with high initial fitness may need a higher stimulus (intensity) to achieve a training effect.[55]

The components of a typical training session are shown in Table 15–2. The warm-up, although often neglected, is of particular importance. The gradual increase in activity will raise muscle temperatures and metabolic rate and thus increase the speed of muscle contraction. There is also an increase in cardiac output and perfusion of both coronary arteries and muscle capillary beds that enhances circulation and oxygen delivery systems before more intense activity begins. Activities suitable for the warm-up period include low-level calisthenics, dynamic and static stretching exercises, and light aerobic activities.

The muscular-conditioning period should last from 15 to 30 minutes. The pur-

**Table 15–2.** Comparison of Training Session Components
for Healthy Adults, Cardiac Patients, and the Elderly*

| Component | Healthy Adult | Phase I | Phase II | Phase III | Elderly |
|---|---|---|---|---|---|
| Warm-up | 10 min | 15–20 min | 10–15 min | 10–15 min | 10–15 min |
| Muscular conditioning | 15–30 min | ROM† | 10–20 min | 10–20 min | 15–20 min |
| Aerobic exercise | 20–60 min | 5–20 min | 10–60 min | 30–60 min | 30–60 min |
| Cool-down | 5–10 min | 15 min | 15 min | 15 min | 10–15 min |

*Adapted from Pollock and Wilmore.[7]
†ROM = Range-of-motion exercise.

pose of this component of the exercise session is to train all the major muscle groups, that is, arms, shoulders, trunk, lower back, abdomen, hips, and legs. The effect of exercise training is specific to the area of the body being trained. As indicated in Table 15–1, 8 to 10 exercises performed a minimum of 2 d/wk is recommended. The recent addition of a resistance training component to the ACSM's recommendations underlines the importance of a well-rounded fitness program while addressing the issue of specificity of training.

Both muscular strength and endurance are developed by the overload principle, that is, by gradually increasing the resistance, volume, frequency, or duration of the activity. Muscular strength is best developed by using heavy weights and few repetitions whereas muscular endurance is best developed by using lighter weights with a greater number of repetitions.[47] The ACSM recommendation of 8 to 12 repetitions represents a middle ground whereby both muscular strength and endurance will be enhanced.[26]

The recommended time for the aerobic conditioning phase is from 20 to 60 minutes. As already mentioned, the duration of the exercise session is inversely related to the intensity. When the intensity is in the lower end of the recommended range (i.e., 50% to 70% $HRR_{max}$), the duration should be longer (i.e., 40 to 60 minutes). This type of program is more suitable for elderly, the obese, the cardiac patient, or the low-fit subject. Higher intensity programs (e.g., 75% to 85% $HRR_{max}$) can be conducted for a shorter duration (e.g., 20 to 30 minutes); this type of program would be more suitable for the healthy, more fit individual, who is at low risk for precipitating a cardiovascular event or for incurring an orthopedic injury. The important factor is the total amount of energy expended: the recommended minimum is 250 to 300 kcal per exercise session or 1000 kcal/wk.[7,26]

The cool-down is the final component of an exercise session. Like the warm-up, it is vitally important yet frequently neglected. Usually stretching and light aerobic activity, for example, walking, are recommended. Continued light activity enhances venous return in the face of peripheral dilation. In addition, stretching of the active muscles with long, static stretches (minimum of 20 to 30 seconds) may minimize soreness and stiffness and enhance flexibility.

## MODIFICATIONS FOR EXERCISE TRAINING IN CARDIAC REHABILITATION

Successful cardiac rehabilitation includes patient education, risk factor modification, and exercise. Generally, the exercise portion of cardiac rehabilitation is divided into three phases. Phase I, the inpatient program, begins as soon after the event as the patient is stable (generally 2 to 4 days for an uncomplicated MI and 1 to 2 days for a postsurgical patient) and extends over the entire hospital stay. The outpatient program (phase II) is an intermediate phase, which can be hospital-, private clinic-, or community-based; it begins when the patient is discharged from the hospital and can last an additional 8 to 12 weeks. The long-term program (phase III) is generally a community-based gymnasium program that admits patients after their initial convalescence from their event when they are more stable medically and stronger physically.

There are some differences between the prescriptions for post-MI and coronary artery bypass graft surgery (CABG) patients: 1) Surgical patients begin rehabilitation sooner and usually ambulate on the first or second treatment day;[56] 2) surgical patients progress more rapidly in intensity and duration; and 3) upper extremity range-of-motion (ROM) exercise is emphasized more with the surgical patient.[7]

There are also differences among patients regarding the level of risk for future events; this factor determines the type and duration of supervision and frequency of electrocardiographic monitoring during rehabilitation. The level of risk (i.e., low, moderate, high) is estimated using data from the patient's medical history and clinical course. Functional capacity, ventricular function, presence of ischemia or significant dysrhythmia, extent of ST-segment depression, and adverse blood pressure or heart rate response to exercise are among the variables to be considered in stratifying patients for rehabilitative treatment.[57] Guidelines for risk stratification are available through the AHA,[51] the American Association of Cardiovascular and Pulmonary Rehabilitation,[5] and the ACSM.[58]

The basic components of a training session for cardiac patients are the same as for healthy adults, but the time allotted to each component varies during the rehabilitation process as the medical status and physical abilities of the patient change. As shown in Table 15–2, the cardiac patient generally needs a longer warm-up period during phases I and II. The adverse effects of bed rest and/or surgery necessitate the use of special stretching and joint readiness exercises. This is particularly true of the CABG patient because of damage to the chest wall and chest and shoulder musculature that occurs during surgery. The use of ROM exercise may forestall the development of adhesions and help maintain muscle integrity (strength and flexibility) during early convalescence. Without ROM exercise, patients often limit their upper body activity, which can accentuate future problems with poor posture, decreased strength, and limited ROM. The warm-up during phase III is similar to that of the lower-fit healthy adult or elderly participant.[7]

The aerobic conditioning component for the phase I patient begins with self-care and short ambulation activities performed two to three times daily and progresses to longer and more continuous exercise in the later phases. Muscular conditioning does not begin until the phase II program, and the emphasis is on dynamic and rhythmic exercises that do not impede normal breathing or cause a significant increase in afterload. Performance of the Valsalva maneuver during sustained muscular contractions can dramatically increase the diastolic blood pressure (DBP), a condition to be avoided with cardiac patients.

In cardiac populations, a longer cool-down period is recommended. Although cardiac events are rare in cardiac rehabilitation programs, approximately 30% to 40% of recurrent events take place during the recovery period after exercise. Therefore a 15-minute cool-down/observation period is the recommended minimum.[59,60]

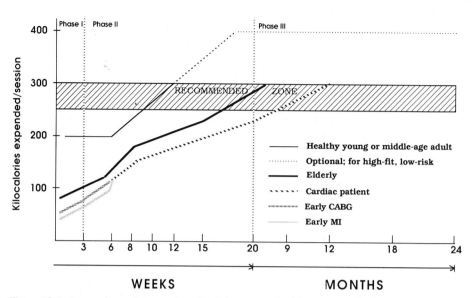

**Figure 15–1.** Comparison of progression of training among healthy young and middle-aged adults, cardiac patients, and the elderly.

The rate of progression in training will be slower in the cardiac patient owing to the lower initial training load. Figure 15–1 compares the rate of progression of healthy adults with that of post-MI and CABG patients. As shown, normal participants usually start at 150 to 200 kcal per exercise session and progress to 250 to 300 kcal per session within 8 to 12 weeks. The cardiac patient in phase I may begin at less than 50 kcal per session and will require weeks to months longer to reach the recommended level of 250 to 300 kcal.[7,61] The high-risk, more fragile patient, however, may not reach this level of energy expenditure. As noted earlier, CABG patients are initially progressed slightly faster than post-MI patients during phase I. After the medical status of the MI patient has been clarified, low-risk and most moderate-risk patients may then be progressed at the same rate as the CABG patient. This usually occurs by the third or fourth week postevent. The maintenance phase of training will take many months longer to reach for the cardiac patient than for the normal adult.

The ACSM recommendations regarding frequency, intensity, duration, and mode of training also apply to the cardiac patient; again, however, modifications are necessary for the cardiac patient to accommodate each patient's medical status and physical abilities (Table 15–3). The following guidelines are offered in making modifications.

## Phase I

In the phase I program there are two common methods of determining intensity. The first involves using a fixed, low-level heart rate (e.g., 110 to 120 beats/min) whereas the second involves using a fixed increment above the standing, resting heart rate (e.g., 20 beats/min or less). Pollock and Wilmore[7] recommend the latter method in light of the large interindividual variation in resting heart rates (i.e., ranging from 50 to 120 beats/min). The use of a fixed, low-level heart rate would

**Table 15–3.** Comparison of the Exercise Prescription for
Cardiac Patients and Healthy Adults*

| Prescription | Healthy Adult | Phase I | Phase II | Phase III |
|---|---|---|---|---|
| Intensity | 50%–85% HRR$_{max}$ | RHR + 20 | RHR + 20†; RPE 13 | 50%–85% HRR$_{max}$ |
| Frequency | 3–5 d/wk | 2–3 times/d | 1–2 times/d | 3–5 times/wk |
| Duration | 20–60 min | MI: 5–20 min CABG: 10–20 min | 20–60 min | 30–60 min |
| Mode, Activity | walk, jog, run, bike, swim, cal, weights, endurance sports | ROM, TDM, bike, 1 flight stairs | ROM, TDM, bike, arm erg, cal, weights | walk, bike, jog, swim, cal, weights, endurance sports |

*Adapted from Pollock and Wilmore.[7]

†3–6 wk after surgery or MI, a symptom-limited exercise test is recommended after which intensity can be based on 60%–70% of maximal heart rate reserve.

‡MI = myocardial infarction patient; CABG = coronary artery bypass graft surgery patient; HRR$_{max}$ = maximal heart rate reserve; RHR = standing resting heart rate; ROM = range-of-motion exercise; TDM = treadmill; arm erg = arm ergometer; cal = calisthenics; RPE = rating of perceived exertion.

preclude patients with high resting heart rates from exercising whereas those with very low resting heart rates (e.g., patients on beta blockers) would be allowed to double their resting heart rate during exercise. Data from symptom-limited graded exercise tests (SL-GXT) at hospital discharge have shown that 30 to 40 beats/min above standing rest is near maximum for most patients and that 20 beats/min above standing rest generally corresponds to a rating of perceived exertion (RPE) of 13 (somewhat hard).[62,63]

Initially, heart rates increase only 5 to 10 beats above standing rest for either ROM or ambulation, but within approximately 10 days, patients' heart rates increase between 10 and 15 beats. Systolic blood pressure (SBP) rises 5 to 10 mmHg during the early ambulation activities and up to 15 mmHg at 14 days postevent. The RPE scale also can be used to monitor exercise intensity; a rating of 11 to 12 (light) has been found for ROM, stair climbing, and ambulation activities.[56,61]

Phase I patients are generally weak from the effects of the cardiac event, surgery, or bed rest and therefore cannot initially tolerate long periods of activity. Thus, several short activity bouts may be used in the beginning stages of rehabilitation. During the hospital stay, activities progress from self-care activities and ROM exercises to low-level ambulation and stair climbing. The workload is raised primarily by gradually increasing the duration of activity while keeping the intensity low. Metabolic cost of the activities range from 1.5 to 3 METs (5.25 to 10.5 ml·kg$^{-1}$·min$^{-1}$).[61] A detailed step program for ambulation, ROM and stair-climbing activities, and education/risk reduction programs is described elsewhere.[7]

## PHASE II

This phase of rehabilitation is a transitional phase in which the patient progresses from a restricted, low level program to a less restricted, moderate-level training program. This phase can take place in a formal, organized program; at home; or some combination thereof. Initially, the intensity of training is similar to that used at the end of the inpatient program but generally increases to 20 beats above standing rest by the third or fourth week post-MI or surgery. Once a SL-GXT is administered (3 to 6 weeks after surgery or MI), the intensity can be based on 60% to 70% of the maximal heart rate reserve ($HRR_{max}$). The program will be progressed first by increasing duration, then intensity. Frequency and duration of training will vary, depending on the patient's level of tolerance. Daily activity is encouraged and, if exercise tolerance is low, it may be necessary to plan two shorter training sessions per day. Duration of aerobic activity usually begins at 10 to 20 minutes; these times may vary depending on the medical and fitness status of the patient. The ultimate goal is for the patient to expend 250 to 300 kcal per exercise session, or 1000 kcal per week. At the low-to-moderate walking speeds used by cardiac patients, this will ultimately necessitate walking for a minimum of 45 minutes per session. Most patients will not reach this goal until phase III or later (3 to 12 months; Fig. 15–1).

The phase II patient has a wider variety of activities to choose from. In addition to ROM, walking, and bike activities, arm ergometry and calisthenics can be safely used. After the sternum is generally healed and scar tissue has formed for the postsurgery or post-MI patient, more activity restrictions can be lifted. In conjunction with the 3 to 6 week SL-GXT, risk classification can be determined. Thus, low-risk CABG and MI patients who have normal left ventricular function can be cleared for light-to-moderate weight training exercise.

Jogging can be initiated in patients without complication who have completed the SL-GXT and who have a MET capacity greater than 8 and/or who can walk on a treadmill at 3.5 mph and 5% grade for up to 20 minutes. The jogging program is usually introduced by using interval training, for example, alternating time or distance intervals at walking speeds (3 to 4 mph) with intervals at jogging speeds (4.75 to 5.5 mph).[64] Beginning intervals can be as short as 1 minute.

Swimming is not recommended until after the SL-GXT and 6-week convalescence period to allow for adequate healing of the sternum and leg incisions of the surgery patient and of the myocardial tissue of the MI patient. It is also not recommended for the patient lacking adequate swimming skill. Swimming has many advantages for the cardiac patient. It is an aerobic activity that can use both arm and the leg musculature, depending on the stroke. Additional emphasis on leg musculature can be obtained during the crawl stroke (front or back) by using swim fins. Because exercise takes place in a nongravity situation, there may be fewer musculoskeletal injuries; this will benefit those who are overweight. Patients with arthritis, intermittent claudication, amputation, or paralysis also will benefit from the nongravity exercise environment. For this reason, some programs use walking in chest-deep water while alternately paddling the arms as an alternate activity in the later stages of phase II and phase III programs.

It is important to note that the maximal heart rate achievable while swimming is approximately 10 to 13 beats/min lower than that which would be obtained on a treadmill.[65,66] Therefore, the training heart rate for swimming (prone or supine positions) needs to be formulated by subtracting this value from the treadmill maximal heart rate before calculating the percent $HRR_{max}$. If this is not done, the training heart rate established using the treadmill SL-GXT will overestimate the swimming training heart rate.

## PHASE III

Patients in a phase III program are generally 8 to 12 weeks past their surgery or event and are more stable medically and stronger physically. This is reflected in the exercise prescription, which is similar to that of the healthy adult. The main difference is that the cardiac patient is generally training at the lower end of the intensity range (60% to 70% $HRR_{max}$). Some patients may in time progress to 85% $HRR_{max}$, particularly when they are able to jog. Although the prescription for frequency is the same as for healthy adults, the minimum recommended duration is slightly longer owing to the fact that most patients will not reach the higher intensity levels. Thus, to reach the goal of expending 1000 kcal/wk, longer and more frequent training sessions are needed. If the patient is able to reach higher exercise intensities, then the duration and frequency can be modified appropriately.

More activities are available to the phase III patient, particularly those who are low-risk or those who have successfully participated in a walk/jog or jog regimen. These individuals may safely participate in walking, cycling, swimming, and weight training activities. Endurance sports and games are not recommended without physician clearance and until after 6 months of rehabilitation, including proper aerobic and musculoskeletal preparatory activities. Extensive examples of exercise programs for all three phases of rehabilitation are available in other sources.[7]

## PHYSIOLOGIC BENEFITS OF CARDIAC REHABILITATION

Although some early studies showed that there was a significant decrease in mortality and morbidity in post-MI patients who exercised as compared with those who did not exercise,[67,68] other studies could not reproduce this finding.[69-75] However, the lack of significant findings in the latter studies can be traced to several methodologic problems. The small number of subjects in these studies decreased the power of the statistical tests and made achieving statistical significance difficult. For example, Oberman and Naughton,[76] in discussing the results from the National Exercise and Rehabilitation Project, stated that 4000 patients would be needed to properly test the hypothesis that exercise rehabilitation will significantly affect mortality from CHD. Most studies had only 200 to 300 patients enrolled. In addition, there were large numbers of dropouts and crossovers from either the control or the exercise intervention groups. Finally, there was an insufficient training stimulus used in some of the studies. To overcome these shortcomings, May and associates[23] and, more recently, Oldridge[24] and O'Connor[25] and their colleagues pooled the data from a large number of studies and found a significant reduction in mortality from CHD with exercise and diet intervention.

It is interesting to note that both the Oldridge and associates[24] and O'Connor and coworkers[25] reports included more than 4000 patients. May and colleagues[23] found that the effectiveness (i.e., reduction in CHD mortality) of pooled exercise trials was 19%, comparable with the 23.5% effectiveness of beta blockers, 22.6% of anticoagulants, and 17.8% of lipid-lowering interventions. Even though the more recent pooled studies showed promising results concerning the effects of cardiac rehabilitation on mortality, there was not a significant effect on morbidity. Also, the data were nonconclusive regarding exercise alone as an intervention because most studies used a multi-interventional approach. Inasmuch as most cardiac rehabilitation programs use this approach (i.e., exercise, diet modification, and smoking cessation), the effectiveness of exercise alone may be academic.

Although the effect of exercise training on morbidity from CHD is nonconclusive, its effect on risk factors associated with CHD is convincing. Exercise training results in reductions in both SBP and DBP[77] and body weight/fat and triglycerides, and increases in high-density lipoproteins[78] and glucose tolerance.[79,80] Other benefits include a reduction in the tendency to smoke,[81] a reduction in circulating catecholamines at rest and at submaximal exercise,[82] a reduction in blood-clotting tendencies, and an improved psychologic profile.[83]

Quite apart from decreased mortality and/or risk-factor profile, there are many physiologic benefits that accrue from exercise training in post-MI and CABG patients. These benefits include a reduction of resting heart rates, heart rate and SBP at submaximal exercise (rate-pressure product), and myocardial oxygen requirement at rest and submaximal exercise, and an increase in physical working capacity ($\dot{V}O_2$max). There may also be a decrease in the incidence of angina and ST-segment depression at a given workload.[84-90] Although some authors have attributed these changes to adaptations in skeletal muscle and the autonomic nervous system,[91] there is recent evidence that intense exercise training in CHD patients can bring about improvement in left ventricular function and myocardial oxygen supply.[92-94]

## MODIFICATION OF EXERCISE TRAINING FOR THE ELDERLY

As with the cardiac patient, the components of the exercise prescription (see Table 15-1) and the exercise session (see Table 15-2) for the elderly are the same as those for the healthy adult; the difference again is in the application of the principles (see Table 15-3). The special needs and goals of the elderly participant together with the greater heterogeneity in the elderly population make exercise prescription for this age group more challenging.

The older individual generally attains steady-state levels of heart rate, blood pressure, and ventilatory response more slowly than the younger person.[95] Thus, there should be an enhanced emphasis on the warm-up period. This portion of the training session should last from 10 to 15 minutes and could include stretching, low-level calisthenics, or low-level aerobic activities such as slow walking, cycling, or swimming. Similarly, because of potential problems with orthostatic hypotension[96] and heat dissipation,[97] there should be a greater emphasis on the cool-down period. This should last 10 to 15 minutes and include low-level aerobic activities as well as exercises for the enhancement of flexibility. Exercising in a cooler environment also will be beneficial in this regard.

The muscular conditioning component can be done before or after the aerobic exercise period and should include 15 to 20 minutes of moderate-intensity calisthenics or resistance training. The addition of resistance training to a fitness program for the elderly helps provide a more well-rounded program. The use of strength exercises can improve the ability of the older person to perform activities of daily living and provide the stimulus for the development/maintenance of both muscle and bone.[98,99]

Although calisthenics can provide enough overload to produce increases in strength in the elderly,[100,101] moderate weight training can be safe and produce better results.[99,102-104] The development of new equipment such as variable resistance exercise devices makes this type of training particularly suitable and safe for the elderly population.[7,105] Advantages of such resistance training machines include:[105]

1. Weight (intensity) can be applied at a low level and adjusted in small increments.

2. Most of the equipment is designed to place an individual into a proper and supported position to protect the lower back. Thus, the potential for injury is lessened.
3. The variable resistance allows the stimulus to be applied more evenly through the full ROM.
4. Many exercise devices are designed to avoid hand gripping, which can cause dramatic increases in blood pressure during exercise.[106]
5. Much of the equipment can be double-pinned so that the subject's ROM can be limited. This is particularly important in elderly participants who have arthritis and other joint problems. Thus, the elderly participants can be exercised within the ROM at which they do not experience discomfort or pain. Limited ROM exercise can provide near full range benefits to a training program.[107]
6. Most resistance exercise devices do not require the individual to balance or control the weights as would be required with barbells and dumbbells. Therefore, those with balance problems can safely engage in resistance exercise.

The aerobic exercise period should last from 30 to 50 minutes and can use a variety of endurance activities such as fast walking, swimming, cycling, stair climbing, or rowing. Because of the association between high-impact activities and injuries,[108–112] low-impact activities should be emphasized.

The principles of frequency, intensity, and duration also may require some modification for use in an exercise prescription for the elderly. Intensity is calculated in the same manner as for young and middle-aged participants and is based on the elderly participant's individualized exercise test results. However, compared with the younger, healthy adult, the prescription for intensity will be for more moderate activity, with the emphasis being on added duration and frequency of exercise. Some recent data from our own (unpublished) and another laboratory[113] suggest that the %$HRR_{max}$ method of determining exercise heart rate underestimates the %$\dot{V}O_2max$ in older persons. Thus, the recommended %HRR for the elderly may be in the range of 40% to 65% $HRR_{max}$. The RPE scale has the same relation to relative oxygen uptake and heart rate in older individuals as in younger individuals so this also can be used in conjunction with heart rate to regulate exercise both physiologically and perceptually. An RPE of 12 to 13 corresponds to "moderate" exercise at approximately 50% to 75% $\dot{V}O_2max$.

Progression of training may take longer in the elderly individual (see Fig. 15–1). It has been suggested that for each decade after age 30, a 40% increase in time should be allowed for adaptation to training.[7,105] Thus, if a 30 year old progresses every week, a 50 year old will progress every 2 weeks and a 70 year old every 3 to 4 weeks. Although this recommendation seems to work empirically, it has not been scientifically tested. An alternative method of determining progression is by RPE: if the participant is rating the training at 10 to 11 (fairly light), then weekly increases in intensity are acceptable. Once a rating of 12 to 13 (somewhat hard) is achieved, progression will be slower, perhaps every 2 to 3 weeks.

Because elderly individuals appear to be at greater risk for injuries during high-impact activities such as jogging,[112] low-impact activities such as walking, swimming, cycling, rowing, or stair climbing should be emphasized. In addition, older exercisers may have other physical or medical problems such as poor vision or an unsteady gait that must be taken into account when designing exercise programs to maximize safety, program adherence, and enjoyment.

## LIFE-STYLE MODIFICATION

Risk factors for cardiovascular disease such as hypertension, elevated cholesterol, diabetes, obesity, and physical inactivity are still prevalent in the elderly and still continue to be predictive for CHD in this population.[114,115] On the other hand, the decline in cardiovascular mortality since the 1960s is evident in the elderly: between 1963 and 1981, coronary mortality declined 37% in the 65- to 74-year-old age group, 30% in the 75- to 84-year-old group, and 25.6% in the older than 85-year-old group.[4] Goldman and Cook[12] have estimated that more than half of the decrease in mortality from CHD in the years 1968 to 1976 was due to changes in life style, specifically to reductions in cholesterol levels and smoking. This suggests that life-style modification is effective in the old as well as the young.

Although risk-factor profiles are effective in distinguishing older persons at high risk for CHD,[115] the strength of the association between some of the individual risk factors and CHD appears to change somewhat as one ages. Total serum cholesterol loses its predictive weight, but increased low density and decreased high density lipoprotein fractions are significant CHD predictors in older persons.[6,115] Cigarette smoking loses its strength as a predictor of CHD with age,[115] but it still remains a risk factor for stroke and intermittent claudication for older men and women.[114] Substantial obesity, particularly with a central fat distribution (android or male-pattern fat distribution), predisposes to cardiovascular disease in the elderly.[114] A convenient index of the extent of central fat distribution is the waist-to-hip ratio: an index greater than 1.0 for men and 0.8 for women indicates an increased risk.[7] Obesity also aggravates other atherogenic traits such as diabetes, hyperlipidemia, and hypertension.[115] The incidence of diabetes increases with age and is an independent cardiovascular risk factor in the elderly, particularly in elderly women.[115] Finally, elevated blood pressure, either systolic or diastolic, remains a strong predictor of cardiovascular disease in the elderly.[114] In light of the increased incidence of hypertension in the elderly, this remains an important area for intervention.

Life-style modification to reduce the risk from these factors involves a multifactorial approach that includes dietary modification, weight control, blood pressure control, smoking cessation, and endurance exercise training. The role of the latter component has been discussed already.

Reduction in cholesterol and saturated fat consumption are important components of a plan for dietary modification. Data from the Oslo Heart Study[116] showed that a dietary plan consisting of fewer than 30% of calories coming from fat and fewer than 10% of calories coming from saturated fat, together with <300 mg of cholesterol per day resulted in a 13% decrease in plasma cholesterol during 5 years. For every 1% decline in serum cholesterol, it is estimated that there is a 2% decline in the risk of CHD.[117]

The National Cholesterol Education Program has recommended a two-step program of dietary change for reducing plasma cholesterol.[118] In the Step-One diet, fat intake should be no more than 30% of the total calories, with a maximum of 10% of the calories coming from saturated fats. Polyunsaturated fats can comprise up to 10% of calories with the remainder of the fat calories coming from monounsaturated fats. The recommendation for cholesterol consumption is no more than 300 mg/d. The AHA estimated that plasma cholesterol should be reduced by 10% to 15% with this diet. In the Step-Two diet, fewer than 7% of calories come from saturated fat with a 200 mg/d limit for dietary cholesterol. Step-Two should be used if further cholesterol lowering is needed. Lipid-lowering drugs should be used if this diet fails to lower LDL-cholesterol to below 130 mg/dl after 6 months.

In addition to reducing serum cholesterol, a fat- and salt-modified diet also will benefit body fat and/or weight reduction and blood pressure control. A 20% to 40% reduction in salt intake can reduce DBP by 2 to 8 mmHg, and a 10 to 15 lb reduction in body weight can reduce DBP by 4 to 10 mmHg and serum cholesterol by 30 to 60 mg/dl.[9] Weight reduction will further enhance HDL cholesterol levels.[6] A fat-modified diet also can help diabetics achieve better control of blood glucose and hypertensives better control of blood pressure.[6]

Clinically, diet composition is assessed either with the food diary or with a food pattern questionnaire.[9,119] The food diary is a detailed record of all food eaten during a 3-day period, usually encompassing at least 1 nonworking day. The patient is asked to recall not only what was eaten, but also the amount of food eaten and the estimated calorie content of the food. Although there is a danger that patients will alter their eating patterns during these days, the food diary still remains a good information-gathering tool as well as a tool for inducing behavioral change. The food questionnaire is designed to elicit information on overall eating patterns and may be more instructive than the 3-day diary. The types of food eaten and how often they are eaten will provide additional information to the practitioner for formulating a plan for change.

By looking over the food diary and the food pattern questionnaire, areas of concern (e.g., high-fat, high-salt, or excessive alcohol consumption) can be identified and discussed. A discussion with the patient of his/her willingness to modify eating habits is also warranted; barriers to change also must be identified. Patients may be willing to change some aspects of their diet but not others. For example, a patient may be agreeable to substituting a bagel for a sweet roll at breakfast but may be unwilling to give up a particular dinner favorite. It is important for the practitioner to remember that eating patterns are ingrained habits that often represent social and emotional issues quite apart from nutritional concerns. Therefore any proposed dietary changes must be negotiated with and agreed to by the patient. The patient may be more comfortable with small, gradual changes than with sweeping dietary reform. The short-term goals therefore must be adjusted to the comfort level of the patient.

Long-term blood pressure control by nonpharmacologic means is an area of risk factor intervention under current investigation. Weight reduction and salt restriction have been shown to reduce blood pressure;[6,9] these measures, when effective, also can be assumed to be safer than drug therapy. Exercise and control of heavy drinking also can be effective in blood pressure control.[6,77] A reduced dependence on drug therapy has benefits in an older population due to a decrease in potential drug side effects and drug interactions. The subsequent financial savings also will aid those on a fixed income. However, studies to determine the long-term adherence to such nonpharmacologic programs need to be conducted.

In light of the continued risk for stroke, intermittent claudication, and lung cancer posed by smoking, strategies for eliminating or reducing smoking behaviors are still warranted in the elderly. The information and advice given to the patient must be tailored to the age, sex, and social background of the patient. The relation of smoking to any underlying disease also can be addressed. Cohen[9] advocates patient-oriented counseling with a seven-step approach that includes such strategies as assessment of the desire and motivation to change, assessment of past experiences with and barriers to change, and negotiation of a plan for change.

Weight control is another component of life-style modification that can help reduce cardiovascular risk factors. In particular, weight reduction has been shown to be one of the most effective measures for reducing high blood pressure;[120] blood cholesterol and blood glucose can also be reduced with weight loss.[121] Although dieting by itself may reduce body weight, a substantial portion of the weight that is lost may be lean mass (muscle). Regular endurance exercise in conjunction with diet will help to maintain muscle mass and increase the proportion of weight loss that is fat.

## SUMMARY

The projected growth of the elderly population in the United States in the coming years underlines the importance of assuring that the quality of life for older persons is maintained. Because CHD is prevalent in this population, measures for preventing disease as well as for optimizing the abilities of those with disease will assume greater significance. Exercise training is a key component in achieving and maintaining optimal capacities in the elderly cardiac and noncardiac populations. These groups can safely undergo exercise training with proper screening and program design. Modifications in the components of the exercise prescription (i.e., frequency, intensity, duration, and activity mode) must be individualized according to the abilities, needs, and goals of each person.

Risk factors for CHD still prevail in the elderly, although the predictive value of some risk factors may change with age. For this reason, efforts to control risk factors in older individuals should still be effective in reducing risk from CHD. Dietary modification, weight control, blood pressure control, smoking cessation, and endurance exercise training are several of the interventions used in concert to control risk for CHD.

## REFERENCES

1. Abrams, WB and Berkow, R (eds): The Merck Manual of Geriatrics. Merck & Co., Inc., Rahway, NJ, 1991.
2. Beck, J: General principles of aging: Demography of aging. In Beck, J (ed): Geriatrics Review Syllabus: A Core Curriculum in Geriatric Medicine. American Geriatrics Society, New York, 1989, pp 1–5.
3. Gersh, B, Kronmal, R, Frye, R, et al: Coronary arteriography and coronary artery bypass surgery: Morbidity and mortality in patients age 65 years or older. A report from the Coronary Artery Surgery Study. Circulation 67:483, 1983.
4. Walker, WJ: Changing U.S. life style and declining vascular mortality—A retrospective. N Engl J Med 308:649, 1983.
5. American Association of Cardiovascular and Pulmonary Rehabilitation: Guidelines for Cardiac Rehabilitation Programs. Human Kinetics Books, Champaign, IL, 1991, pp 1–8.
6. Kannel, WB, Doyle, JT, Ostfield, AM, et al: Optimal resources for primary prevention of atherosclerotic diseases. Circulation 70:157A, 1984.
7. Pollock, ML and Wilmore, JH: Exercise in Health and Disease: Evaluation and Prescription for Prevention and Rehabilitation, ed 2. WB Saunders, Philadelphia, 1990, p 741.

8. American Heart Association: 1991 Heart and Stroke Facts. American Heart Association, Dallas, TX, 1990, pp 20–22.
9. Cohen, JD (ed): New Approaches to Cardiovascular Risk Management. Advanced Therapeutics Communications International, Hasbrouck Heights, NJ, 1988, p 59.
10. Kannel, WB: Epidemiologic insights into atherosclerotic cardiovascular disease from the Framingham Study. In Pollock, ML and Schmidt, DH (eds): Heart Disease and Rehabilitation, ed 2. John Wiley & Sons, New York, 1986, pp 3–28.
11. Burke, GL, Sprafka, JM, Folsom, AR, et al: Trends in CHD mortality, morbidity and risk factor levels from 1960 to 1986: The Minnesota Heart Survey. Int J Epidemiol 18(3 Suppl 1):S73, 1989.
12. Goldman, L and Cook, EF: The decline in ischemic heart disease mortality rates. An analysis of the comparative effects of medical interventions and changes in lifestyle. Ann Intern Med 101:825, 1984.
13. Morris, JM, Adam, C, Chave, SPW, et al: Vigorous exercise in leisure-time and the incidence of coronary disease. Lancet 1:333, 1973.
14. Morris, JN, Pollard, P, Everitt, MG, et al: Vigorous exercise in leisure-time: Protection against coronary disease. Lancet 2:1207, 1980.
15. Paffenbarger, RS, Hale, WE, Brand, RJ, et al: Work-energy level, personal characteristics, and fatal heart attack: A birth cohort effect. Am J Epidemiol 105:200, 1977.
16. Paffenbarger, RS, Hyde, RT, Hyde, RT, et al: A natural history of athleticism and cardiovascular health. JAMA 252:491, 1984.
17. Leon, AS, Connett, J, Jacobs, DR, Rauramaa, R: Leisure-time physical activity levels and risk of coronary heart disease and death. JAMA 258:2388, 1987.
18. Ekelund, LG, Haskell, WL, Johnson, JL, et al: Physical fitness as a predictor of cardiovascular mortality in asymptomatic North American men. N Engl J Med 319:1379, 1988.
19. Blair, SN, Koh, HW, Paffenbarger, RS, et al: Physical fitness and all-cause mortality: A prospective study of healthy men and women. JAMA 262:2395, 1989.
20. Morris, JN, Clayton, DG, Everitt, MG, et al: Exercise in leisure time: Coronary attack and death rates. Br Heart J 63:325, 1990.
21. Paffenbarger, R, Hyde, R, Wing, A, et al: Physical activity and all-cause mortality, and longevity of college alumni. N Engl J Med 314:605, 1986.
22. Caspersen, CJ: Physical inactivity and coronary heart disease. Physician and Sportsmedicine 15:43, 1987.
23. May, GS, Eberlein, KA, Furberg, CD, et al: Secondary prevention after myocardial infarction: A review of long-term trials. Prog Cardiovasc Dis 24:331, 1982.
24. Oldridge, NB, Guyatt, GH, Fischer, ME, et al: Cardiac rehabilitation after myocardial infarction: Combined experience of randomized clinical trials. JAMA 260:945, 1988.
25. O'Connor, GT, Buring, JE, Yusaf, S, et al: An overview of randomized trials of rehabilitation with exercise after myocardial infarction. Circulation 80:234, 1989.
26. American College of Sports Medicine: The recommended quantity and quality of exercise for developing and maintaining cardiorespiratory and muscular fitness in healthy adults. Med Sci Sports Exerc 22:265, 1990.
27. Kilbom, A: Physical training in women. Scand J Clin Lab Invest 199(Suppl):1, 1971.
28. Pollock ML, Miller, H, Janeway, R, et al: Effects of walking on body composition and cardiovascular function of middle-aged men. J Appl Physiol 30:126, 1972.
29. Burke, EJ and Franks, BD: Changes in $\dot{V}O_2$max resulting from bicycle training at different intensities holding total mechanical work constant. Res Q 46:31, 1975.
30. Kearney, JT, Stull, AG, Ewing, JL, et al: Cardiorespiratory responses of sedentary college women as a function of training intensity. J Appl Physiol 41:822, 1976.
31. Gaesser, GA and Rich, RG: Effects of high- and low-intensity exercise training on aerobic capacity and blood lipids. Med Sci Sports Exerc 16:269, 1984.
32. Wenger, HA and Bell, GJ: The interactions of intensity, frequency, and duration of exercise training in altering cardiorespiratory fitness. Sports Med 3:346, 1986.
33. Santiago, MC, Alexander, JF, Stull, GA, et al: Physiological responses of sedentary women to a 20-week conditioning program of walking or jogging. Scand J Sports Sci 9:33, 1987.
34. Pollock, ML, Gettman, LR, Mileses, CA, et al: Effects of frequency and duration of training on attrition and incidence of injury. Med Sci Sports 9:31, 1977.
35. Barry, AJ, Daly, JW, Pruett, EDR, et al: The effects of physical conditioning on older individuals.

I. Work capacity, circulatory-respiratory function, and work electrocardiogram. J Gerontol 21:182, 1966.

36. Hanson, JS, Tabakin, BS, Levy, AM, et al: Long-term physical training and cardiovascular dynamics in middle-aged men. Circulation 38:783, 1968.

37. Hartley, LH, Grimby, G, Kilbom, A, et al: Physical training in sedentary middle-aged and older men. Scand J Clin Lab Invest 24:335, 1969.

38. Ribisl, PM: Effects of training upon the maximal oxygen uptake of middle-aged men. Int Z Angew Physiol 26:272, 1969.

39. Shephard, RJ: Intensity, duration, and frequency of exercise as determinants of the response to a training regimen. Int Z Angew Physiol 26:272, 1969.

40. Wilmore, JH, Royce, J, Girandola, RN, et al: Physiological alternatives resulting from a 10-week jogging program. Med Sci Sports 2:7, 1970.

41. Davies, CTM and Knibbs, AV: The training stimulus, the effects of intensity, duration and frequency of effort on maximum aerobic power output. Int Z Angew Physiol 29:299, 1971.

42. Pollock, ML, Broida, J, Kendrick, Z, et al: Effects of training two days per week at different intensities on middle-aged men. Med Sci Sports 4:192, 1971.

43. Ismail, AH, Corrigan, D, McLeod, DF: Effect of an eight-month exercise program on selected physiological, biochemical, and audiological variables in adult men. Br J Sports Med 7:230, 1973.

44. Pollock, ML: The quantification of endurance training programs. In Wilmore, JH (ed): Exercise and Sports Sciences Reviews. Academic Press, New York, 1973, pp 155–188.

45. Leon, AS, Conrad, J, Hunninghake, DB, et al: Effects of a vigorous walking program on body composition, and carbohydrate and lipid metabolism of obese young men. Am J Clin Nutr 32:1776, 1979.

46. Seals, DR, Hagberg, JM, Hurley, BF, et al: Endurance training in older men and women. I. Cardiovascular responses to exercise. J Appl Physiol 57:1024, 1984.

47. Fleck, S and Kraemer, W: Designing Resistance Training Programs. Human Kinetics Publishers, Champaign, IL, 1987, pp 25–26.

48. Hagberg, JM, Graves, JE, Limacher, M, et al: Cardiovascular responses of 70–79 year old men and women to exercise training. J Appl Physiol 66:2589, 1989.

49. Gettman, LR, Pollock, ML, Durstine, JL, et al: Physiological responses of men to 1, 3, and 5 day per week training programs. Res Q 47:638, 1976.

50. Pollock, ML, Miller, HS, Linnerud, AC, et al: Frequency of training as a determinant for improvement in cardiovascular function and body composition of middle-aged men. Arch Phys Med Rehabil 56:141, 1975.

51. Fletcher, GF, Froelicher, VF, Hartley, H, et al: Exercise standards: A statement for health professionals from the American Heart Association. Circulation 82:2286, 1990.

52. Lieber, DC, Lieber, RL, Adams, WC: Effects of run-training and swim-training at similar absolute intensities on treadmill $\dot{V}O_2$max. Med Sci Sports Exerc 21:655, 1989.

53. Pollock, ML, Dimmick, J, Miller, HS, et al: Effects of mode of training on cardiovascular function and body composition of middle-aged men. Med Sci Sports 7:139, 1975.

54. Saltin, B, Hartley, L, Kilbom, A, et al: Physical training in sedentary middle-aged men, II. Scand J Clin Lab Invest 24:323, 1969.

55. Gledhill, N and Eynon, RB: The intensity of training. In Taylor, AS and Howell, ML (eds): Training, Scientific Basis and Application. Charles C. Thomas, Springfield, IL, 1972, pp 97–102.

56. Dion, FW, Grevenow, P, Pollock, ML, et al: Medical problems and physiologic responses during supervised inpatient cardiac rehabilitation: The patient after coronary bypass grafting. Heart Lung 11:248, 1982.

57. DeBusk, RF, Blomqvist, CG, Kouchoukos, NT, et al: Identification and treatment of low-risk patients after acute myocardial infarction and coronary-artery bypass graft surgery. N Engl J Med 314:161, 1986.

58. American College of Sports Medicine. Guidelines for Exercise Testing and Prescription, ed 4. Lea & Febiger, Philadelphia, 1991, pp 122–125.

59. Haskell, WL: Cardiovascular complications during exercise training of cardiac patients. Circulation 57:920, 1978.

60. Van Camp, SP and Peterson, RA: Cardiovascular complications of outpatient cardiac rehabilitation programs. JAMA 256:1160, 1986.

61. Silvidi, GE, Squires, RW, Pollock, ML, et al: Hemodynamic responses and medical problems asso-

ciated with early exercise and ambulation in coronary artery bypass graft surgery patients. J Cardiac Rehabil 2:355, 1982.

62. Rod, JL, Squires, RW, Pollock, ML, et al: Symptom-limited graded exercise testing soon after myocardial revascularization surgery. J Cardiac Rehabil 2:199, 1982.

63. Borg, GAV: Psychophysical bases of perceived exertion. Med Sci Sports Exerc 14:377, 1982.

64. Pollock, ML: Exercise regimens after myocardial revascularization surgery. In Wenger, NK (ed): Exercise and the Heart, ed 2. FA Davis, Philadelphia, 1985, pp 159–174.

65. Thompson, DL, Boone, TW, Miller, HS: Comparison of treadmill exercise and tethered swimming to determine validity of exercise prescription. J Cardiac Rehabil 2:363, 1982.

66. Holmer, I, Stein, EM, Saltin, B, et al: Hemodynamic and respiratory responses compared in swimming and running. J Appl Physiol 37:49, 1974.

67. Kallio, V, Hamalainen, H, Hakkila, J, et al: Reduction in sudden deaths by a multifactorial intervention programme after acute myocardial infarction. Lancet 2:1091, 1979.

68. Vermueulen, A, Lie, KI, Durrer, D: Effects of cardiac rehabilitation after myocardial infarction: Changes in coronary risk factors and long-term prognosis. Am Heart J 105:798, 1983.

69. Kentala, E: Physical fitness and feasibility of physical rehabilitation after myocardial infarction in men of working age. Ann Clin Med Suppl 9:1, 1972.

70. Wilhelmsen, L, Sanne, H, Elmfeldt, D, et al: A controlled trial of physical training after myocardial infarction. Prev Med 4:491, 1975.

71. Palatsi, I: Feasibility of physical training after myocardial infarction and its effect on return to work, morbidity and mortality. Acta Med Scand 599(Suppl):1, 1976.

72. Shaw, LW: Effects of a prescribed supervised exercise program on mortality and cardiovascular morbidity in patients after a myocardial infarction. The National Exercise and Heart Disease Project. Am J Cardiol 48:39, 1981.

73. Carson, P, Phillips, R, Lloyd, M, et al: Exercise after myocardial infarction: A controlled trial. J Roy Coll Phys Lond 16:147, 1982.

74. Roman, O, Gutierrez, M, Luksic, I, et al: Cardiac rehabilitation after acute myocardial infarction. Cardiology 70:223, 1983.

75. Rechitzer, PA, Cunningham, DA, Andrew, GM, et al: Relation of exercise to the recurrence rate of myocardial infarction in men. Ontario Exercise Heart Collaborative Study. Am J Cardiol 51:65, 1983.

76. Oberman, A and Naughton, J: The National Exercise and Heart Disease Project. In Pollock, ML and Schmidt, DH (eds): Heart Disease and Rehabilitation, ed 2. Churchill Livingstone, New York, 1986, pp 369–385.

77. Hagberg, J and Seals, D: Exercise training and hypertension. Acta Med Scand 711(Suppl):131, 1986.

78. Huttunen, JK, Lansimies, E, Voutilainen, E, et al: Effect of moderate physical exercise on serum lipoproteins: A controlled clinical trial with special reference to serum high-density lipoproteins. Circulation 60:1220, 1979.

79. Holloszy, JO, Schultz, J, Kusnierkiewiez, J, et al: Effects of exercise on glucose tolerance and insulin resistance. Acta Med Scand 711(Suppl):55, 1987.

80. Leon, AS: Scientific evidence of the value of cardiac rehabilitation services with emphasis on patients following myocardial infarction—Section 1: Exercise conditioning component. Journal of Cardiopulmonary Rehabilitation 10:79, 1990.

81. Paffenbarger, RS and Hyde, RT: Exercise as protection against heart attack (Editorial). N Engl J Med 302:1026, 1980.

82. Cousineau, D, Ferguson, R, deChamplain, J, et al: Catecholamines in coronary sinus during exercise in man before and after training. J Appl Physiol 43:801, 1977.

83. Hartley, LH: The role of exercise in the primary and secondary prevention of atherosclerotic coronary artery disease. In Wenger, NK (ed): Exercise and the Heart, ed 2. FA Davis, Philadelphia, 1985.

84. Ades, PA, Grunvald, MH, Weiss, RM, et al: Usefulness of myocardial ischemia as predictor of training effect in cardiac rehabilitation after acute myocardial infarction or coronary artery bypass grafting. Am J Cardiol 63:1032, 1989.

85. Naughton, J, Bruhn, JG, Lategola, MT: Effects of physical training on physiologic and behavioral characteristics of cardiac patients. Arch Phys Med Rehabil 49:131, 1968.

86. Clausen, JP and Trap-Jensen, J: Effects of training on the distribution of cardiac output in patients with coronary artery disease. Circulation 42:611, 1970.

87. Laslett, LJ, Paumer, L, Amsterdam, EA: Increase in myocardial oxygen consumption indexes by exercise training at onset of ischemia in patients with coronary artery disease. Circulation 71:958, 1985.

88. Detry, JM and Bruce, RA: Effects of physical training on exertional S-T segment depression in coronary heart disease. Circulation 44:390, 1971.

89. Rogers, MA, Yamamoto, C, Hagberg, JM, et al: The effect of 7 years of intense exercise training on patients with coronary artery disease. J Am Coll Cardiol 10:321, 1987.

90. Shephard, RJ: Exercise regimens after myocardial infarction. Rationale and results. In Wenger, NK (ed): Exercise and the Heart, ed 2. FA Davis, Philadelphia, 1985, pp 145–157.

91. Clausen, JP: Circulatory adjustments to dynamic exercise and effect on physical training in normal subjects and in patients with coronary artery disease. Prog Cardiovasc Dis 18:459, 1976.

92. Ehsani, AA, Heath, GW, Hagberg, JM, et al: Effects of 12 months of intense exercise training on ischemic ST-segment depression in patients with coronary artery disease. Circulation 64:1116, 1981.

93. Ehsani, AA, Biello, DR, Schulta, J, et al: Improvement of left ventricular contractile function by exercise training in patients with coronary artery disease. Circulation 74:350, 1986.

94. Hagberg, JM, Ehsani, AA, Holloszy, JO: Effect of 12 months of intense exercise training on stroke volume in patients with coronary artery disease. Circulation 67:1194, 1983.

95. Smith, JJ and Kampine, JP: Circulatory Physiology: The Essentials, ed 2. Williams & Wilkins, Baltimore, 1984, pp 239–241.

96. Robbins, AS and Rubenstein, LZ: Postural hypotension in the elderly. JAGS 32:769, 1984.

97. Irion, G, Wailgum, T, Stevens, C, et al: The effect of age on the hemodynamic response to thermal stress during exercise. In Cristafalo, V, Baker, G, Adelman, R, et al: (eds): Altered Endocrine States During Aging. HA Liss, New York, 1984, pp 187–195.

98. Smith, EL, Reddan, W, Smith, PE: Physical activity and calcium modalities for bone mineral increase in aged women. Med Sci Sports Exerc 13:60, 1981.

99. Fiatarone, M, Marks, E, Ryan, N, et al: High intensity strength training in nonagenarians. JAMA 263:3029, 1990.

100. deVries, H: Physiological effects of an exercise training program upon men aged 52 to 88. J Gerontol 24:325, 1970.

101. Agre, J, Pierce, L, Raab, D, et al: Light resistance and stretching exercise in elderly women: Effect upon strength. Arch Phys Med Rehabil 69:273, 1988.

102. Kauffman, T: Strength training effect in young and aged women. Arch Phys Med Rehabil 66:223, 1985.

103. Moritani, T and deVries, H: Potential for gross muscle hypertrophy in older men. J Gerontol 35:672, 1980.

104. Perkins, L and Kaiser, H: Results of short term isotonic and isometric exercise programs in persons over sixty. Phys Ther Rev 41:633, 1961.

105. Pollock, ML: Exercise prescriptions for the elderly. In Spirduso, W and Eckert, H (eds): Physical Activity and Aging. Human Kinetics Books, Champaign, IL, 1988, pp 163–174.

106. Lind, A and McNicol, G: Muscular factors which determine the cardiovascular responses to sustained and rhythmic exercise. Can Med Assoc J 96:706, 1967.

107. Graves, J, Pollock, M, Jones, A, et al: Specificity of limited range of motion variable resistance training. Med Sci Sports Exerc 21:84, 1989.

108. Kilbom, A, Hartley, LH, Saltin, B, et al: Physical training in sedentary middle-aged and older men. Scand J Clin Lab Invest 24:315, 1969.

109. Mann, GV, Garrett, LH, Farhi, A, et al: Exercise to prevent coronary heart disease. Am J Med 46:12, 1969.

110. Oja, P, Teraslinna, P, Partanen, T, et al: Feasibility of an 18 months' physical training program for middle-aged men and its effect on physical fitness. Am J Public Health 64:459, 1974.

111. Richie, DH, Kelso, SF, Bellucci, PA: Aerobic dance injuries: A retrospective study of instructors and participants. Physician and Sportsmedicine 14:100, 1985.

112. Pollock, ML, Carroll, JF, Graves, JE, et al: Injuries and adherence to walk/jog and resistance training programs in the elderly. Med Sci Sports Exerc 23:1194, 1991.

113. Malley, MT, Kohrt, WM, Coggan, AR, et al: Exercise prescription in healthy older adults. Med Sci Sports Exerc 22(Suppl):S23, 1990.

114. Kannel, WB, Koyle, JT, Shephard, RJ, et al: Prevention of cardiovascular disease in the elderly. J Am Coll Cardiol 10:25A, 1987.

115. Gordon, T, Castelli, WP, Hjortland, MC, et al: Predicting coronary heart disease in middle-aged and older persons. The Framingham Study. JAMA 238:497, 1977.

116. Hjermann, I, Velve Byre, K, Holme, I, et al: Effect of diet and smoking intervention on the incidence of coronary heart disease: Report from the Oslo Study Group of a randomised trial in healthy men. Lancet 2:1303, 1981.

117. Lipid Research Clinics Program: The Lipid Research Clinics Coronary Primary Prevention Trial Results. II. The relation of reduction in incidence of coronary heart disease to cholesterol lowering. JAMA 251:365, 1984.

118. National Cholesterol Education Program. Report on the National Cholesterol Education Program Expert Panel on Detection, Evaluation, and Treatment of High Blood Cholesterol in Adults. Arch Intern Med 148:38, 1988.

119. Blackburn, H: Coronary risk factors. How to evaluate and manage them. Eur J Cardiol 2/3:249, 1975.

120. Dustan, HP: Obesity and hypertension. Ann Intern Med 103:1047, 1985.

121. Ashley, FW and Kannel, WB: Relation of weight change to changes in atherogenic traits: The Framingham Study. J Chronic Dis 27:103, 1974.

# PART 4

# Socioeconomic Considerations

# CHAPTER 16

# The Relationship Between Socioeconomic Status and Coronary Heart Disease in Older Patients: Implications for Health Care

*Raymond T. Coward, MSW, PhD*
*Claydell Horne, RN, MSN*

During the past decade, research with coronary heart disease (CHD) patients of all ages has identified a range of major risk factors, which include clinical, social, and biologic determinants.[1,2] However, these generally, widely recognized risk factors account for only a portion of the variation in CHD that has been observed.[3] As a consequence, the search for other correlates continues.

Within this quest for a better understanding of the risk factors associated with CHD, the examination of psychosocial and socioeconomic factors has received increasing attention.[2–4] Indeed, the link between the behavioral norms of different social classes, the existence of certain risk factors, and the incidence of CHD has been a fertile area of research with *working-age adults.*[2] The precise manner in which these factors operate and interrelate in *older persons,* however, is not well understood and remains the subject of empiric investigation.[5]

In the sections that follow, the research on socioeconomic factors that are associated with CHD is summarized and briefly discussed. Then, using data from the Supplement on Aging of the 1984 National Health Interview Survey,[6] the link between socioeconomic variables and the higher odds of an *older person* reporting CHD is examined among middle-aged subjects and different age groups of older subjects. Finally, the implications of socioeconomic risk factors for the care and rehabilitation of older persons with CHD is discussed.

## THE LINK BETWEEN SOCIOECONOMIC STATUS AND CORONARY HEART DISEASE

Recent research has demonstrated that an individual's social environment and life style influences the incidence of cardiovascular events through health-related

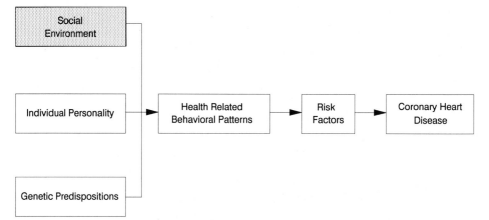

**Figure 16–1.** An illustration of the Interaction of Social Environment, Personality, and Genetic Predisposition in the Formulation of Health-Related Behavioral Patterns, Risk Factors, and Coronary Heart Disease.

behaviors and other risk factors.[7-9] Figure 16–1 depicts this general association by suggesting that an individual's social environment (determined in large part by socioeconomic status) interacts with personality and genetic predisposition to account for variations in health-related behaviors. These health-related behaviors, often referred to as life-style variables, in turn influence the presence of risk factors (e.g., diet, smoking, and sedentariness). As risk factors increase in number, so does the individual's probability of manifesting CHD.

For example, there is evidence that, despite a decline in overall smoking rates, a higher proportion of people from lower socioeconomic backgrounds continue to smoke and use tobacco.[10] Smoking, as is well documented, increases the risk of CHD. Thus, the higher incidence of heart disease among lower socioeconomic classes can be attributed, at least in part, to the higher concentration of smokers in that group. Smoking, however, is only one example from an extensive profile of health-related behaviors that is associated with the life styles of lower income persons. The higher incidence of heart disease among persons from lower socioeconomic backgrounds also has been attributed to their poorer diets and nutrition (e.g., higher amounts of solid fat, calories, and salt), less exercise, and the infrequent use of preventive and specialized medical services.[11,12] Indeed, Fraser[3] has suggested that, in today's modern society, upper-class people tend to be "better educated about the new-found connection between life style, diet, and cardiovascular health," and their health-related behaviors reflect that greater sophistication.

Three primary indicators of socioeconomic status are occupation, education, and income. Each of these factors has been associated with a higher risk of CHD. For example, Rose and Marmot[8] followed 17,520 male government employees in London for a period of more than 7 years and found large occupational differences in cumulative mortality from ischemic heart disease. Their data indicated that unskilled manual workers had age-adjusted mortality rates that were nearly four times that of administrative personnel. Similarly, Ilmarinen,[13] from a longitudinal study of municipal workers in Finland (n = 5556), reported that the highest rates of CHD were found among those manual laborers who had performed heavy and very heavy physical work for a period of 20 years or more.

Education also has been associated with mortality from CHD. For example, Hoffmans and associates[14] examined the health records of 78,612 men born in the Netherlands in 1932 and linked them to the death certificates of all men born that year who had died between 1950 and 1981. They then compared the prevalence of risk factors between those who had died from CHD (n = 648) and a control group randomly selected from those who were at risk, but had not died. Compared with the control group, they found that those men who had died from CHD were more likely to have attended only primary school (the lowest level of education attainment measured). This work is consistent with other research by Ruberman and associates[15] that demonstrated that men with lower education levels were twice as likely to die following a myocardial infarction than were men with more education.

Finally, income has been related to CHD. For example, Wielgosz and colleagues[16] examined the association between annual household income and the risk of acute myocardial infarction. The sample they studied included 100 patients with a confirmed diagnosis of acute myocardial infarction and a control sample from the same community matched for age and sex. Individuals with higher annual incomes were much less likely to have had a myocardial infarction—low-income individuals experienced four times the risk. Some have suggested, however, that there may be a slight up-turn in the prevalence of CHD among the very highest income groups (increasing over the prevalence rates of middle-income populations but *not* reaching the levels observed among low-income groups).[2]

Nevertheless, Hahn and associates,[17] working with 9-year survival data from the Alameda County Human Population Laboratory, were able to demonstrate that persons with incomes above the poverty threshold had significantly higher rates of survival from CHD compared with persons with incomes below the poverty line. Moreover, these income differentials persisted even after controls were introduced to account for a wide range of other individual characteristics (e.g., age, sex, race, income, smoking, alcohol consumption, physical activity, sleep, chronic health conditions, and disabilities).

## THE ASSOCIATION BETWEEN SOCIOECONOMIC STATUS AND CORONARY HEART DISEASE AMONG OLDER PERSONS

Among the elderly, the association between socioeconomic status and CHD may reflect the cumulative effects, during a large number of years, of a higher risk profile for those individuals from lower socioeconomic classes. That is, for many elders who have spent their lives in poverty or among the "near poor" (those with incomes just above the official poverty threshold), the years of poor health habits, inadequate diet, and insufficient health care may exact a toll on their health in later life.

Alternatively, the health of older populations is affected by the characteristics of the individuals who *survive* to old age. Thus, some of the differences in disease prevalence that are observed in younger populations (e.g., differences between males and females) are *not* present among older populations. This "leveling" or "survivor" effect (i.e., two groups becoming more alike as age increases) is a function of the removal from older age comparisons of those individuals who did not *survive* earlier illness and who may have accounted for most of the variation at earlier ages. Maddox[18] has called such elderly survivors "elites of one sort or another." Thus, as a consequence of the higher mortality rates from CHD among lower socioeconomic working-age adults, a reduction, or leveling, of the distinction between classes may ensue among older aged survivors.

Simultaneously, this process of survivorship may account for part of the variability that is observed *within* the cohort of people in our society who are described as "elderly." Geriatric research during the past two decades, for example, has illustrated the dramatic differences in health status and health care use between the "young-old" (those 65 to 74 years of age) and the "old-old" (those older than the age of 85).[18] As a consequence, some degree of "leveling" may occur after the age of 65. Thus, significant differences that exist among the young-old (aged 65 to 74 years), may not be present among the old-old.

Finally, when "leveling" does occur, sometimes the correlates of disease that are significant in younger cohorts are no longer important among older age groups. Thus, in comparisons of different groups of elders, "leveling" may cause certain factors that are significant predictors of disease among the "young-old" (e.g., socioeconomic characteristics) to be insignificant, or negligible, correlates of illness among the "old-old."

There is still much to be learned about the association between socioeconomic factors and CHD—especially among older persons.[19] Although age is certainly one of the major correlates of heart disease, and there is reason to believe that lower socioeconomic status is associated with the greater prevalence of heart disease among *working-age adults,* we do not have a clear understanding of the influence of socioeconomic factors in predicting heart disease among older aged populations, especially among groups of elders of different ages. In the section that follows, the relationship between socioeconomic status and age is explored using data from the Supplement on Aging of the 1984 National Health Interview Survey.

## THE INFLUENCE OF SOCIOECONOMIC FACTORS ON THE ODDS OF REPORTING CORONARY HEART DISEASE AMONG THE ELDERLY

The National Health Interview Survey (NHIS) is an annual survey, completed continuously since 1957, of the civilian noninstitutionalized U.S. population conducted by the National Center for Health Statistics. Based on a multistage probability sampling design and using specially trained interviewers from the U.S. Bureau of the Census, personal interviews are conducted each year with members of about 42,000 households. (For additional, and more detailed, information on the design of the survey, the sampling procedures, and the conduct of the interviews, consult materials from the National Center for Health Statistics).[5]

In 1984, the Supplement on Aging was added to the NHIS questionnaire to obtain information about persons 55 years of age and older who were living in the community (n = 16,148). The general content areas of the survey included physical limitations, chronic health conditions, housing, retirement status, interactions with family and community organizations, the use of formal community-based social and medical services, and other health-related information. When possible, the supplement was administered to all household members aged 65 years and older and to half of those 55 to 64 years of age. Information was obtained from proxies in cases in which physical or mental impairments, or extended absence from the household, precluded interviews with the eligible respondent (n = 1265 or 8.5%).

In the present analysis, some respondents from the original data set were not included because they had missing values on the variables of interest (n = 2658 or 16.5%). Most of these were eliminated because they lacked information about income. Thus, the sample used in this analysis comprises 13,490 persons (or 83.5% of the original sample). These respondents were distributed among the following age categories: 55 to 64 years (3978 or 29.5%); 65 to 74 years (5989 or 44.4%); 75 to 84 years (2911 or 21.5%); and 85 years of age and older (612 or 4.5%).

## Variable Definition

Five variables were included as indicators of the socioeconomic status of the respondents: gender, race, marital status, education, and income below the poverty threshold. All five of these variables have been previously associated with the higher risk of heart disease and were coded into dichotomies (the specific coding of variables is presented in Table 16–1). The distribution of these five socioeconomic

**Table 16–1.** Demographic Characteristics of the Sample of Middle-Aged and Elderly Respondents by Age (n = 13,490)

| Respondent Characteristics | Complete Sample (13,490) 100.0% | 55–64 yr (3978) 29.5% | 65–74 yr (5989) 44.4% | 75–84 yr (2911) 21.6% | 85+ yr (612) 4.5% |
|---|---|---|---|---|---|
| *Gender:* | | | | | |
| 0 Female | 7735 | 2134 | 3362 | 1814 | 425 |
| | (57.3) | (53.7) | (56.1) | (62.3) | (69.4) |
| 1 Male | 5755 | 1844 | 2627 | 1097 | 187 |
| | (42.7) | (46.4) | (43.9) | (37.7) | (30.6) |
| *Race:* | | | | | |
| 0 Non-black* | 12,487 | 3682 | 5527 | 2704 | 574 |
| | (92.6) | (92.6) | (92.3) | (92.9) | (93.8) |
| 1 Black | 1003 | 296 | 462 | 207 | 38 |
| | (7.4) | (7.4) | (7.7) | (7.1) | (6.2) |
| *Marital status:*† | | | | | |
| 0 Married | 8351 | 3064 | 3831 | 1325 | 131 |
| | (61.9) | (77.0) | (64.0) | (45.5) | (21.4) |
| 1 Not married | 5139 | 914 | 2158 | 1586 | 481 |
| | (38.1) | (23.0) | (36.0) | (54.5) | (78.6) |
| *Education:* | | | | | |
| 0 High school and above | 7078 | 2596 | 3133 | 1161 | 188 |
| | (52.5) | (65.3) | (52.3) | (39.9) | (30.7) |
| 1 Less than high school | 6412 | 1382 | 2856 | 1750 | 424 |
| | (47.5) | (34.7) | (47.7) | (60.1) | (69.3) |
| *Poverty level:*‡ | | | | | |
| 0 Above | 11624 | 3568 | 5233 | 2358 | 465 |
| | (86.2) | (89.7) | (87.4) | (81.1) | (76.0) |
| 1 Below | 1866 | 410 | 756 | 553 | 147 |
| | (13.8) | (10.3) | (12.6) | (19.0) | (24.0) |

*Source:* 1984 Supplement on Aging, National Health Interview Survey (National Center for Health Statistics, 1985).

*Includes Whites; Aleut, Eskimo, or American Indians; Asian/Pacific Islanders; Other; and those of Multiple Race.

†Includes never married, presently divorced, separated.

‡Based on family size, number of children, 18 years of age, and family income using the 1983 poverty levels published by the Census Bureau in August, 1984.

characteristics is presented in Table 16–1 for the total sample and each of the four specific age groups. The data indicate that as age increased, a smaller proportion of the respondents were male, fewer were married, fewer had a high school diploma or higher, and more had incomes that placed them below the official poverty line. In contrast, there was no significant fluctuation by age in the proportion of each sample that was black.

The dependent variable, self-reported CHD, was created from responses to four questions on the original survey. Respondents were classified as having CHD if, during the original interview, they reported having CHD, angina pectoris, myocardial infarction, or any other heart attack.

**Results**

A total of 1909 persons, or 14.2% of the sample of elders, were classified as having CHD—approximately one in seven of this nationally representative sample of community-dwelling middle-aged and elderly persons. There was a steady increase in the percentage of elders reporting CHD among older cohorts; that is, the smallest percentage with CHD was observed among middle-aged respondents aged 55 to 64 years (10.1%), and linear increases were observed among the three elderly groups—65 to 74 years (15.3%), 75 to 84 years (16.7%), and 85 years and older (17.0%). The role of socioeconomic factors in accounting for these age group differences, however, is not straightforward given that such factors *also* vary by age (see the data in Table 16–1). Thus, to portray more accurately the relationship between these socioeconomic factors and CHD, it is necessary to use a multivariate analytic framework.

Thus, Table 16–2 contains a series of logistic regression models that estimate the relationship between the socioeconomic characteristics of the population and the odds of a person reporting CHD. Separate models were estimated for the complete sample and individually for each of the four age groups (55 to 64, 65 to 74, 75 to 84, 85+). The odds for each respondent characteristic represents the influence of that factor above and beyond the influences of the other factors in the model.

Among the complete sample (all persons 55 years of age or older), all five of the socioeconomic variables were significantly associated with reporting CHD. Race exerted the most powerful influence. Blacks were about half as likely as non-blacks to have reported CHD (0.55). Gender was the next most formidable factor—males were 1.54 times more likely than females to have reported having CHD. Beyond those two factors, respondents with incomes below poverty had higher odds (1.23) as did those with less than a high school education (1.21) and those who were not married (1.16).

However, none of the five respondent characteristics significantly affected the odds of reporting CHD across all four age groups. Race was the most uniformly significant—reaching statistical significance in three of the four age groups. Using the implied coefficient to calculate the odds, we can estimate that non-blacks in the youngest three age categories had odds of reporting CHD that were nearly twice as high as blacks (1.90, 1.72, and 2.03, respectively). However, among persons 85 years of age and older, there were no statistically significant racial differences in the odds of reporting CHD.

Similarly, there were statistically significant gender differences in the odds of reporting CHD among younger age groups, but those differences did not exist

**Table 16–2.** Logit Models for Predicting the Likelihood of Reporting Coronary Heart Disease by Age (n = 13,490)*

| Sociodemographic Predictors | Complete Sample (13,490) β ($x^2$ Prob) | Odds Ratio | 55–64 yr (3978) β ($x^2$ Prob) | Odds Ratio | 65–74 yr (5989) β ($x^2$ Prob) | Odds Ratio | 75–84 yr (2911) β ($x^2$ Prob) | Odds Ratio | 85+ yr (612) β ($x^2$ Prob) | Odds Ratio |
|---|---|---|---|---|---|---|---|---|---|---|
| Intercept | −2.14 | | −2.69 | | −2.05 | | −1.53 | | −1.61 | |
| *Respondent characteristics:* | | | | | | | | | | |
| Gender | 0.43 (<0.01) | 1.54 | 0.66 (<0.01) | 1.93 | 0.50 (<0.01) | 1.65 | 0.16 (0.17) | 1.17 | −0.10 (0.72) | 0.90 |
| Race | −0.59 (<0.01) | 0.55 | −0.64 (<0.01) | 0.53 | −0.54 (<0.01) | 0.58 | −0.71 (<0.01) | 0.49 | −0.07 (0.89) | 0.93 |
| Marital status | 0.15 (<0.01) | 1.16 | 0.19 (0.14) | 1.21 | 0.05 (0.55) | 1.05 | −0.20 (0.09) | 0.82 | 0.49 (0.14) | 1.63 |
| Education | 0.19 (<0.01) | 1.21 | 0.23 (0.04) | 1.26 | 0.18 (0.01) | 1.20 | 0.03 (0.81) | 1.03 | −0.59 (<0.01) | 0.55 |
| Income | 0.21 (<0.01) | 1.23 | 0.59 (<0.01) | 1.80 | 0.22 (0.05) | 1.25 | −0.03 (.81) | 0.97 | 0.17 (0.51) | 1.19 |
| $x^2$ = | 115.40 | | 59.59 | | 63.59 | | 19.85 | | 10.98 | |
| DF = | 5 | | 5 | | 5 | | 5 | | 5 | |
| −2 Log Likelihood | 10,884.32 | | 2549.55 | | 5057.02 | | 2609.21 | | 546.90 | |

*Source:* 1984 Supplement on Aging, National Health Interview Survey (National Center for Health Statistics, 1985).
*A respondent was classified as having coronary heart disease if they self-reported coronary heart disease, angina pectoris, myocardial infarction, or any other heart attack.

among the two oldest age groups. Specifically, at ages 55 to 64, males were about twice as likely as females to report CHD (1.93) and between 65 and 74 they were slightly more than one-and-a-half times as likely (1.65). However, among the two oldest age categories (i.e., those 74 to 84 and those 85 years of age and older) there were no statistically significant differences by gender.

Among the other three variables (education, income, and marital status), no consistent pattern of results was observed. For example, education was significantly related to CHD among two of the four age groups—but the direction of the association reversed itself across age groups. That is, those who had less than a high school education had significantly higher odds of reporting CHD among those aged 64 to 74 (1.20 times more likely). Yet, among the oldest-old (85+), those who had a high school diploma or more had greater odds of CHD. (Using the implied coefficient, the odds were 1.80 higher.)

Among the income comparisons, only one of the age groups reached statistical significance. (Because of the large sample size used in the analysis, we used the 0.01 level of probability to define significance.) Middle-aged persons (55 to 64 years) with incomes below poverty had odds of reporting CHD that were 1.80 times greater than those persons with incomes above the official poverty line.

Finally, although marital status was significantly associated with CHD in the complete sample (i.e., those who were not married had odds of CHD that were 1.16 greater), none of the comparisons in the individual age groups were statistically significant. The presence of the significant association in the large aggregated complete sample, although not observed among the individual age groups, is probably a function of the fact that a very small difference in the aggregated group would be statistically significant because of the very large sample size (i.e., 13,490).

To facilitate the interpretation of these data, one perspective on the manner in which the findings are presented needs to be stressed. By definition, the models estimated in Table 16–2 represent the direct relationship between each individual socioeconomic variable and self-reported CHD controlling for the influence of the other variables. In reality, life is seldom so mutually exclusive. In the real world, these socioeconomic factors are likely to be observed contemporaneously (e.g., people with little formal education are more apt to have incomes that are below the poverty line; and, older females are more likely to have incomes below the poverty line). As a consequence, when these factors are considered in real-world combinations, they are likely to create risk profiles that are particularly onerous. For example, non-black males with low incomes and little education who are between the ages of 65 and 74 years may be at particular risk of CHD. In contrast, among those who have lived to be 85 years of age or older, the socioeconomic factors that were observed in this research do not appear to be good predictors of who will, or will not, report CHD.

Given this caveat, the analyses and data in Table 16–2, nevertheless, illustrate two important findings. First, the socioeconomic characteristics of a population can be significant predictors of higher rates of CHD—especially among middle-aged and young elderly persons. But, second, the effects of such forces are not uniform across different age cohorts of elders. That is, leveling was observed and, as a consequence, those socioeconomic factors that were significant correlates of CHD among the middle-aged and young-old (aged 65 to 74), were not consequential among the old-old (85+).

# IMPLICATIONS OF SOCIOECONOMIC FACTORS IN THE CARE OF THE ELDERLY WITH CORONARY HEART DISEASE

Even among older patients, many of the risk factors that are associated with CHD are modifiable through appropriate interventions. The limitation and control of risk factors not only reduces the CHD mortality of middle-aged persons, but those persons older than 65 also can benefit from preventive measures.[20] Health care providers must consider prevention programs, as well as treatment, when caring for elders who are potential candidates, or current victims, of CHD. Moreover, the data presented previously suggest that women may lose their CHD risk advantage over men in their later years (due to "leveling") and, as a consequence, could represent prime candidates for CHD risk prevention programs.

As persons with CHD age, or as aged persons develop CHD, varying degrees of chronicity and disability can be observed. Yet, the diagnosis of CHD, in and of itself, is a poor predictor of a person's disability or functional capacity (i.e., the ability to perform personal and instrumental care for yourself). Without an evaluation of the elder's capacity to function in everyday settings and situations, stereotypes of the older "cardiac cripple" may yield false impressions of the person's limitations. For example, out of 13 chronic conditions experienced by the elderly, Verbrugge and colleagues[21] found ischemic heart disease to rank fifth in prevalence, but seventh for impact of illness. A functional view approach to disease in the elderly may lessen the perceived impact of the disease by focusing attention on what can, and cannot, be done by the patients for themselves. Therefore, a comprehensive appraisal of the health and disability of an older person with CHD should include an assessment of functional ability as well as medical diagnosis.

Persons do not lose the desire to function independently with age and neither does the onset of chronic illness alter a person's value for an independent life style. Rather than label a person as physically or mentally disabled, due to the inability to perform certain self-care measures, a careful functional assessment may show that the disability results from lack of knowledge, lack of proper equipment or facilities, or lack of motivation. For instance, an older widower may not take proper care of his clothes because he does not have access to, or know how to use, a washer and dryer. He may not eat properly because he has not had to cook for himself before. He may be depressed and, therefore, give the appearance of not being able to perform certain self-care activities, when, truly, these abilities are still intact. Thus, a *functional* assessment may represent an opportunity for the elder, as well as the family and health caregivers, to recognize the capabilities that do still exist.

A plan of care for an elder with CHD cannot be successfully implemented without a consideration of the person's social environment and life style. How can the socioeconomic status of an elder with CHD be altered or compensated? Can elders make needed changes in life style, such as, ceasing to smoke, dietary changes, weight reduction, and alterations in stress-producing activities? To answer these questions and implement a plan of care for the elder with CHD, education and economic status as well as social support and patient education are topics in which healthcare providers need to be interested and can be influential.

For example, little or no formal education may cause some older persons to feel inadequate in their ability to understand and to carry out prescribed treatment plans, thus, resulting in feelings of dependence, fear, or depression. Some fears and feelings of dependence may be avoided by offering explanations of the illness and treatment plan in a manner and style that is understandable by the elder and family. Feelings of control and independence can be enhanced and, perhaps, maintained if the elder is directly addressed, rather than talked over or avoided, when health information and instructions are given.

Although most older persons have incomes above the poverty threshold, the impact of chronic illness can create economic burdens both in the form of direct costs (such as medical care, drugs, and other health services) as well as indirect costs (through the loss of productivity). Some elders bring a lifelong history of economic problems to old age, such as minorities, whereas others lose economic status during these years, such as older, widowed women (especially those older than 85 years).[22] Elders with CHD who are either economically disadvantaged or vulnerable (i.e., have fixed or marginal incomes that do not keep pace with inflation) may find it difficult to attain the needed treatment or counseling for their illness, and may fail to purchase the necessary medications or services for their care. Thus, health care providers and agencies always must be aware of the economic impact of the treatments they prescribe and the burdens and hardships such expenses may cause.

Stress is increasingly related to the etiology of illness, particularly cardiovascular illness.[23] Although retirement is anticipated to be a time of relaxation and freedom from worries of the work world, persons age 65 and older are not immune to stress resulting from changes in economic status, occupational roles, family structures, and sometimes residence. It has been shown that heart disease mortality will increase following economic downturns and decrease during more prosperous periods.[24] Fraser[3] also has reported that persons who experience a decrease in socioeconomic status are more prone to have an increased incidence of coronary events. Therefore, stress management programs may be a helpful part of the plan of care for CHD patients by increasing their personal contact with health care providers, encouraging compliance with treatment plans, and enhancing their social support system.

With many elders experiencing the effects of CHD, as well as less formal education, economic hardships, and life stress, family and social support is a necessary ingredient to care and to the maintenance of independence. The family, a critical and primary source of elder support, can significantly influence the quality of an elder's life by contributing to their motivation and ability to adhere to a plan of care. According to Fraser,[3] as social support increases, CHD mortality rates decrease across studies for both genders and for all ages.

Finally, to maintain a sense of independence and self-control for elders in the health care arena, patient and family education are increasingly important. With health care cost-containment strategies in place, families are faced with more intense health care responsibilities for their elderly members. To meet the challenge of this added responsibility, the patient and family must not be disadvantaged by a lack of opportunity to learn about the disability, causes, and plan of care. Elders place a high priority on health care and can benefit from health education. Most elders have time for visits to health care facilities for treatment and teaching sessions and can change lifelong practices with sufficient education, support, and positive reinforcement.[25] To maximize the effects of patient education for elders, health care providers need to give special consideration to providing shorter learning sessions and more frequent visits, assisting with transportation, and offering alternative methods of learning for those with visual or hearing deficits. A plan of care considering medical needs as well as educational, economic, and social support needs will likely result in a more self-sufficient, compliant, and functionally capable older patient.

## REFERENCES

1. Wenger, NK, Furberg CD, Pitt, E: Coronary heart disease in the elderly: Review of current knowledge and research recommendations. In Wenger, NK, Furberg, CD, and Pitt, E (eds): Coronary Heart Disease in the Elderly. Elsevier, New York, 1986, pp 1–7.

2. Kyle, EH: Socioeconomic factors. In Blocker, WP and Cardus, D (eds): Rehabilitation in Ischemic Heart Disease. SP Medical and Scientific Books, New York, 1983, pp 31–43.

3. Fraser GE: Preventive Cardiology. Oxford University Press, Oxford, 1986.

4. Krantz, DS and Raisen, SE: Environmental stress, reactivity and ischemic heart disease. Br J Med Psychol 61:3–16, 1988.

5. Kannel, WB, and Vokonas, PS: Primary risk factors for coronary heart disease in the elderly: The Framingham study. In Wegner, NK, Furberg, CD, and Pitt, E (eds): Coronary Heart Disease in the Elderly. Elsevier, New York, 1986, pp 60–95.

6. National Center for Health Statistics. Aging in the eighties: Preliminary data from the Supplement on Aging to the National Health Interview Survey, United States, January-June, 1984. Advance Data from Vital and Health Statistics, No. 115, 1984, U.S. Government Printing Office, Washington, DC.

7. Salonen, JT: Oral contraceptives, smoking and risk of myocardial infarction in young women. Acta Med Scand 212:141–144, 1982.

8. Rose, G and Marmot, MG: Social class and coronary heart disease. Br Heart J 45:13–19, 1981.

9. Koskenvuo, M, Kaprio, J, Kesaniemi, A, et al: Differences in mortality from ischemic heart disease by marital status and social class. J Chronic Dis 33:95–106, 1980.

10. Escabedo, LG, Anda, RF, Smith, PF, et al: Sociodemographic characteristics of cigarette smoking initiation in the United States: Implications for smoking prevention policy. JAMA 264(12):1550–1555, 1990

11. Kigagawa, EM and Hauser, PM: Differential Mortality in the United States: A Study in Socioeconomic Epidemiology. Harvard University Press, Cambridge, Mass., 1973.

12. Pratt, L: The relationship of socioeconomic status to health. Am J Public Health 61(2):281–291, 1971.

13. Ilmarinen, J: Work and cardiovascular health: Viewpoint of occupational physiology. Ann Med 21:209–214, 1989.

14. Hoffmans, MDAF, Kromhout, D, de Lezenne Coulander, C: Body mass index at the age of 18 and its effects on 32-year-mortality from coronary heart disease and cancer. J Clin Epidemiol 42(6):513–520, 1989.

15. Ruberman, W, Weinblatt, E, Goldberg, JD, et al: Psychosocial influences on mortality after myocardial infarction. N Engl J Med 311:552–559, 1984.

16. Wielgosz, AT, Wielgosz, M, Biro, E, et al: Risk factors for myocardial infarction: The importance of relaxation. Br J Med Psychol 61:209–217, 1988.

17. Hahn, MN, Kaplan, GA, Camachho, I: Poverty and health: Prospective evidence from the Alameda County Study. Am J Epidemiol 125:989–998, 1987.

18. Maddox, GL: Aging differently. The Gerontologist 27(5):557–564, 1987.

19. Maschewsky-Schneider, U Greiser, E: Primary prevention of coronary heart disease versus health promotion—a contradiction? Ann Med 21:215–218, 1989.

20. Kannel, WB, Doyle, JT, Shephard, RJ, et al: Prevention of cardiovascular disease in the elderly. J Am Coll Cardiol, 10(2):25A–28A, 1987.

21. Verbrugge, LM, Lepkowski, JM, Imanaka, Y: Comorbidity and its impact on disability. The Milbank Quarterly 67(3–4):450–484, 1989.

22. Neugarten, BL: Social and psychological characteristics of older persons. In Cassel, CK, Riesenberg, DE, Sorensen, LB, et al (eds): Geriatric Medicine. Springer-Verlag, New York, 1990, pp 28–37.

23. Graney, MJ: Interpersonal support and health of older people. In Peterson, WA and Quadagno, J (eds): Social Bonds in Later Life: Aging and Interdependence. SAGE Publications, Beverly Hills, California, 1985, pp 287–304.

24. Brenner, MH: Economic change and heart disease mortality. J Public Health 61(3):606–611, 1971.

25. Rosen, RC, Kostis, JB, and Brondolo, E: Nondrug treatment approaches for hypertension. Clin Geriat Med 5(4):791–802, 1989.

# CHAPTER 17

# Ethical Considerations and Quality of Life

*Nannette Hoffman, MD*

The Hippocratic Oath guiding the principles of medical practice states, "To protect life, to maintain and support it, to restore it to wholeness and certainly not to destroy it is the common principle." However, implicit in medical practice and perhaps of greater importance is the physician's endeavor to improve quality of life. For many patients, quality, rather than quantity of life, is the core issue. Physicians caring for the elderly often use quality-of-life considerations when making decisions regarding technologic interventions for their patients.

Despite this frequent use of quality-of-life considerations in medical decision making, the concept, quality of life, remains undefined. This has been illustrated in two studies that examined physicians' and patients' perceptions of quality of life as it impacted upon medical decision making. These studies showed that physicians' quality-of-life assessments differed from those of patients. Furthermore physicians' quality-of-life judgments about the same patient's clinical situation also differed.[1,2] One explanation for these differences in the quality-of-life assessment is that physicians' decision making can be influenced by personal values, unconscious motivations, inner conflicts, unrealistic expectations, and fear of professional failure when there is an unsuccessful patient outcome. Also influential is medical training and the availability of complex technology that fosters the use of aggressive life supportive treatments. Likewise, diagnostic and prognostic uncertainty of some diseases can cause physicians to err on the side of "doing more," when in fact, their patients "want less." Finally, fear of legal liability drives physicians to recommend therapies that may be life prolonging.[3,4] Equally if not more difficult to contend with, are patients who demand "everything be done" when in fact "everything" may not be medically justified or indicated.

Inasmuch as the most common cause of death in those older than 65 years old is ischemic heart disease and the elderly population is growing, the practicing cardiologist will increasingly encounter quantity versus quality-of-life dilemmas in medical decision making. This situation is complicated by the fact that elderly individuals are more likely than younger ones to have dementing illnesses and other disorders that temporarily or permanently impair their decision-making ability.[5]

How should physicians adequately deal with ethical issues in their practice? Many who are reading this, owing to daily experience, are already adept at clarifying and resolving ethical issues with their patients. Nevertheless, it is useful to understand and reinforce the background and formal principles guiding ethical decision making.

## BACKGROUND ON ETHICAL AND LEGAL PRINCIPLES

Before patient autonomy became the prevailing medical ethic, physicians historically made medical decisions according to the principles of beneficence and paternalism. These latter principles encouraged physicians, by virtue of their special knowledge, to make decisions for their patients without soliciting patient or family input. This presumption that physicians always knew what was "best" for their patients was readily challenged in the 1900s such that autonomy replaced paternalism and autonomy is now the current mode of medical ethical practice.[6]

The principle of patient autonomy in medical decision making has been legally recognized since 1914 when Justice Cardozo rendered the legal opinion: "Every human being of adult years and sound mind has the right to determine what shall be done with his own body." This opinion has been termed the common law right of self-determination. Another legal concept recognizing autonomy is the constitutional right of privacy. In the past, this right has been upheld by the U.S. Supreme Court to protect individuals from governmental intrusion in fundamental and personal medical decisions.[5] Hence, it is accepted and practiced that once properly informed, patients have the right to refuse treatment as long as they are mentally capable of 1) understanding the treatment and 2) consenting to the treatment. When an individual's wishes regarding a treatment are unknown or unclear, societal interest in the preservation of life with the presumption for life generally prevails, and physicians act accordingly in their decision making.[6]

Physicians also have a professional ethic to maintain the integrity of the medical profession. We are not obligated to render useless care just because patients demand it. In fact, when we acquiesce to patients' requests for unnecessary or harmful treatment to respect their autonomy, our own autonomy is reciprocally undermined.[6,7] When there is conflict between the respective autonomies of physicians and patients, it is usually recommended to transfer the patient's care to a physician willing to honor the patient's wishes. However, in practice this is often unfeasible and sometimes impossible to accomplish especially when patients request treatments that are clearly inappropriate or contraindicated. Thus, it is reassuring that the courts have upheld physicians' professionalism and autonomy in certain circumstances. One example has been when physicians have withheld cardiopulmonary resuscitation (CPR) when the likelihood for recovery was remote and the decision was based on sound medical judgment.[8,9]

In conclusion, the ethical principle of autonomy has legal basis, such that mentally capable patients have the right to refuse treatment and this right must be respected. Likewise, the physician has an ethical duty to maintain professional integrity and not render useless care. Occasionally, these two ethical tenets oppose one another and, in this instance, medical decision making must be guided by sound professional practice.

## DECISION MAKING, INFORMED CONSENT, AND
## INCOMPETENT PATIENTS

Sometimes patients obviously mentally capable of making decisions decline recommended beneficial treatments even after hearing their physicians' convincing arguments about the treatment's merits. When this occurs, physicians should try to determine the basis for their patients' seemingly irrational decision. One reason for an irrational decision is a bias toward the present and near future such that patients do not appreciate the full import of a treatment if its effects are not noted until years later. Another reason is magical thinking by patients that the deleterious consequences of treatment refusal will not happen to them. Finally, patients may have a marked fear of the treatment, especially if it entails pain and disability. Upon discovering the reasons for their patients' irrational decision, physicians should explore these reasons and attempt to persuade their patients to reconsider their choice.[10] In the end, however, although mentally capable patients do have the right to refuse treatment, they do not have the right to receive inappropriate treatment upon demand. It should be understood that patients' irrational decisions do not necessarily imply their incompetence. If there is any question as to a patient's decision-making ability, psychiatric consultation should be obtained.

How does one determine a patient's mental capability to make decisions? Even the Alzheimer's disease patient in the late stages of illness is considered legally competent, if he or she has not been declared incompetent by a court of law. Nevertheless physicians and caregivers readily recognize that such a patient is mentally incapable of decision making. Because legal competency determinations are not the norm in practice, the patient's ability to consent is routinely assessed by physicians without legal guidance. The physician has the primary responsibility to determine whether a patient lacks the capacity to make decisions. This determination is one that an informed lay person might make: that a patient lacks the ability to understand a situation and to make a choice in light of the lack of understanding. A patient should be able to weigh the risks and benefits of a proposed treatment and understand the outcomes of its acceptance or refusal. Patients should be able to communicate their choices and paraphrase information told to them. Even for those patients with legal guardians, if possible, the opinions of the former should be solicited and considered in the final treatment decision.[6,11,12] Again, when there is doubt as to the patient's abilities to make decisions, psychiatric consultation may be useful. Physicians should be careful not to automatically assume that a diagnosis of dementia or stroke connotes decision-making impairment. Although some mildly demented or stroke patients have difficulty with certain tasks, like balancing a checkbook or completing their activities of daily living, they may be capable of making simple treatment decisions. It is important for physicians to take the time to talk to their patients to determine their patients' decision-making capabilities. Not infrequently, the next of kin acts as the spokesperson for the patient and consequently physicians do not attempt to personally discuss with the patient his or her wishes. Supporting this observation in the literature is the fact that at least in the hospital, the "do not resuscitate" (DNR) order is more often discussed with the patient's family rather than the patient, even when the patient is capable of involvement in the decision making.[13–17]

Of interest is a recent study examing elderly patients' decision-making capacity, which suggested that elderly medically ill patients who appear competent may deyelop unrecognized decisional impairment during hospitalization for acute illness. Thus, the validity of informed consent in these settings must be questioned.[18]

If the patient is definitely incompetent, to whom does the physician turn for informed consent and decision making? Generally, the physician should consult the patient's legal guardian first, if one exists. In most instances, however, there is no legal guardian, and the physician should then consult the surrogate decision maker who has preferably been designated in writing. This individual is not always the next of kin. When designated in writing, the surrogate decision maker is usually empowered as the patient's spokesperson by the authority of a legal document called a durable power of attorney. All states have durable power of attorney statutes that permit individuals to delegate a proxy to act on his or her behalf and this is indicated in the power of attorney. This durable power of attorney is "durable" because it remains valid after the patient becomes incompetent. Not all states explicitly allow the power of attorney to be used for medical decisions, although no court has ruled that a durable power of attorney cannot be used for this purpose. Some states have specific statutes for a durable power of attorney for healthcare. California was one of the first states to enact such a statute.[5] Some states with living will or natural death acts allow the surrogate to be designated in the living will. When the patient has not designated a surrogate, the physician usually consults the available next of kin. Your institution's policy or state law, when the state has a natural death act, may determine the particular relative selected as the final decision maker. This relative may not necessarily be the family member who knows the patient best or has the patient's best interests at heart. It is incumbent upon all practicing physicians to be familiar with the natural death act of their state. When in doubt how to proceed, physicians should consult their hospital attorney for advice.

When surrogates are making decisions for patients, the decisions should be based upon the patients' values and not those of the surrogates. There are situations in which financial interests on the part of the surrogate may unduly bias decisions toward those that are not in the patients' best interests. If the physician truly believes this is the case, then the matter may have to be settled in the courts.

Finally, when physicians practice medicine responsibly and respect the preferences of their patients or patients' surrogates, judicial precedent supports discontinuing life supportive treatments that are not in the patients' best interests. Physicians need not fear civil or criminal culpability in these circumstances. To the contrary, we may face greater legal liability, if we use life-prolonging treatments in patients who clearly do not want them.[19]

## ADVANCE DIRECTIVES AND LIVING WILLS

The terms advance directives and living wills are often used interchangeably. *Advance directives* are statements, usually written by competent individuals, indicating their wishes regarding life-sustaining treatments in the event of future decision-making inability. *Living wills* are directives that specify in the event of a terminal illness, if incompetence precludes participation in decision making, that individuals do not want life-sustaining treatments to postpone death. Legal recognition of living wills is embodied in states' natural death acts. Currently more than 80% of the states in the United States have natural death acts. The purposes of these natural death acts are to facilitate patient autonomy and to protect physicians from legal liability when they withhold or withdraw life-sustaining treatments.[20]

Two common criticisms of living wills are that they are not specific enough to direct decision making for many treatment options, and they may not be applicable in emergency situations. Nonetheless, they can spare a patient from life-prolonging procedures in many instances. Unfortunately, physicians in general are not proactive in initiating discussions with their patients about advance directives.[21] Several studies show that DNR orders are generally written while patients are in an acute care setting and late in the patient's clinical course. In one of these studies, only 4% of the patients were admitted to the hospital with preexisting DNR orders.[16,17,22] The acute care setting is not the optimal place for discussion of advance directives as elderly patients are often very ill, anxious, and may be too confused to participate in discussions about life-prolonging procedures. The ideal time for these discussions is during routine office visits. Many patients welcome a chance to discuss their feelings about life-prolonging treatments.

Currently, the Joint Commission for Accreditation of Healthcare Organizations requires for certification that hospitals, psychiatric facilities, and nursing homes have policies regarding withholding of resuscitative services. New regulations for Medicare and Medicaid certified nursing homes include in their initial patient assessment requirements that the status of advance directives and durable power of attorneys be ascertained.[23-26] Congress has recently approved legislation requiring hospitals to advise patients upon admission about the importance of advance directives.[27]

To avoid crisis decision making about life-prolonging procedures in the acute care setting, when patients may be too impaired to participate, physicians should routinely discuss advance directives with their elderly patients during office visits. Local medical societies should be able to provide information as to where copies of advance directives for your patients may be obtained that are applicable to your state. Choice in Dying, Inc. will provide copies of living wills for your state upon request (250 W. 57th St., New York, NY 10107). Discussions regarding life-prolonging procedures with patients should be documented in the medical record, and it is advisable for physicians to keep copies of the advance directives in their patients' medical records.

Another practical matter to consider is that not all ambulance services honor advance directives, and some require a physician's order along with the advance directive, otherwise full CPR is attempted if necessary. Physicians or their patients should inquire with their local ambulance service as to the policies regarding the honoring of advance directives.

## CARDIOPULMONARY RESUSCITATION AND DO NOT RESUSCITATE ORDERS

"The purpose of CPR is the prevention of sudden, unexpected death. CPR is not indicated in certain situations, such as in cases of terminal irreversible illness where death is not unexpected." This quote is from the National Council on Cardiopulmonary Resuscitation and Emergency Cardiac Care. Despite the National Council's recommendation, in the 1970s and 1980s CPR was often performed indiscriminately in hospitals on all patients regardless of the diagnoses. Only recently has there been a trend for physicians to write DNR orders for patients who are terminally ill or refuse resuscitation, and for institutions to implement policies about DNR orders.

There are three general indications for writing DNR orders: no medical benefit, poor quality of life after CPR, and poor quality of life before CPR. The latter two should involve the patient or surrogate directly in the decision-making process. The former theoretically should not involve the patient and is a medical determination by the physician such that the physician would not offer CPR in the absence of its benefit.[28]

The decision that the physician does not offer CPR when it lacks efficacy, although supported ethically and judicially, remains controversial. Some practitioners believe patients desiring CPR have the right to have CPR performed, and others believe physicians should at least discuss with their patients the rationale for not offering it.[4,29] Nevertheless, it should be remembered that ultimately, physicians are not obligated to perform procedures offering no benefit, and to do so, breaches the professional ethic.[29-31]

One state, New York, has legislated the conditions under which CPR can be withheld. This resulted when a grand jury found a New York hospital permitted the use of DNR orders that were neither recorded in the patients' medical records nor discussed with the patients. Hence, legally, the patient's or surrogate's consent is required to withhold CPR, otherwise CPR must be performed. Unfortunately, the problem arising when CPR is not medically indicated but the patient insists upon its use, is not addressed by this legislation.[32]

One reason for disagreement about how to proceed when CPR lacks medical benefit and the patient demands it is the precept that physicians can accurately predict which patients would not benefit from CPR. Clinical determinations of CPR futility are difficult because of inconclusive evidence about CPR efficacy for certain patients and conflict about the therapeutic goals for the patient among physician, patient, and family members. In addition, a "1% likelihood" of a successful CPR outcome may represent futility to some and not to others.[33] Although not everyone would agree, physicians should make a "reasonable" determination as to whether CPR is offered if its efficacy is low. The physician, not the patient, must sort out the possibilities, weigh risks and benefits, and recommend a therapeutic plan. This responsibility should not be shifted to the patient in the guise of respect for patient autonomy. Again not all would concur; the use of CPR should be justified by a realistic expectation of prolonged benefit, and a treatment plan could exclude CPR in some instances.[34,35]

Is CPR futile for some patients? The literature does support that CPR is relatively ineffective for certain patient populations. Survival to hospital discharge following unwitnessed cardiac arrest is approximately 1%.[36-39] Sepsis uniformly predicts virtually no survival to discharge with an overall survival rate of less than 1%, with 0% reported in many series.[36,38,40-43] Malignancy, especially when widespread, is also a predictor of a poor CPR outcome. In documented studies to date, no patient with metastatic cancer survived CPR to discharge.[36,40,43-45] Survival rates for patients with renal failure ranges from 0% to 6%.[37,38,40,41,46,47] Progressive systemic acidosis secondary to respiratory or circulatory failure predicts abysmal survival.[48] Other conditions associated with a poor CPR outcome of less than 10% survival to discharge include congestive heart failure, cerebrovascular accidents, and severe physical impairment.[37,38,40,44,47,49]

The overall success rate of CPR is usually less than 20% in hospital patients and less than 10% in nursing home patients. The elderly appear to fare less well than their younger counterparts with respect to CPR outcome, which is probably related to concomitant illness and to disability.[36-62] In particular, the "old-old" have the lowest survival rates. One study reported 0% survival to discharge in all patients 90 years of age or older. On the other hand, relatively healthy elderly individuals suffering witnessed cardiac arrests with an initial rhythm of ventricular fibrillation have at least approximately a 20% chance of survival to hospital discharge following CPR.[54,60] For some physicians, age may be the sole criteria upon which the decision to perform CPR is based, but the literature does not clearly support this premise.[63]

In summary, there is compelling evidence that CPR is ineffective for certain groups of patients: those with unwitnessed cardiac arrest, metastatic cancer, sepsis, and systemic acidosis when due to irreversible major cardiorespiratory failure. Some believe when physicians decide not to perform CPR in such patient populations owing to a lack of benefit, that this is a "value judgment" in that physicians can never predict with absolute certainty that a patient would not survive CPR to hospital discharge. Furthermore, it may be unacceptable for physicians to make these "value judgments." However, two authorities in this field, Drs. Tomlinson and Brody, in a recent article, have presented what is a very valid concept: that physicians constantly make value judgments in their practice.[64] This is not only inherent in their profession but entirely appropriate even when applied to CPR, which in many respects is like any other medical treatment or procedure with risks and benefits that must be weighed before making a final decision about its use. Drs. Tomlinson and Brody further state, "It is for the sake of patient autonomy, then, that physicians must be able to restrict the alternatives made available to patients and must be able to employ value judgments in doing so." They do believe that patients should be informed when CPR will not be attempted.[64]

## CONCLUSION

Not only should physicians consider their patients' quality of life when making treatment decisions, but they need to actively solicit their patients' desires regarding these decisions. Physicians should remember that their concept of quality of life may not be the same as that of their patients. A sound practice to avoid last minute "crises" is to routinely ask patients during office visits about their wishes for life-prolonging procedures as this is the time when patients usually still have their decision-making abilities. It is helpful for physicians to keep copies of their state's living will form in the office for their patients. Finally, it is ethically appropriate and judicially supported that physicians make judgments based upon professional expertise and the literature as to the futility of CPR. Physicians are not obligated to offer ineffective treatments, although they may wish to discuss with their patients the rationale for not offering such treatments.

## REFERENCES

1. Starr, TJ, Pearlman, RA, Uhlmann, RF: Quality of life and resuscitation decisions in elderly patients. J Gen Intern Med 1:373, 1986.
2. Pearlman, RA and Jonsen, A: The use of quality-of-life considerations in medical decision making. J Am Geriatr Soc 33:344, 1985.
3. Wanzer, SH, Federman, DD, Adelstein JS, et al: The physician's responsibility towards hopelessly ill patients: A second look. N Engl J Med 320:844, 1989.
4. Youngner, S: Futility in context. JAMA 264:1295, 1990.
5. U.S. Congress, Office of Technology Assessment: Life-sustaining Technologies and the Elderly. OTA-BA-306, US Government Printing Office, Washington, DC, July 1987.

6. Marsh, FM: Refusal of treatment. In Jahnigen, EW and Schrier, RW (eds): Ethical Issues in the Care of the Elderly. Clinics in Geriatric Medicine, WB Saunders vol 2, 1986, p 511.

7. Brett, AS and McCullough, LB: When patients request specific interventions: Defining the limits of physician's obligation. N Engl J Med 315:1347, 1986.

8. In re Dinnerstein, 380 NE 2d 134 (Appt Ct. Mass. 1987).

9. Hackler, JC and Hiller, FC: Family consent to orders to not resuscitate: Reconsidering hospital policy. JAMA 264:1281, 1990.

10. Brock, D and Wartman, SA: When competent patients make irrational choices. N Engl J Med 322:1595, 1990.

11. President's Commission for Study of Biomedical Ethics and Behavioral Research: Making Health Care Decisions. US Government Printing Office, Washington, DC, October 1982.

12. Applebaum, PS and Grisso, T: Assessing patient's capacities to consent to treatment. N Engl J Med 319:1635, 1988.

13. Stolman, CJ, Gregory, JD, Dunn, D, et al: Evaluation of the do not resuscitate orders at a community hospital. Arch Intern Med 149:1851, 1989.

14. Evans AL and Brody, BA: The do-not-resuscitate order in teaching hospitals. JAMA 253:2236, 1985.

15. Bedell, SE, Pelle, D, Maher, P, et al: Do-not-resuscitate orders for critically ill patients in the hospital. JAMA 256:233, 1986.

16. Gleeson, K and Wise, S: The do-not-resuscitate order. Arch Intern Med 150:1057, 1990.

17. Jonsson, PV, McNamee, M, Compion, EW: The "do not resuscitate" order. Arch Intern Med 148:2373, 1988.

18. Fitten, JL and Waite, MS: Impact of medical hospitalization on treatment decision-making capacity in the elderly. Arch Intern Med 150:1717, 1990.

19. Weir, RF and Gostin, L: Decisions to abate life-sustaining treatment for nonautonomous patients. JAMA 264:1846, 1990.

20. Lazaroff, AE and Orr, WF: Living wills and other advance directives. In Jahnigen, DW and Schrier, RW (eds): Ethical Issues in the Care of the Elderly. Clinics in Geriatric Medicine, vol 2, 1986, p 521.

21. Franke, D, Oye, RK, and Bellamy, PE: Attitudes of hospitalized patients towards life support: A survey of 200 medical inpatients. Am J Med 86:645, 1989.

22. Bedell, SE and Delbanco TL: Choices about cardiopulmonary resuscitation in the hospital. When do physicians talk with patients? N Engl J Med 310:1089, 1984.

23. Emanuel, LL: Does the DNR order need life-sustaining intervention? Time for comprehensive advance directives. Am J Med 86:87, 1989.

24. Davidson, KW and Moseley, R: Advance directives in family practice. J Fam Pract 22:439, 1986.

25. Morris, JW, Hawes, C, Fries, BE, et al: Designing the national resident assessment instrument for nursing homes. Gerontologist 30:293, 1990.

26. U.S. Congress, Office of Technology Assessment: Institutional Protocols for Decisions about Life-Sustaining Treatments. Special Report, OTA-BA-389, US Government Printing Office, Washington, DC, July 1988.

27. The Danforth-Moynihan Bill (S. 1766) 101st Congress, 1st Session, 1989.

28. Tomlinson, T and Brody, H: Ethics and communication in do-not-resuscitate orders. N Engl J Med 318:43, 1988.

29. Tomlinson, T and Brody, H: Futility and the ethics of resuscitation. JAMA 264:1281, 1990.

30. Brett, AS and McCullough, LB: When patients request specific interventions: Defining the limits of the physician's obligation. N Engl J Med 315:1347, 1986.

31. Blackhall, LJ: Must we always use CPR? N Engl J Med 317:1281, 1987.

32. Sivak, SL: Effect of New York State's do-not-resuscitate legislation on in-hospital cardiopulmonary resuscitation practice. Am J Med 88:108, 1990.

33. Youngner, SJ: Who defines futility? JAMA 160:2094, 1988.

34. Lantos, JD, Singer, PA, Walker, RM, et al: The illusion of futility in clinical practice. Am J Med 87:81, 1989.

35. Paris, JJ, Crones, RK, Rearden, JD: Physician's refusal of requested treatment: The case of Baby L. N Engl J Med 322:1012, 1990.

36. Taffet, GE, Teasdale, TA, Luchi, RJ: In-hospital cardiopulmonary resuscitation. JAMA 260:2069, 1988.

37. Murphy, DJ, Murray, AM, Robinson, BE, et al: Outcomes of cardiopulmonary resuscitation in the elderly. Ann Intern Med 111:199, 1989.

38. Saphir, R: External cardiac massage: Retrospective analysis of 123 cases and review of the literature. Medicine 47:73, 1968.

39. Hershey, CO and Fisher, L: Why outcome of cardiopulmonary resuscitation in general wards is so poor. Lancet 1:31, 1982.

40. Bedell, SE, Delbanco, TL, Cook, EF, et al: Survival after cardiopulmonary resuscitation in the hospital. N Engl J Med 309:570, 1983.

41. Smith, HJ and Anthonisen, NR: Results of cardiac resuscitation in 254 patients. Lancet 1:1022, 1965.

42. Klassen, GA, Broadhurst, C, Peretz, DI, et al: Cardiac resuscitation in 126 medical patients using external cardiac massage. Lancet 1:1290, 1963.

43. Stiles, QR, Tucker, BL, Meyer, BW, et al: Cardiopulmonary arrest: Evaluation of an active resuscitation program. Am J Surg 122:282, 1971.

44. Peatfield, RC, Sillett, RW, Taylor, D, et al: Survival after cardiac arrest in hospital. Lancet 1:1223, 1977.

45. Jeresaty, RM, Godar, TJ, Liss, JP: External cardiac resuscitation in a community hospital: A three-year experience. Arch Intern Med 124:588, 1969.

46. George, AL, Folk, BP, Crecelius, PL, et al: Pre-arrest morbidity and other correlates of survival after in-hospital cardiac arrest. Am J Med 87:28, 1989.

47. Hollingsworth, JM: The results of cardiopulmonary resuscitation: A 3 year university hospital experience. Ann Intern Med 71:459, 1969.

48. Camarata, SJ, Well, MH, Hanashiro, PK, et al: Cardiac arrest in the critically ill: A study of predisposing causes in 132 patients. Circulation 44:688, 1971.

49. Baringer, JR, Salzman, EW, Jones, WA, et al: External cardiac massage. N Engl J Med 265:62, 1961.

50. Linn, BS and Yurt, RW: Cardiac arrest among geriatric patients. Br Med J 2:25, 1970.

51. Lemire, JG and Johnson, AJ: Is cardiac resuscitation worthwhile? N Engl J Med 286:970, 1972.

52. Burns, R, Graney, MJ, Nichols, LO: Prediction of in-hospital cardiopulmonary arrest outcome. Arch Intern Med 149:1318, 1989.

53. Peschin, A and Coakley, C: A five-year review of 734 cardiopulmonary arrests. South Med J 63:506, 1970.

54. Gulati, RS, Hhan, GL, Horan, MA: Cardiopulmonary resuscitation of old people. Lancet 1:267, 1983.

55. Castagna, J, Weil, MH, Shubin, H: Factors determining survival in patients with cardiac arrest. Chest 65:527, 1974.

56. Stemmler, EJ: Cardiac resuscitation: A one-year study of patients resuscitated within a university hospital. Ann Intern Med 63:613, 1965.

57. Himmelhoch, SR, Dekker, A, Cazzaniga, AB, et al: Closed-chest cardiac resuscitation. N Engl J Med 270:118, 1964.

58. Applebaum, GE, King, JE, Finucane, TE: The outcome of CPR initiated in nursing homes. J Amer Geriatr Soc 38:197, 1990.

59. Kaiser, TF, Kayson, EP, Campbell, RG: Survival after cardiopulmonary resuscitation in a long term care institution. J Am Geriatr Soc 34:909, 1986.

60. Longstreth, WT, Cobb, LA, Fahrenbrock, CE, et al: Does age affect outcome of out-of-hospital cardiopulmonary resuscitation? JAMA 264:2109, 1990.

61. Saklayen, MG: Letter to the Editor. Ann Intern Med 111:854, 1989.

62. Gordon, M and Hurowitz, E: Cardiopulmonary resuscitation of the elderly. J Am Geriatr Soc 32:930, 1984.

63. Farber, NJ, Bowman, SM, Major DA, et al: Cardiopulmonary resuscitation (CPR) patient factors and decision making. Arch Intern Med 144:2229, 1984.

64. Tomlinson, T and Brody, H: Futility and the ethics of resuscitation. JAMA 264:1276, 1990.

# INDEX

A "f" following a page number indicates a figure. A "t" following a page number indicates a table.